Atlas of Oncology Imaging

For further volumes:
http://www.springer.com/series/8759

Sasan Karimi
Editor

Atlas of Brain and Spine Oncology Imaging

Springer

Editor
Sasan Karimi
Department of Radiology
New York Presbyterian Hospital/
Weill Cornell Medical College
New York, NY
USA

Neuroradiology Service,
Department of Radiology
Memorial Sloan-Kettering Cancer Center
New York, NY
USA

ISBN 978-1-4614-5652-0 ISBN 978-1-4614-5653-7 (eBook)
DOI 10.1007/978-1-4614-5653-7
Springer New York Heidelberg Dordrecht London

Library of Congress Control Number: 2012954858

Printed on acid-free paper

Springer is part of Springer Science+Business Media (www.springer.com)

The atlas is dedicated to all those suffering from cancer, their families, and loved ones.

Sasan Karimi, M.D.

Preface

Neuroimaging has come far from its early days when plain films of the skull and pneumoencephalography were used to aid the diagnosis of intracranial abnormalities. The steady improvements in computed tomography (CT) and magnetic resonance imaging (MRI) techniques have significantly enhanced our understanding of the human central nervous system (CNS) anatomy and pathology. These techniques are effective tools that neuroradiologists use routinely to better localize CNS lesions and arrive at more precise radiological diagnoses. This, in turn, results in improved patient care. Advancements in neuroimaging have also had a direct impact on how clinicians manage patients. CT angiography and perfusion in managing acute stroke and intraoperative MRI and functional MRI in the surgical management of intracranial neoplasms are only a few examples of the impact that imaging has had on patient management.

This atlas is a compilation of various CNS neoplasms and contains cases that have both classic and atypical imaging features. The chapters are concise yet provide the reader with comprehensive information about each topic. They were also written with an emphasis on detailed graphical representations of the anatomy and pathology.

I am grateful to all those who contributed to this atlas, which we hope will be a useful tool for a wide variety of practitioners involved in the care of patients with CNS neoplasms.

Contents

1 **Adult Brain Tumors** 1
Gitanjali V. Patel, Sasan Karimi, and Robert J. Young

2 **Pediatric Brain Tumors** 63
Gitanjali V. Patel, Robert J. Young, and Sasan Karimi

3 **Sellar and Parasellar Masses** 109
Gitanjali V. Patel, Sasan Karimi, and Robert J. Young

4 **Neoplastic Disease of the Spine** 141
Alan Victor Krauthamer, Sasan Partovi, and John Lyo

Index 233

Contributors

Sasan Karimi Department of Radiology, New York Presbyterian Hospital/Weill Cornell Medical College, New York, NY, USA

Neuroradiology Service, Department of Radiology, Memorial Sloan-Kettering Cancer Center, New York, NY, USA

Alan Victor Krauthamer Neuroradiology Division, Department of Radiology, New York Presbyterian Hospital/Weill Cornell Medical College, New York, NY, USA

Neuroradiology Division, Department of Radiology, Memorial Sloan-Kettering Cancer Center, New York, NY, USA

John Lyo Department of Radiology, New York Presbyterian Hospital/Weill Cornell Medical College, New York, NY, USA

Neuroradiology Service, Department of Radiology, Memorial Sloan-Kettering Cancer Center, New York, NY, USA

Sasan Partovi Department of Radiology, Memorial Sloan-Kettering Cancer Center, New York, NY, USA

Gitanjali V. Patel Department of Radiology, Memorial Sloan-Kettering Cancer Center, New York, NY, USA

Robert J. Young Department of Radiology, New York Presbyterian Hospital/Weill Cornell Medical College, New York, NY, USA

Neuroradiology Service, Department of Radiology, Memorial Sloan-Kettering Cancer Center, New York, NY, USA

Adult Brain Tumors

1

Gitanjali V. Patel, Sasan Karimi, and Robert J. Young

Intra-axial

General

Metastasis. A metastasis arises from the spread of a systemic malignancy or nonadjacent primary central nervous system (CNS) malignancy to the brain or its coverings. Parenchymal metastases account for about half of all brain tumors [1]. The incidence of metastases to brain parenchyma tends to increase with age [2, 3]. Parenchymal metastasis has peak prevalence at 65 years old and a slight predominance in men [1]. Extra-axial metastasis is more common in the pediatric population [3]. Survival of patients with cranial metastasis is dictated by size, number, and location of lesions [2, 3]. Metastasis to the brain parenchyma, however, generally indicates a poor prognosis as most patients who receive whole brain radiation therapy have a median survival of 3–6 months [1].

Imaging features. Parenchymal brain metastases are often found near the gray-white junctions and arterial blood supply within the cerebral hemispheres [3]. Around 15 % of parenchymal metastases are located within the cerebellum and 3 % are located within the basal ganglia [1]. Neoplastic dissemination into the ventricles and leptomeninges is far less common [1, 3]. Half of all parenchymal metastases are solitary lesions, whereas the other half include two or more [2]. Most metastatic brain lesions enhance with contrast imaging. Presence of hemorrhage and edema is variable.

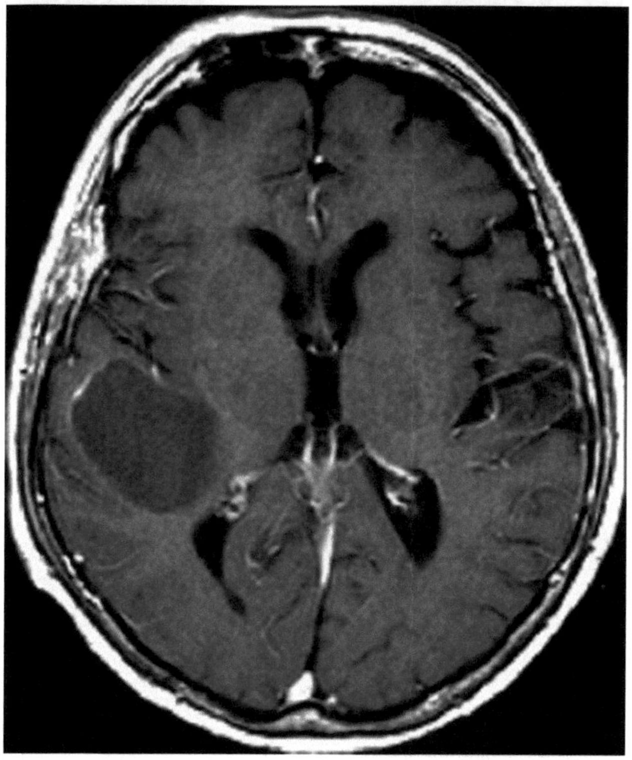

Fig. 1.1 Metastasis. Axial contrast T1-weighted image demonstrates a metastasis at the right temporo-occipital junction with thin enhancing rim

G.V. Patel
Department of Radiology, Memorial Sloan-Kettering Cancer Center, 1275 York Avenue, MRI-1156, New York, NY 10065, USA
e-mail: gita.patel@gmail.com

S. Karimi • R.J. Young (✉)
Department of Radiology, New York Presbyterian Hospital/Weill Cornell Medical College, New York, NY, USA

Neuroradiology Service, Department of Radiology, Memorial Sloan-Kettering Cancer Center, 1275 York Avenue, MRI-1156, New York, NY 10065, USA
e-mail: karimis@mskcc.org; youngr@mskcc.org

S. Karimi (ed.), *Atlas of Brain and Spine Oncology Imaging*, Atlas of Oncology Imaging,
DOI 10.1007/978-1-4614-5653-7_1, © Springer Science+Business Media New York 2013

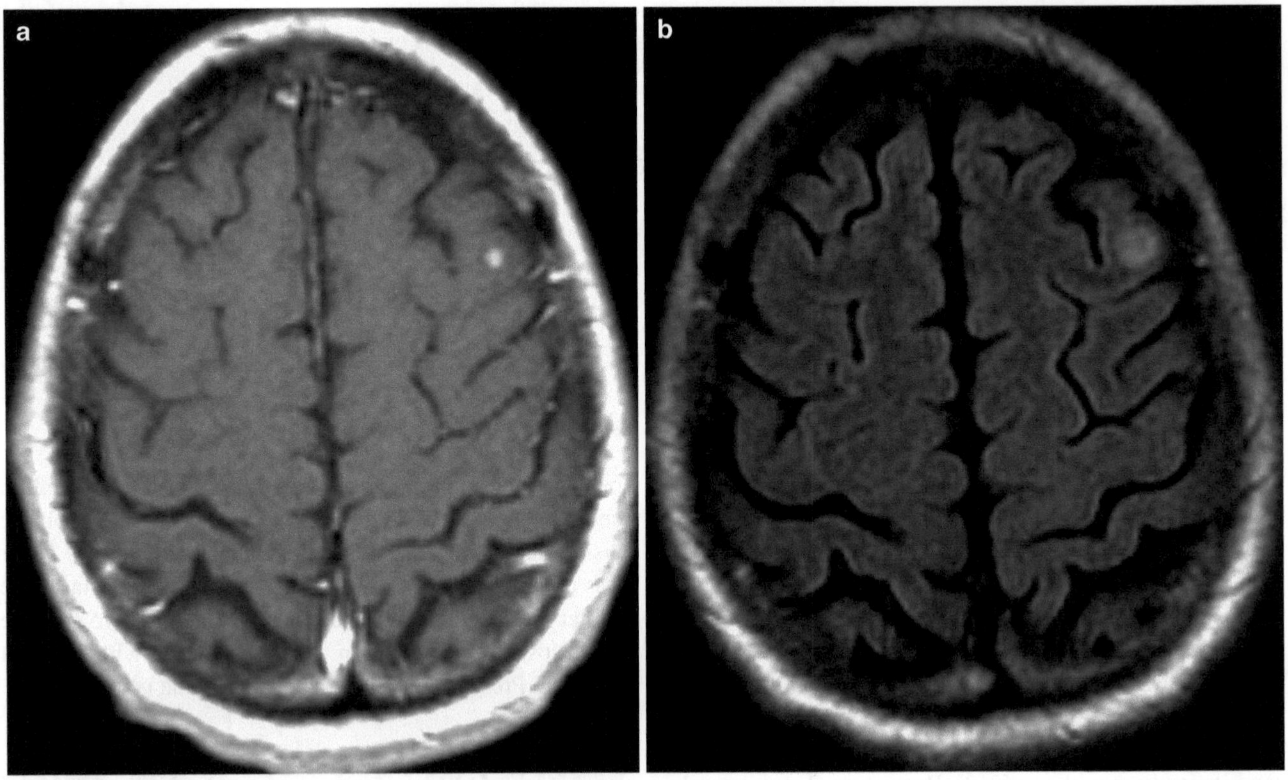

Fig. 1.2 Metastasis. Axial contrast T1-weighted (**a**) and fluid-attenuated inversion recovery (FLAIR) (**b**) images reveal a small metastasis in the left middle frontal gyrus at the gray-white junction with minor surrounding edema as seen on the FLAIR image

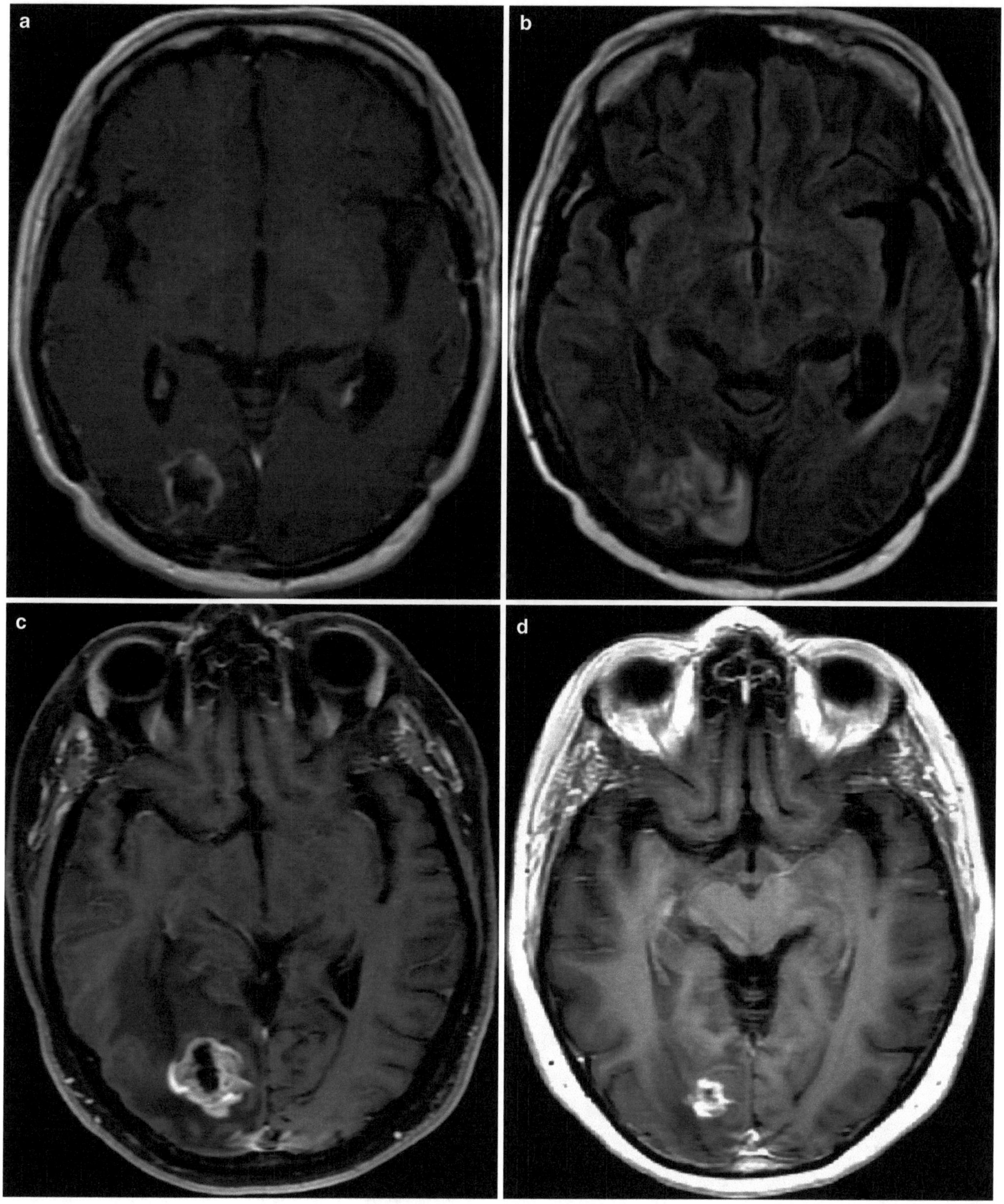

Fig. 1.3 Metastases. Axial contrast T1-weighted (**a**) and FLAIR (**b**) images show a heterogeneously enhancing metastasis in the right occipital lobe. Craniotomy and postoperative changes are partially visualized in the left temporal lobe. Six months after stereotactic radiosurgery (SRS) to the occipital lobe metastasis, fat-suppressed contrast T1-weighted image (**c**) revealed an enlarging heterogeneously enhancing mass in the treated site. Because the patient remained asymptomatic, this was thought to represent radiation necrosis and simply followed without additional therapy. Contrast T1-weighted image (**d**) 9 months after *C* demonstrated a decrease in radiation necrosis

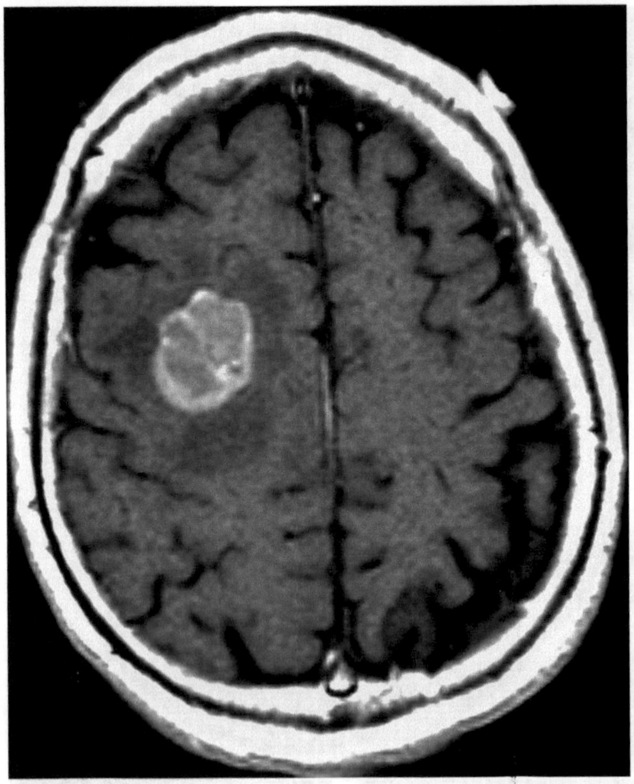

Fig. 1.4 Metastases. Axial contrast T1-weighted image of a large right frontal lobe mass. Surrounding hypointensity is consistent with vasogenic edema

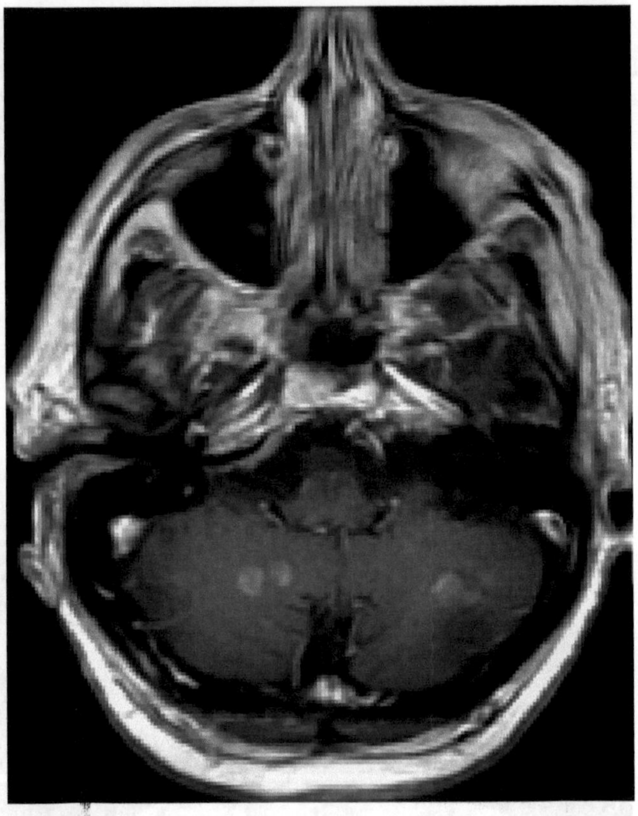

Fig. 1.5 Metastases. Axial contrast T1-weighted image of a patient with non-small-cell lung carcinoma with multiple small cerebellar metastases

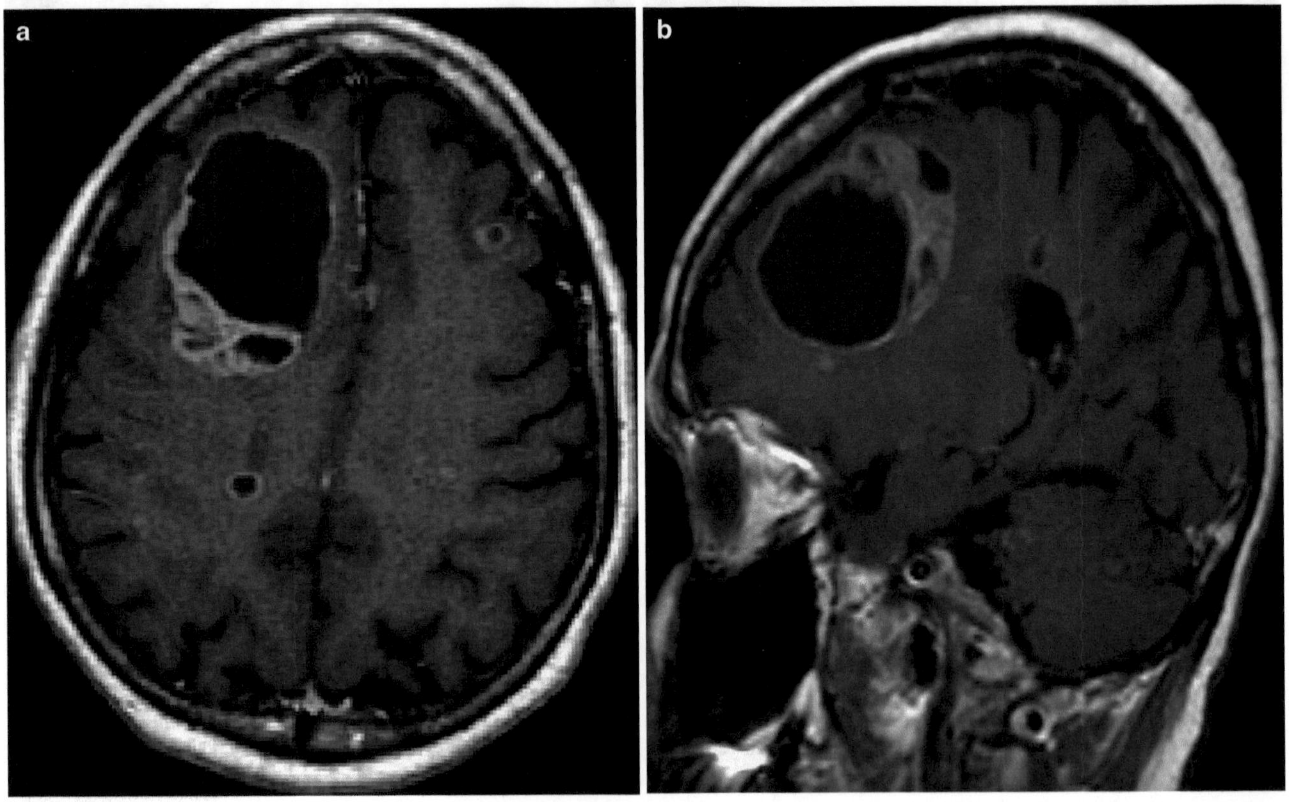

Fig. 1.6 Metastases. Axial (**a**) and sagittal (**b**) contrast T1-weighted images demonstrate complex cystic and solid right frontal lobe metastasis. Note additional small cystic/necrotic rim-enhancing metastases in bilateral frontal lobes

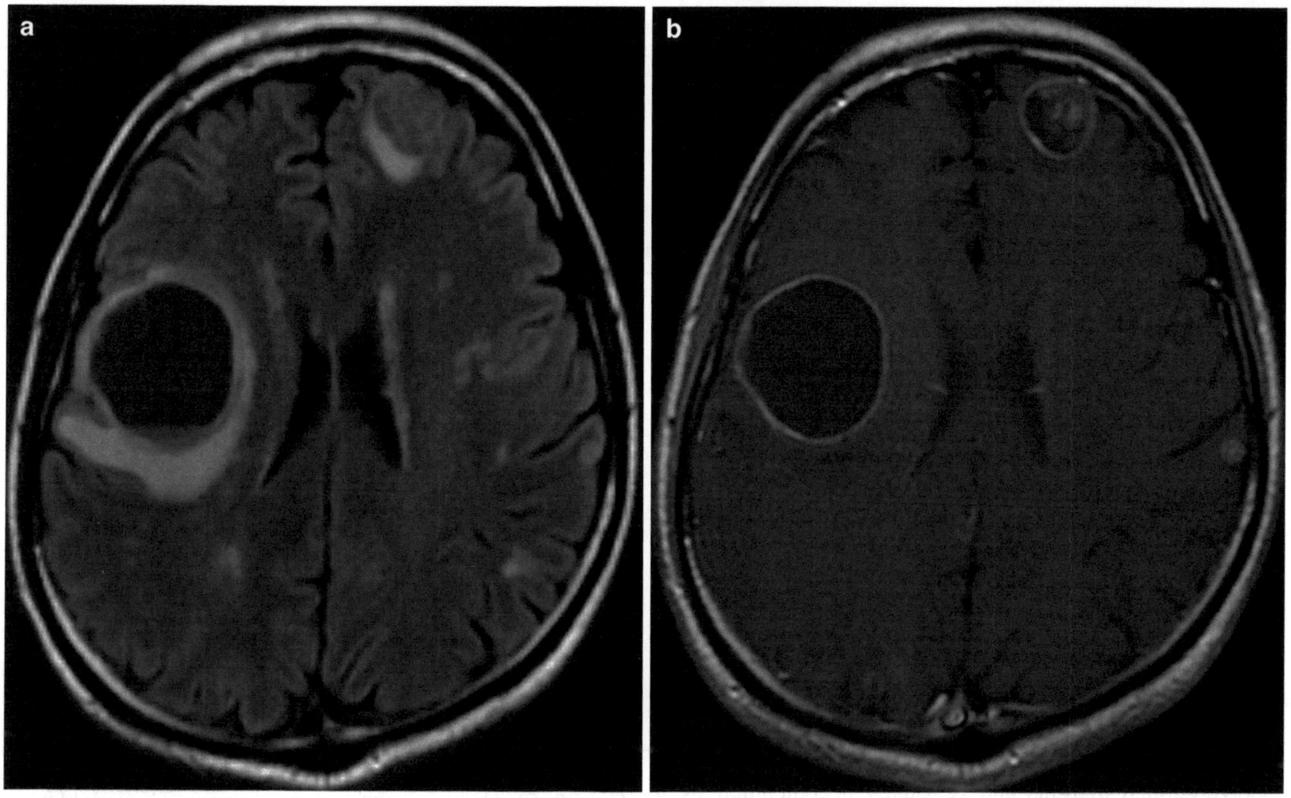

Fig. 1.7 Metastases. Axial FLAIR (**a**) and contrast T1-weighted (**b**) images of a right frontal cystic metastasis with an internal fluid–fluid (hematocrit) level on the FLAIR image, indicating intralesional hemorrhage

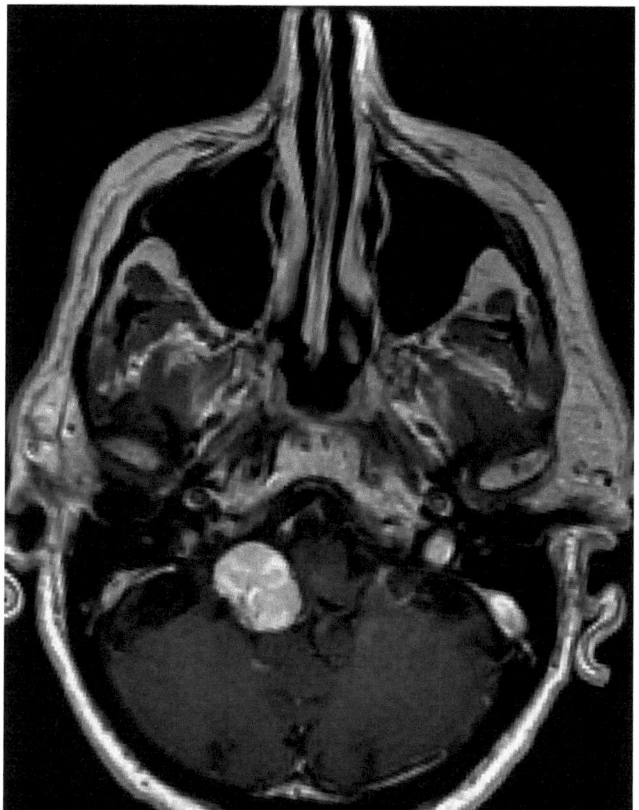

Fig. 1.8 Metastases. Axial contrast T1-weighted image of a patient with renal cell carcinoma and an extra-axial metastasis to the choroid plexus in the right foramen of Luschka

Glioblastoma Multiforme

Glioblastoma multiforme (GBM) is a grade IV glial brain tumor that is characterized by poorly differentiated anaplastic cells surrounding focal areas of necrosis and neovascularity [4, 5]. It is the most common of all primary brain tumors and accounts for 12–15 % of all intracranial malignancies and 50–60 % of all astrocytomas [4]. GBM has an incidence of around 2–3 cases per 100,000 people and has a male to female ratio of 1.6:1 [5, 6]. This tumor typically occurs in adults 40–70 years old but can occur at any age [4]. GBM is a rapidly growing tumor and, as such, carries a poor prognosis; patients usually die within 1 year after diagnosis [7].

Imaging features. GBM can be identified on imaging as an irregular, heterogeneously enhancing mass, usually with areas of necrosis [4]. These tumors are frequently located in the white matter of cerebral hemispheres with relative sparing of the occipital lobe [4, 8]. GBM tumors located in the brain stem and cerebellum are more commonly found in the pediatric population [4, 8]. GBM tumors are often seen crossing white matter tracts to involve the contralateral hemisphere [8]. The term "butterfly glioma" typically refers to GBM that cross the corpus callosum [4, 8]. This tumor has poorly defined margins and is usually accompanied by a great deal of surrounding edema and mass effect [4, 8]. GBM may contain necrosis, cysts, and hemorrhage and rarely contain calcium [4, 8], although mineralization may occur after treatment.

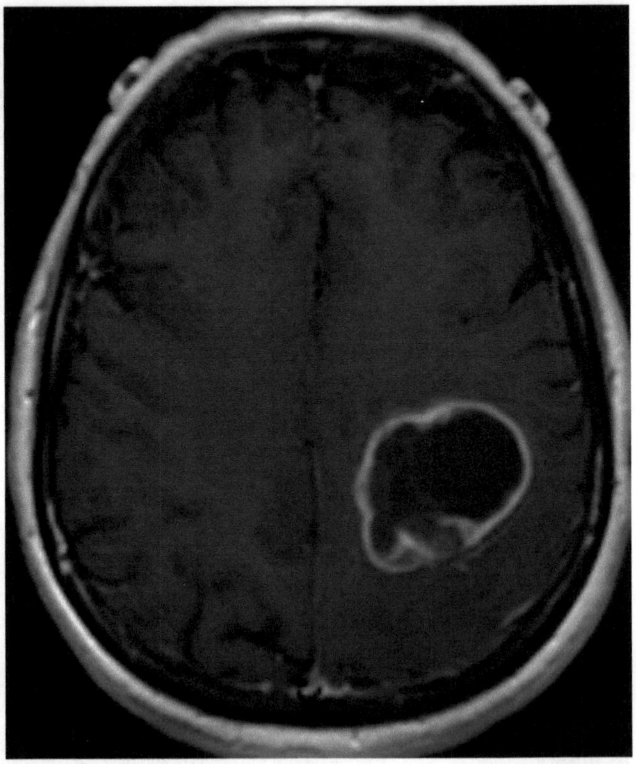

Fig. 1.9 Glioblastoma multiforme. Axial contrast T1-weighted image of left parietal lobe rim-enhancing GBM

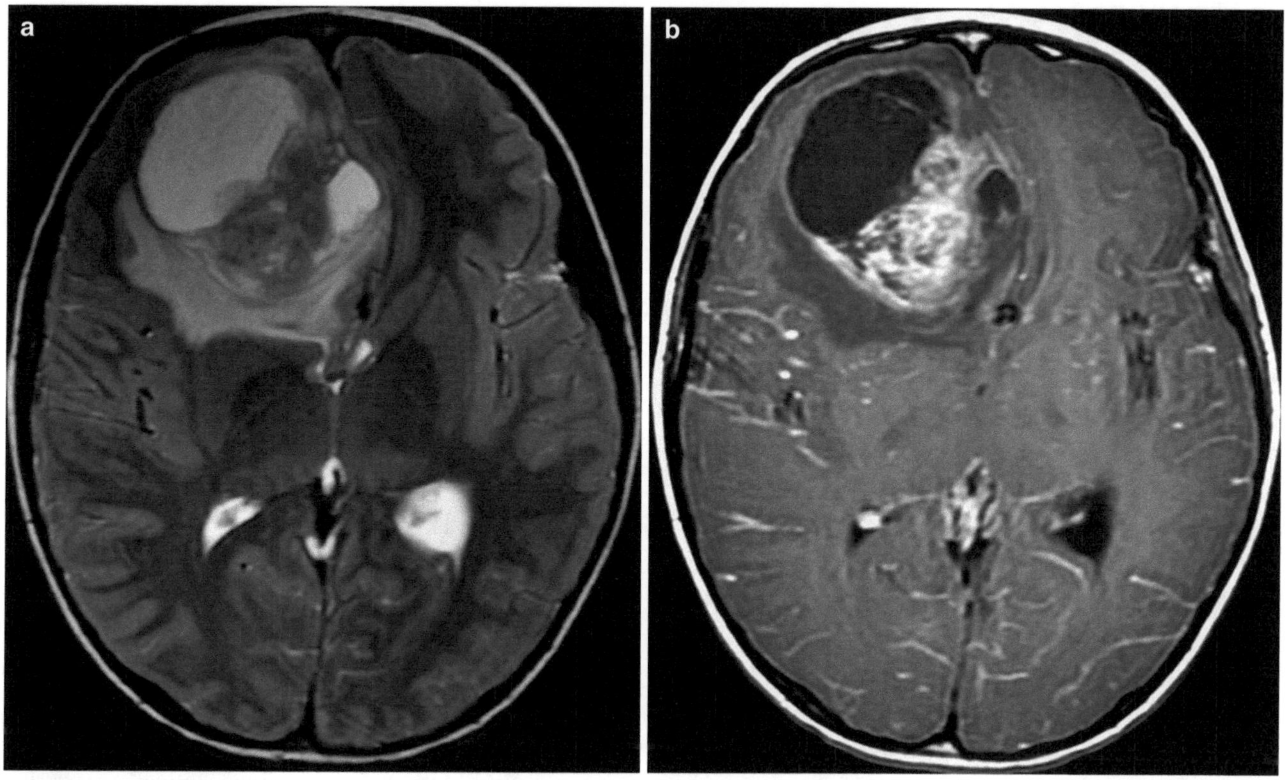

Fig. 1.10 Glioblastoma multiforme. Axial T2-weighted (**a**) and contrast T1-weighted (**b**) images of a patient with GBM reveal a large, heterogeneous, right frontal lobe mass containing cystic and necrotic components. Surrounding T2 hyperintensity is consistent with edema and/or nonenhancing tumor

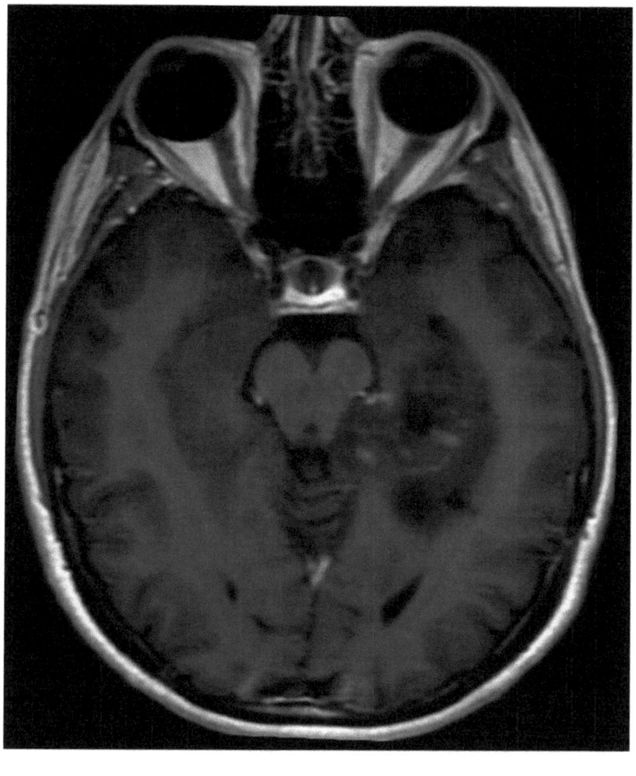

Fig. 1.11 Glioblastoma multiforme. Axial contrast T1-weighted image of a minimally enhancing expansile GBM in the medial left temporal lobe. Most but not all high-grade gliomas show contrast enhancement

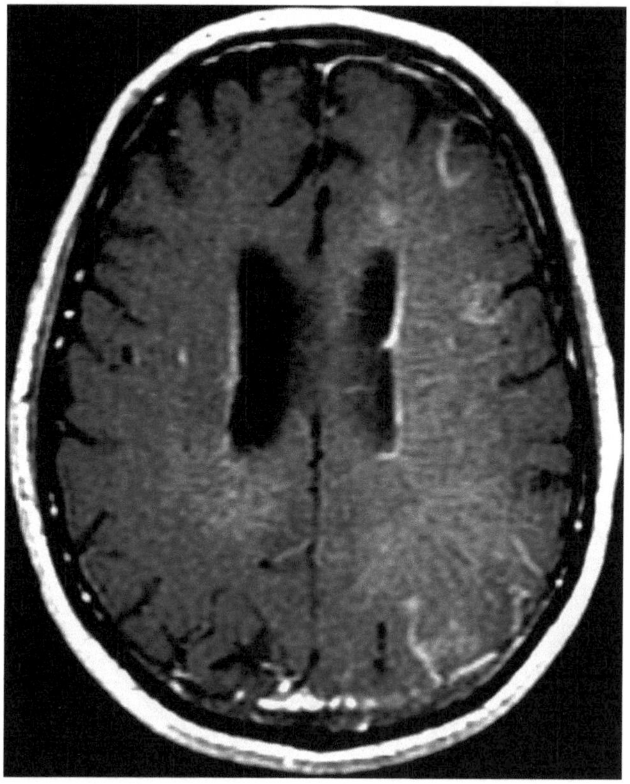

Fig. 1.12 Glioblastoma multiforme. Axial contrast T1-weighted image of a GBM invading along perivascular and leptomeningeal spaces resembling angioinvasive lymphoma. Neurosarcoidosis and tuberculosis are also possibilities

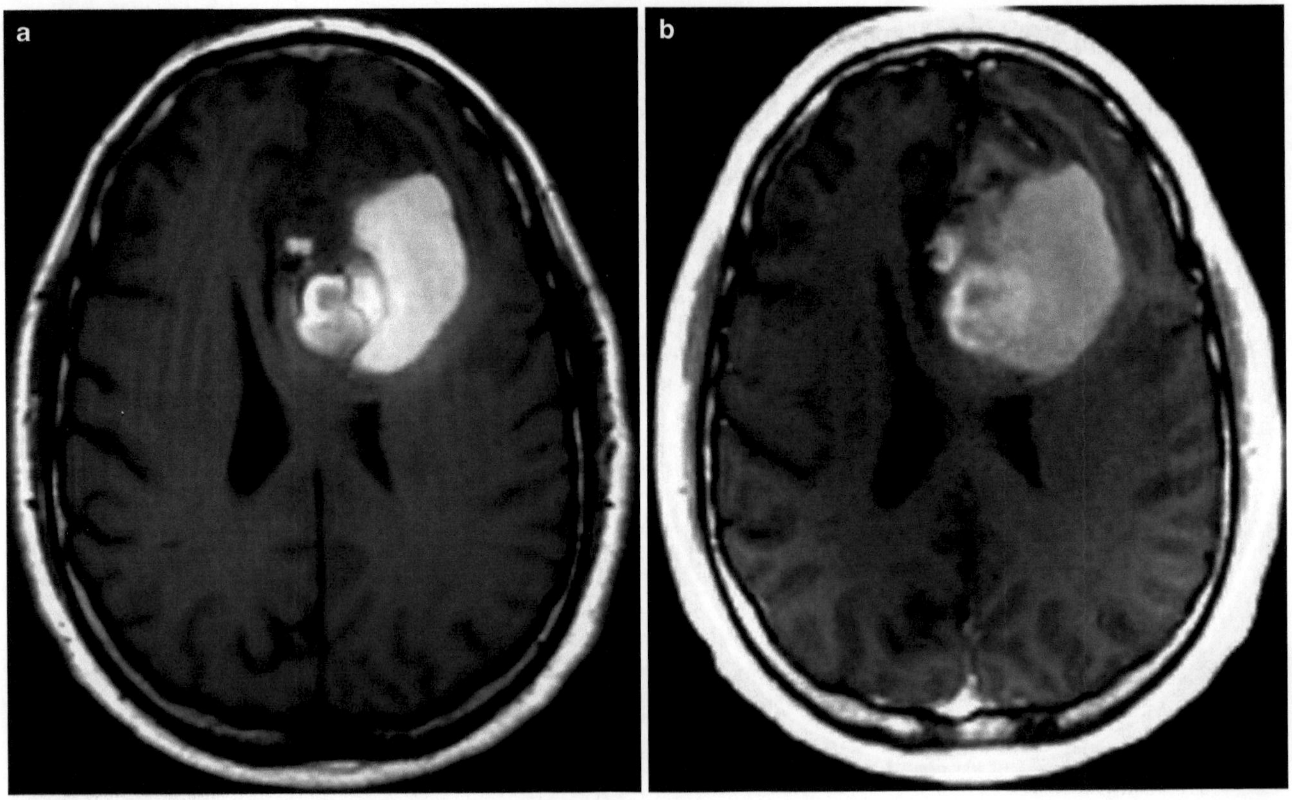

Fig. 1.13 Glioblastoma multiforme. Axial pre- (**a**) and contrast (**b**) T1-weighted images of a large left frontal lobe GBM extending into the corpus callosum containing a large amount of T1 hyperintense subacute blood

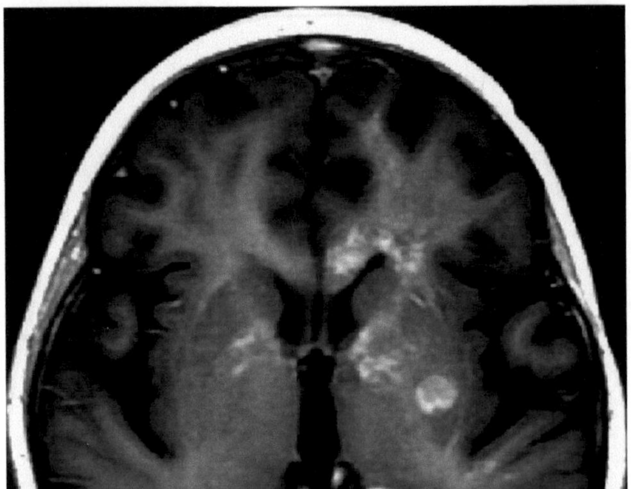

Fig. 1.14 Glioblastoma multiforme. Axial contrast T1-weighted image demonstrates patchy enhancing tumors in the bilateral basal ganglia, periventricular, and corpus callosum in a patient with GBM. The tumor is parenchymal and perivascular in location

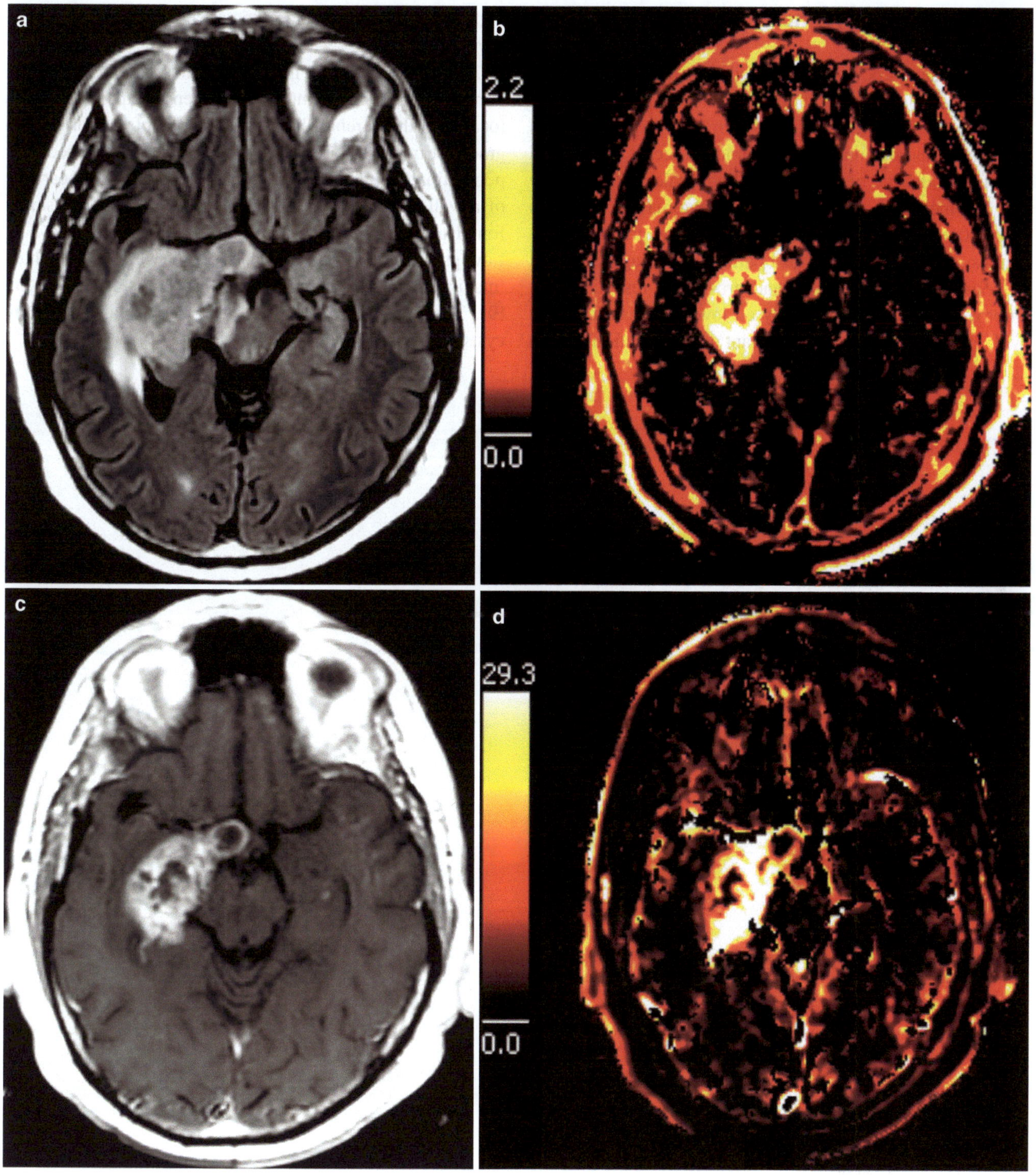

Fig. 1.15 Glioblastoma multiforme. Axial FLAIR (**a**), dynamic contrast-enhanced plasma volume map (**b**), contrast T1-weighted (**c**), and permeability, volume transfer coefficient (Ktrans) maps (**d**) demonstrate a heterogeneously enhancing right medial temporal GBM. Increased vascularity from angiogenesis is demonstrated on the plasma volume map (**b**). Increased permeability (**d**) corresponds with the region of enhancement (**c**)

Low-Grade Astrocytoma

A low-grade astrocytoma is a grade II primary glial brain tumor that is diffusely infiltrating and slow growing [9]. This tumor is responsible for 10–15 % of all astrocytomas [9]. Low-grade astrocytoma most commonly occurs in the third and fourth decade of life with a slight male predominance [9]. The incidence of a low-grade astrocytoma is 0.6 cases in 100,000 person years [10]. Patients with low-grade astrocytoma survive around 6–10 years after initial diagnoses [11]. A younger age at diagnosis and gross total resection may improve prognosis [11]. Nearly all low-grade astrocytomas will eventually undergo malignant transformation into a high-grade glioma, an anaplastic astrocytoma, or a glioblastoma [11, 12].

Imaging features. A majority of these brain tumors are nonenhancing, T2-weighted, hyperintense, expansile lesions located in the cerebral hemispheres [9]. Infratentorial low-grade astrocytomas are more commonly seen in the pediatric population [11]. On imaging, this tumor has the appearance of a well-circumscribed lesion, which on biopsy is usually found to be infiltrating neighboring brain tissue [11, 12]. Low-grade astrocytomas appear hyperintense on T2-weighted imaging sequences and restricted diffusion is usually absent [9]. The presence of enhancement, hemorrhage, calcium, cysts, or edema is rare in this tumor type [9].

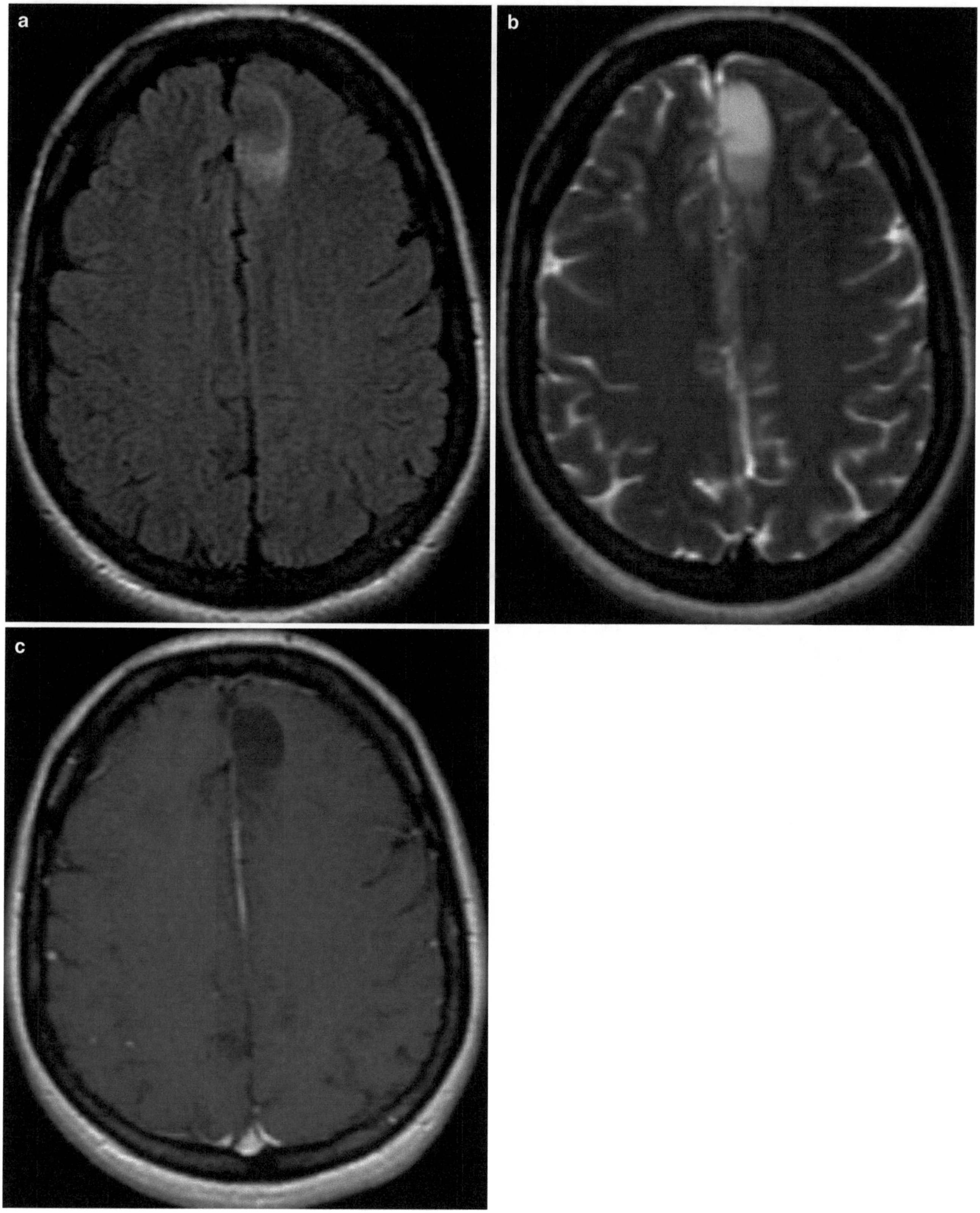

Fig. 1.16 Low-grade astrocytoma. Axial FLAIR (**a**), T2-weighted (**b**), and contrast T1-weighted (**c**) images demonstrate a left anterior paramedian frontal lobe nonenhancing tumor

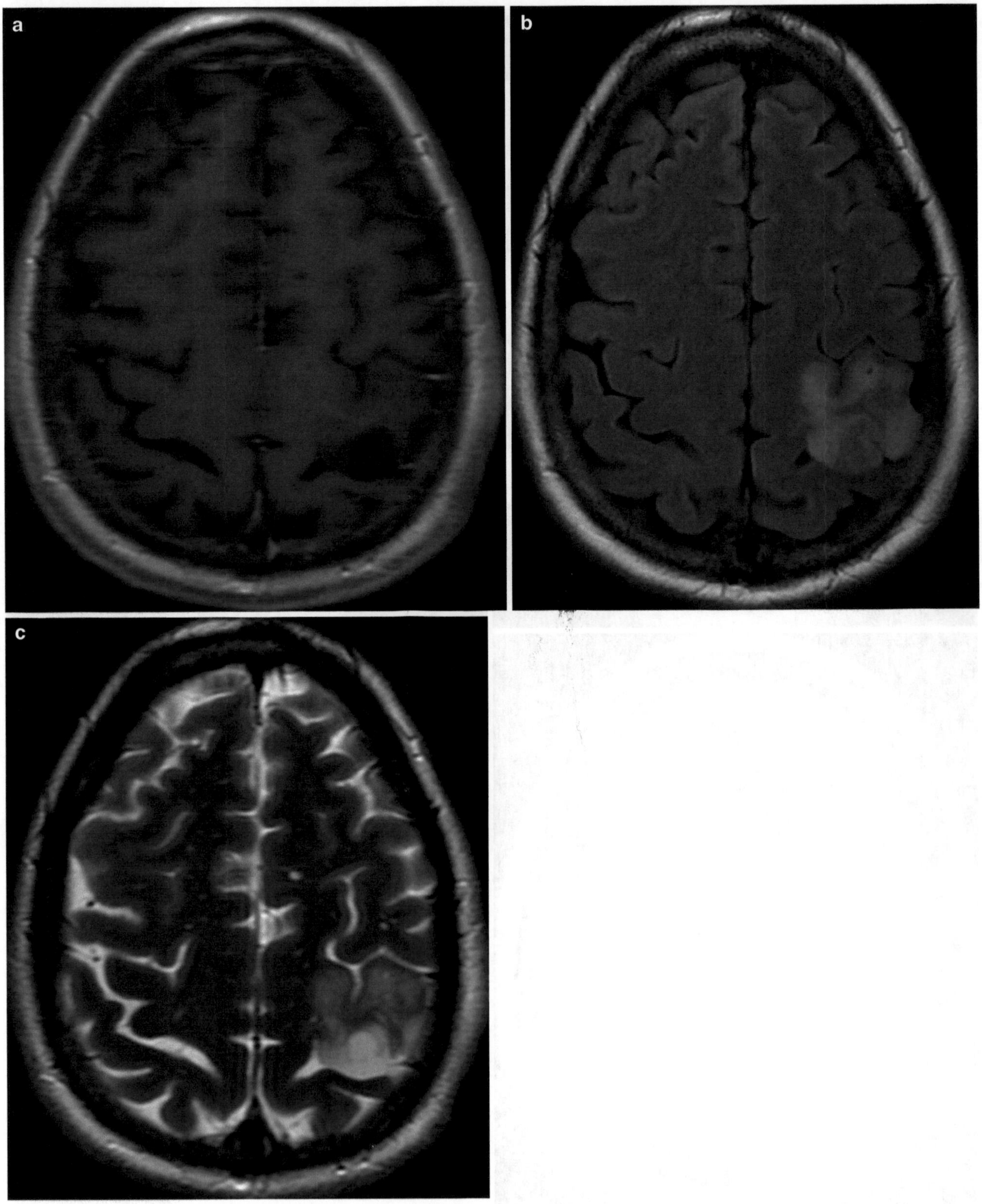

Fig. 1.17 Low-grade astrocytoma. Axial contrast T1-weighted (**a**), FLAIR (**b**), and T2-weighted (**c**) images demonstrate a left posterior frontal lobe nonenhancing expansile tumor involving the motor strip

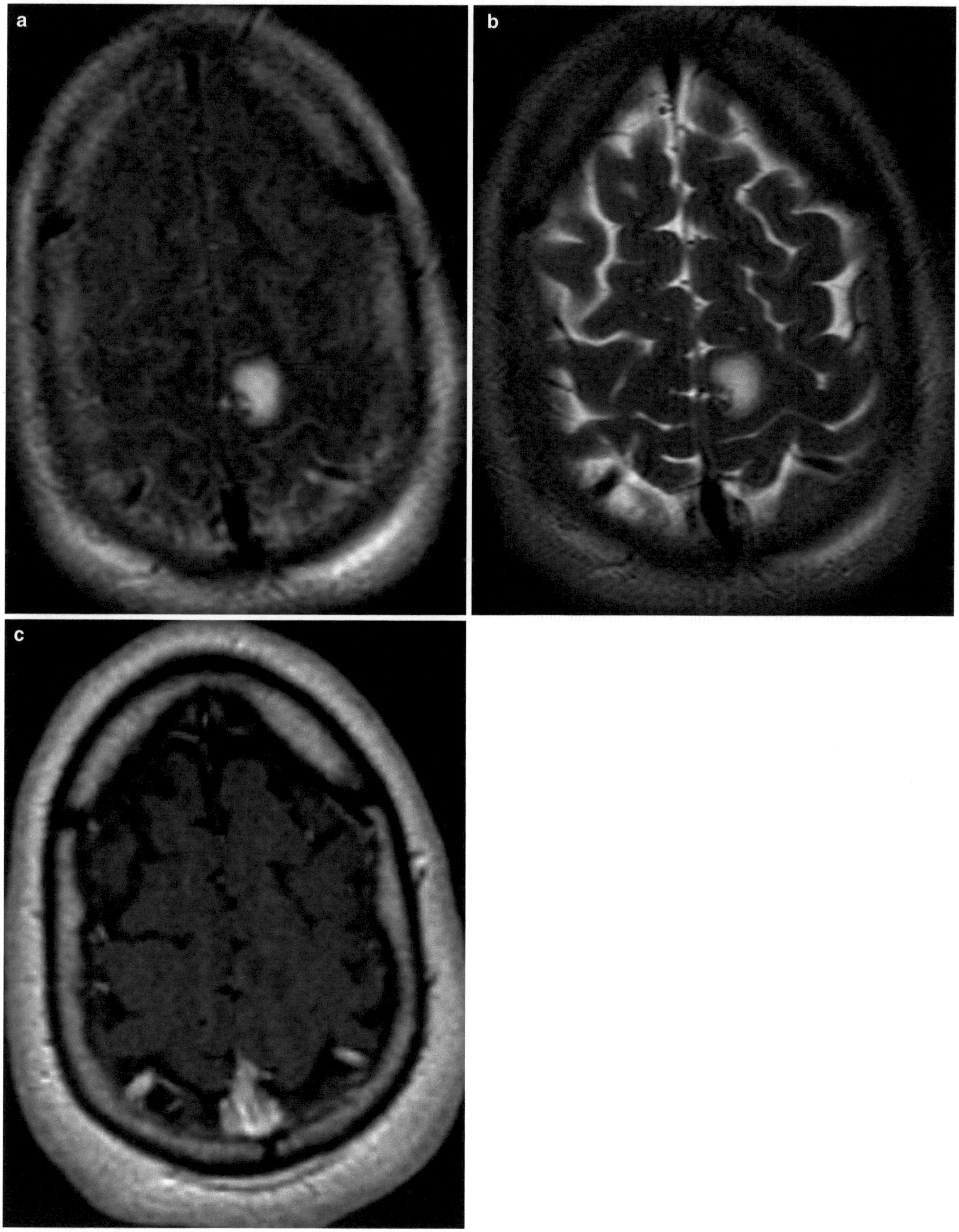

Fig. 1.18 Low-grade astrocytoma. Axial FLAIR (**a**), T2-weighted (**b**), and contrast T1-weighted (**c**) images demonstrate a left posterior paramedian frontal lobe nonenhancing tumor

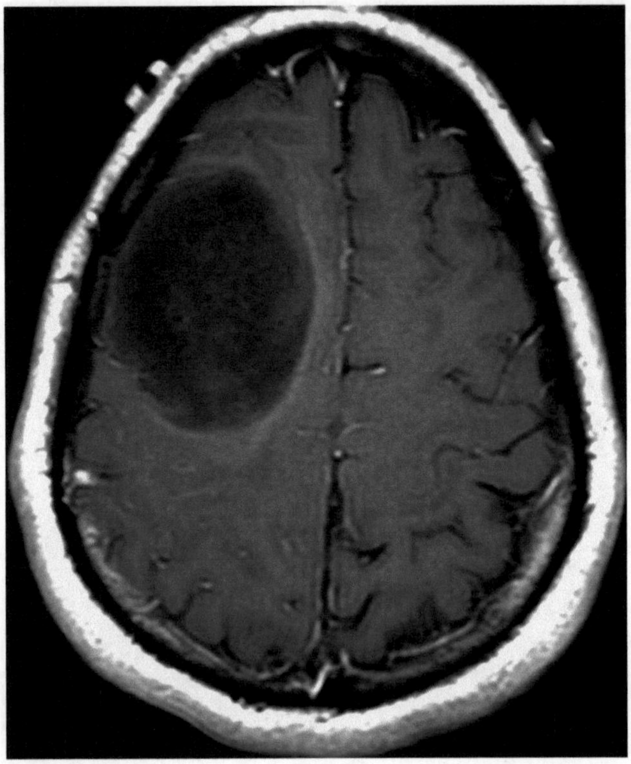

Fig. 1.19 Low-grade astrocytoma. Axial contrast T1-weighted image reveals a large right frontal lobe hypointense nonenhancing tumor

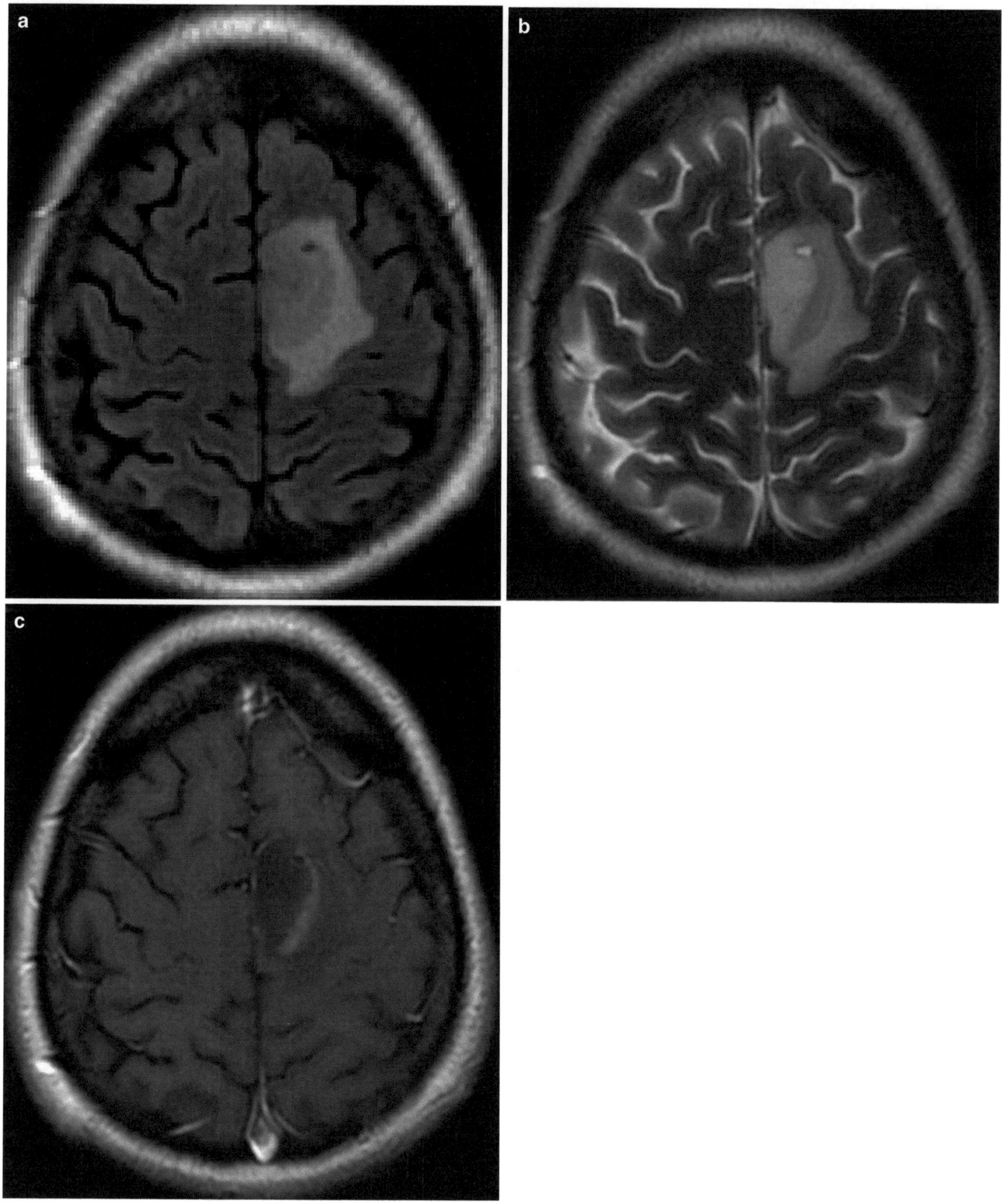

Fig. 1.20 Low-grade astrocytoma. Axial FLAIR (**a**), T2-weighted (**b**), and contrast T1-weighted (**c**) images demonstrate a left posterior paramedian frontal lobe tumor with mild marginal enhancement, involving the supplemental motor area. Notice that the tumor extends posteriorly to involve the medial extent of the motor strip

Supratentorial

Oligodendroglioma

An oligodendroglioma is a grade II primary glial brain tumors that is well differentiated and indolent in nature. This tumor is the most common intracranial mass to calcify [13, 14]. Oligodendrogliomas account for 5–10 % of all primary intracranial neoplasms and 5–25 % of all gliomas [13]. These tumors have an incidence of 0.27 cases in 100,000 person-years and usually occur in the middle-aged adult population [13, 14]. Patients with oligodendroglioma survive around 10 years after diagnosis and have a 5-year survival rate of 50–75 % [13]. Patients with a younger age of diagnosis, lack of enhancement on imaging, and frontal location of tumor tend to have a better prognosis [13, 14].

Imaging features. Oligodendrogliomas are typically calcified frontal lobe lesions that invade the cortex and subcortical white matter [13]. They are well-defined masses that are most commonly located supratentorially [13, 15]. Infratentorial and intraventricular location of oligodendrogliomas are rare [13, 15]. These tumors commonly contain areas of cystic degeneration whereas enhancement, edema, and hemorrhage are rarely seen [13]. New enhancement of a previously nonenhancing lesion usually indicates progression to an anaplastic oligodendroglioma [14].

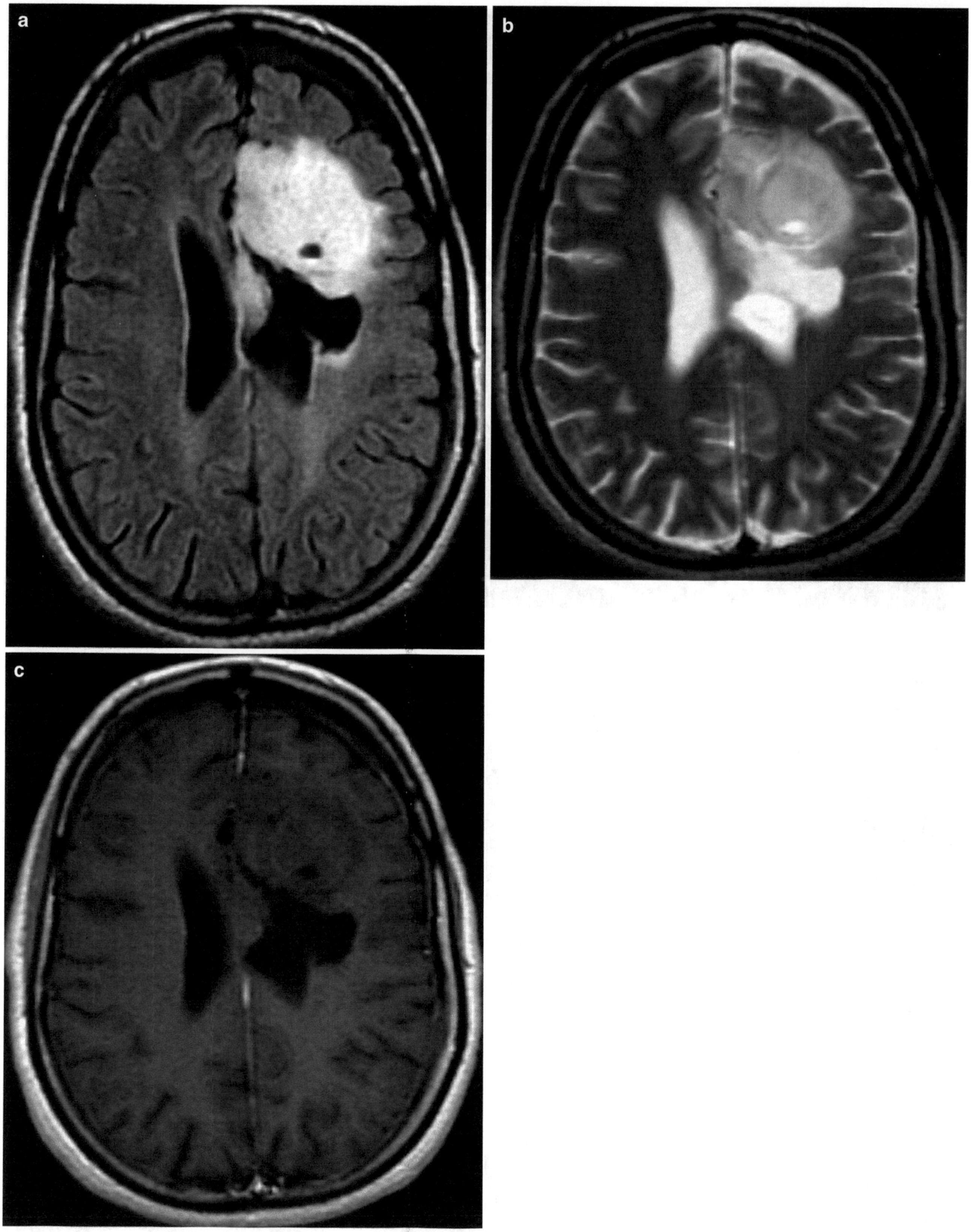

Fig. 1.21 Oligodendroglioma. Axial FLAIR (**a**), T2-weighted (**b**), and contrast T1-weighted (**c**) images of a patient with left frontal oligodendroglioma extending in to the corpus callosum. There is a small cystic-appearing area within the tumor

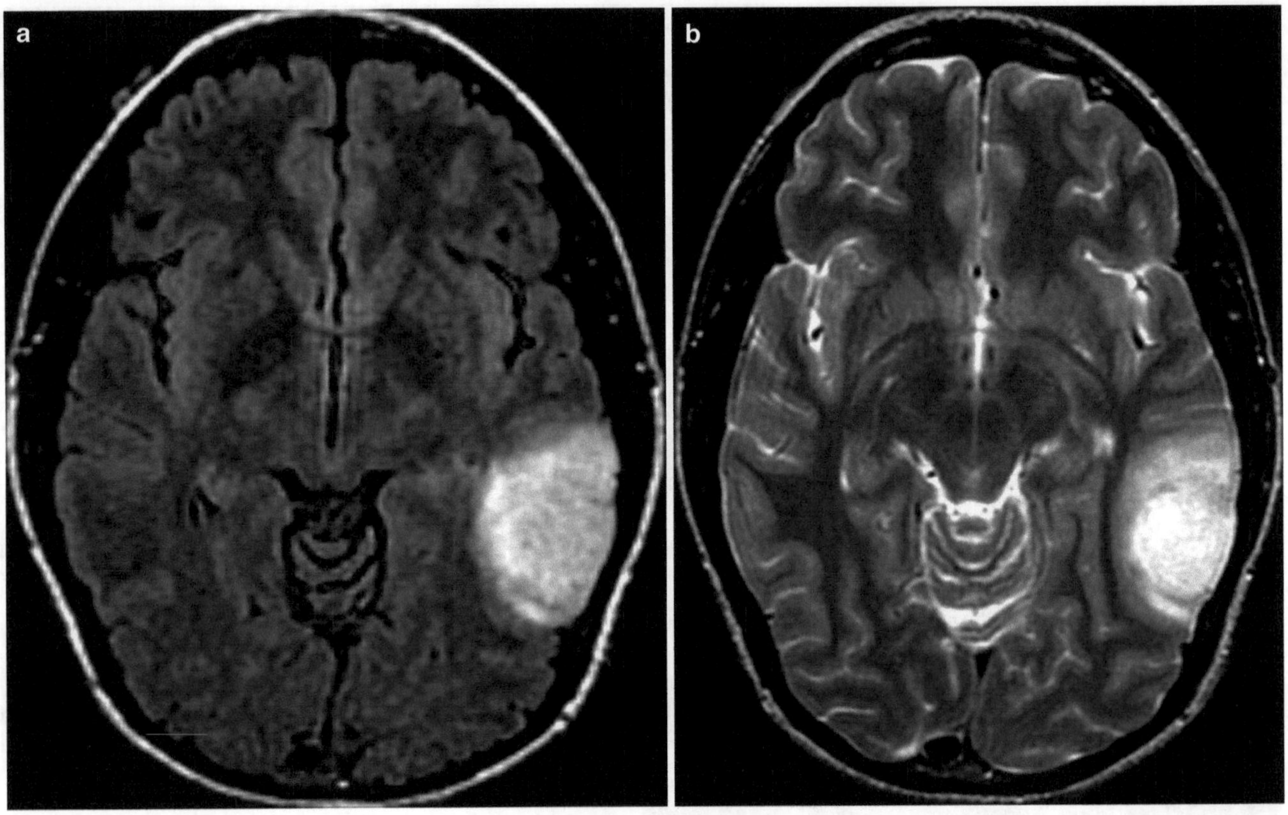

Fig. 1.22 Oligodendroglioma. Axial FLAIR (**a**) and T2-weighted (**b**) images demonstrate a slightly expansile, peripherally based tumor typical for an oligodendroglioma

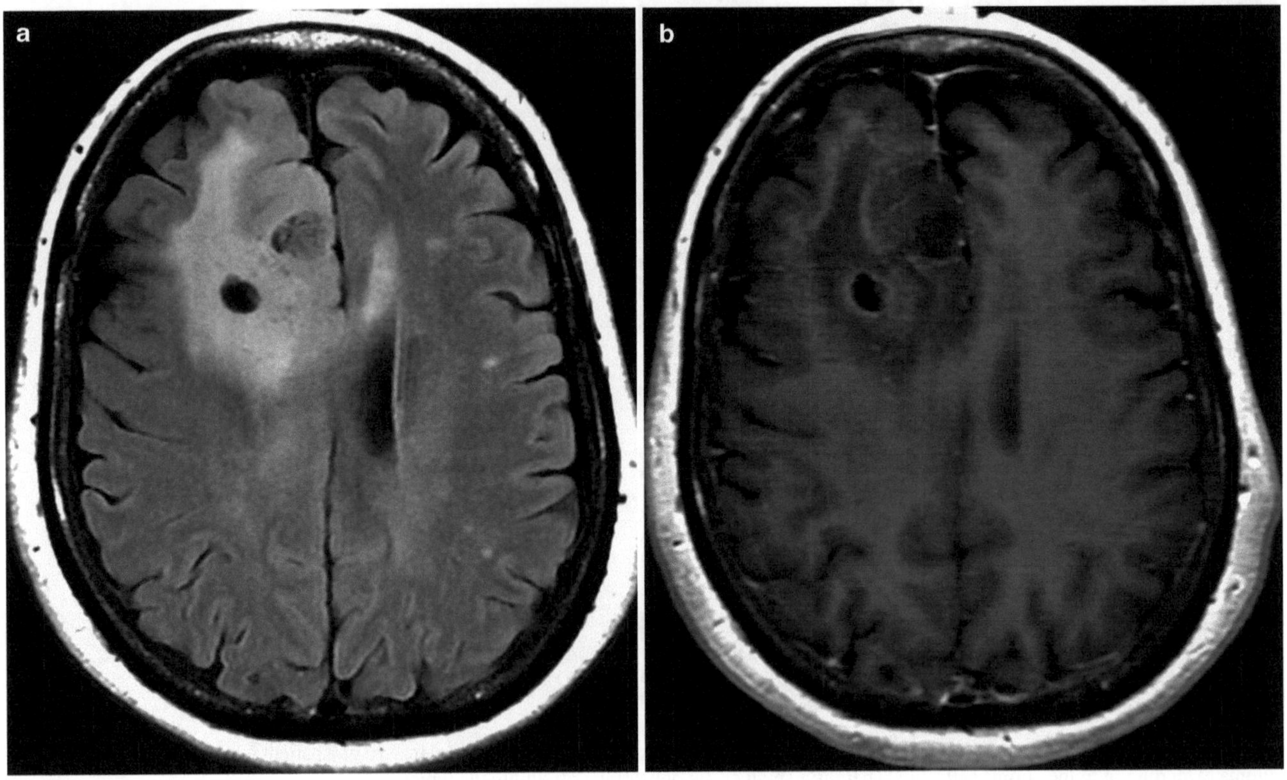

Fig. 1.23 Oligodendroglioma. Axial FLAIR (**a**) and contrast T1-weighted (**b**) images of a patient with a right frontal lobe oligodendroglioma extending through the anterior corpus callosum

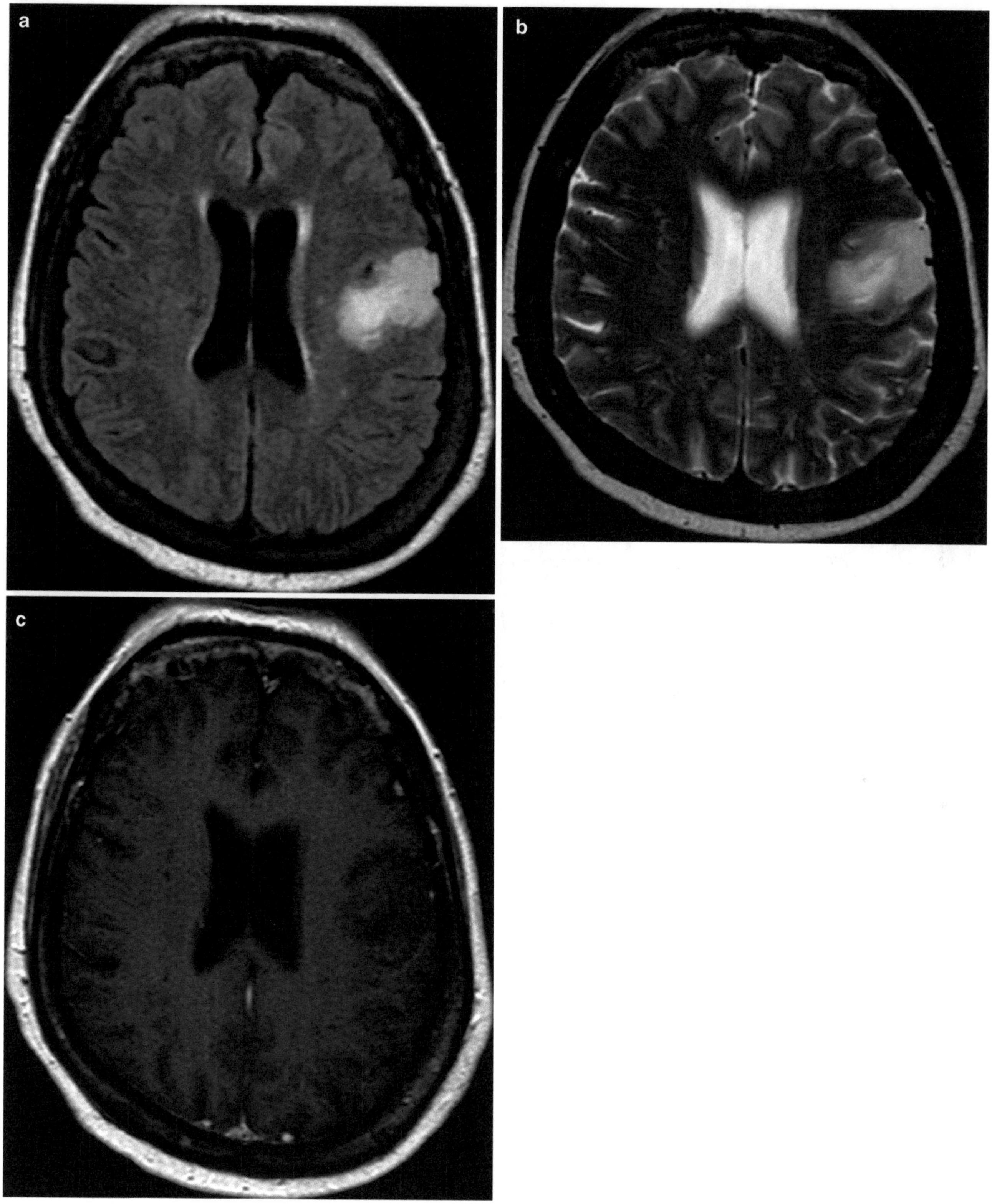

Fig. 1.24 Oligodendroglioma. Axial FLAIR (**a**), T2-weighted (**b**), and contrast T1-weighted (**c**) images of a left posterior frontal nonenhancing oligodendroglioma extending to brain surface

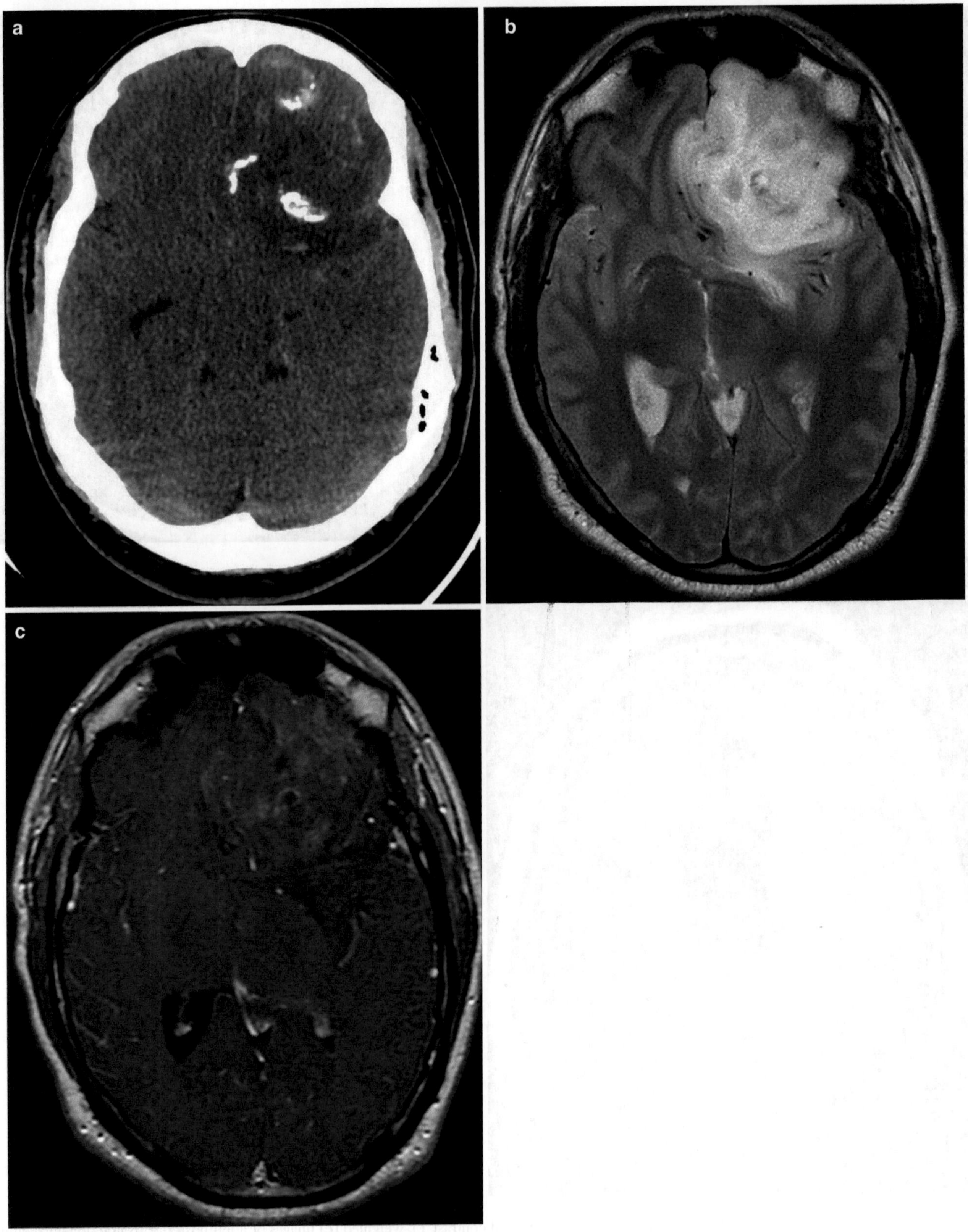

Fig. 1.25 Oligodendroglioma. Axial non-contrast computed tomography (CT) (**a**), T2-weighted (**b**), and contrast T1-weighted (**c**) images of an expansile, left frontal lobe oligodendroglioma containing calcification. Note that the tumor extends to brain surface

Anaplastic Astrocytoma

An anaplastic astrocytoma is a grade III brain tumor that has a focal or diffuse lack of cellular differentiation and has a tendency to invade neighboring brain tissue [16]. These tumors account for about one third of all astrocytomas and have an incidence of 0.4 cases per 100,000 person years [10, 17]. Anaplastic astrocytomas occur most frequently in the sixth decade of life with a male to female ratio of 1.8:1 [17]. They may be primary (de novo anaplastic astrocytoma) or secondary (malignant transformation of a low-grade astrocytoma) in nature [16]. Patients with anaplastic astrocytoma have a median survival of 2–3 years after diagnosis [16, 17].

Imaging features. Anaplastic astrocytomas are ill-defined heterogenous lesions that most frequently involve hemispheric white matter in the frontal or temporal lobes [16, 17]. Most show heterogenous enhancement, and only rarely contain calcium, hemorrhage, or cysts [16, 17]. At pathology, these lack the typical necrosis that is requisite for the diagnosis of grade IV glioblastoma [17]. This tumor may appear discrete but neoplastic cells are often found outside the region of abnormal signal [17].

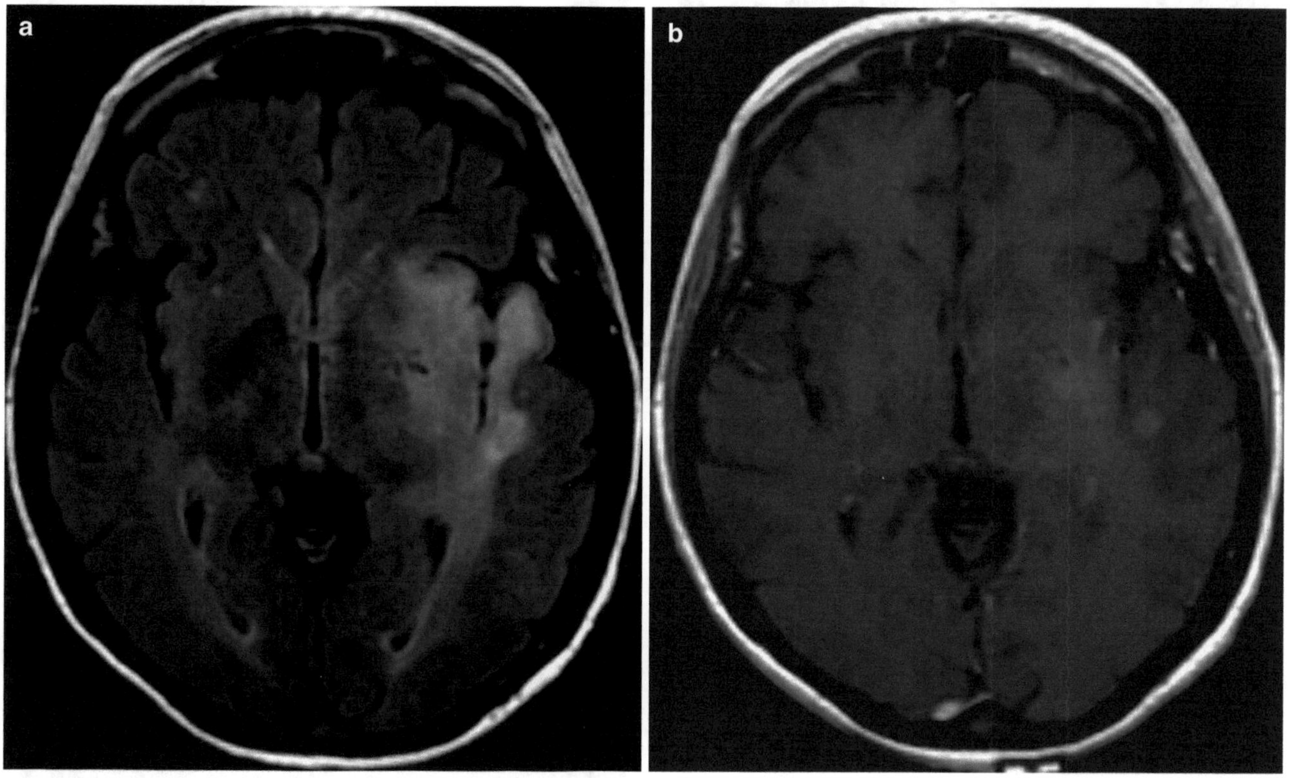

Fig. 1.26 Anaplastic astrocytoma. Axial FLAIR (**a**) and contrast T1-weighted (**b**) images of a patient with anaplastic astrocytoma reveals left insular and peri-insular infiltrating tumor with patchy regions of enhancement

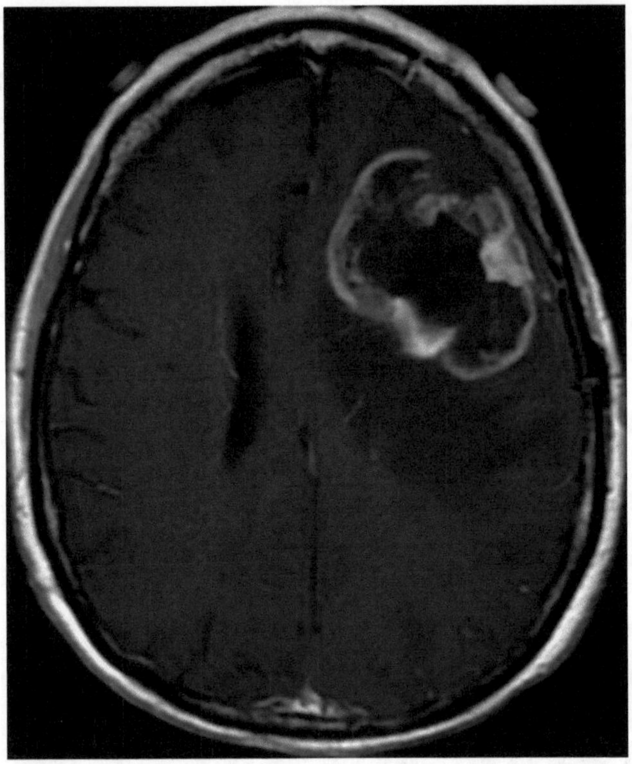

Fig. 1.27 Anaplastic astrocytoma. Axial contrast T1-weighted image demonstrates a peripherally enhancing anaplastic astrocytoma within the left frontal lobe

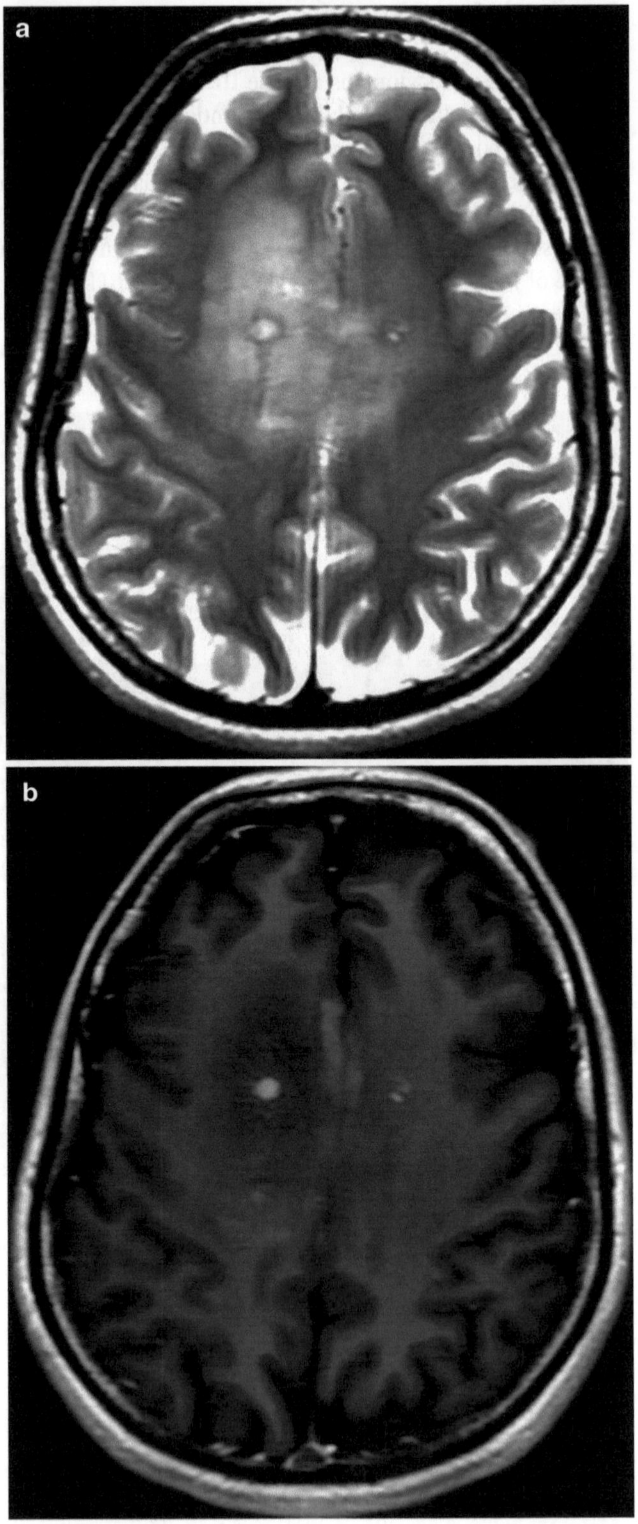

Fig. 1.28 Anaplastic astrocytoma. Axial T2-weighted (**a**) and T1-weighted contrast (**b**) images of a patient with anaplastic astrocytoma reveal bifrontal-transcallosal infiltrating tumor with small foci of enhancement

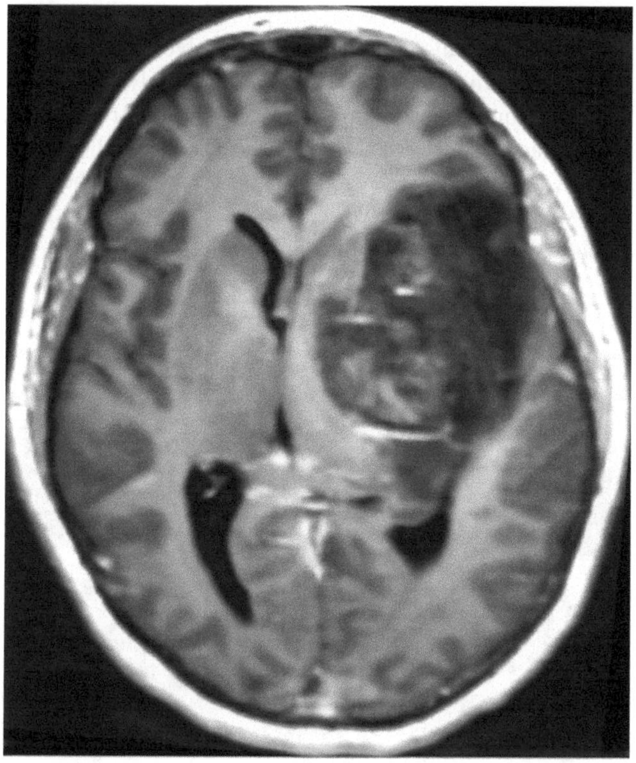

Fig. 1.29 Anaplastic astrocytoma. Axial contrast T1-weighted image demonstrates a large left hemispheric, minimally enhancing, expansile tumor

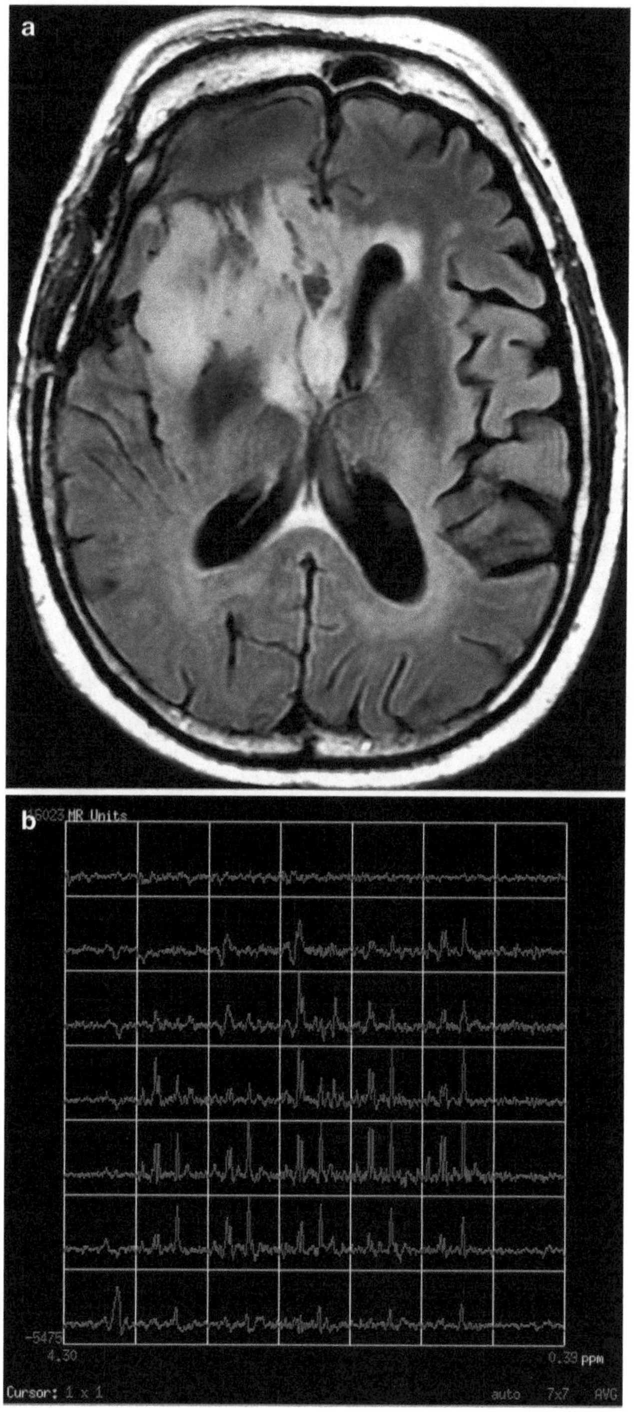

Fig. 1.30 Anaplastic astrocytoma. Axial FLAIR (**a**) and multivoxel spectroscopy (**b**) of the tumor and surrounding normal-appearing brain tissue. Large infiltrating right insular and basal ganglia tumor extending into the genu of corpus callosum and septum pellucidum. Marked elevation of choline to creatine ratio with diminished N-acetylaspartate (NAA) is evident in several voxels consistent with a malignant neoplasm

Anaplastic Oligodendroglioma

An anaplastic oligodendroglioma is a grade III glial brain tumor that is poorly differentiated, very cellular and has a tendency to invade neighboring brain tissue [18, 19]. These tumors are less common than low-grade oligodendrogliomas and most commonly occur in the middle-aged adult population [18, 19]. This tumor carries a poor prognosis with a median survival of 4 years after diagnosis [19].

Imaging features. The majority of anaplastic oligodendrogliomas are calcified masses that involve the cortex and subcortical white matter [19]. This diffusely infiltrative expansile tumor most commonly occurs in the frontal lobe [18]. Anaplastic oligodendrogliomas are typically heterogeneous with variable enhancement patterns [18, 19]. The presence of blood, cystic change, and necrosis in addition to calcium may be present on imaging sequences [18].

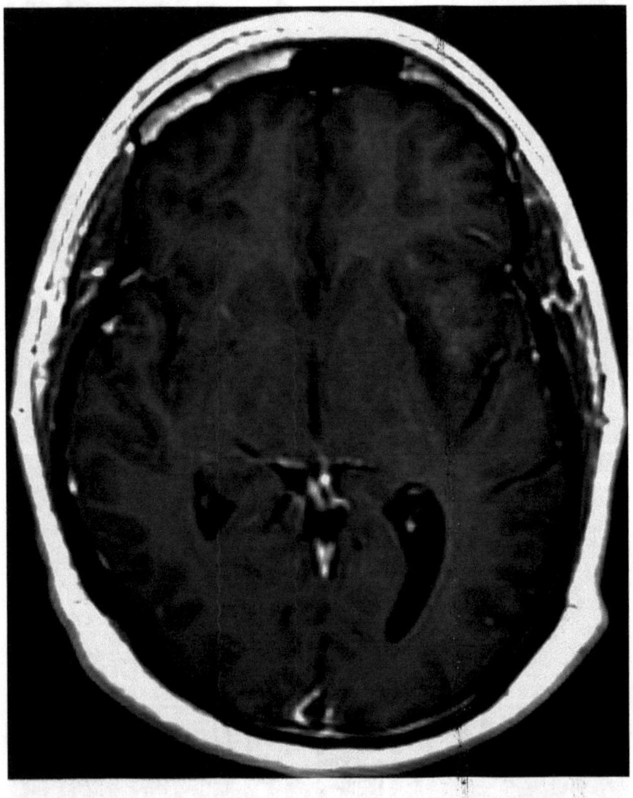

Fig. 1.31 Anaplastic oligodendroglioma. Axial contrast T1-weighted image demonstrates an expansile left insular and basal ganglia minimally enhancing tumor

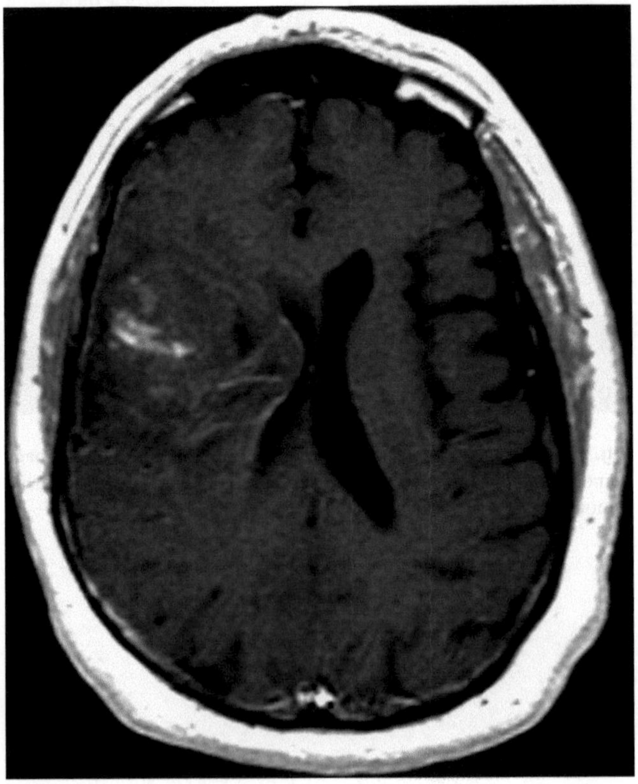

Fig. 1.32 Anaplastic oligodendroglioma. Axial contrast T1-weighted image of a patient with anaplastic oligodendroglioma demonstrates a large, right frontal, predominantly nonenhancing tumor that extends to brain surface

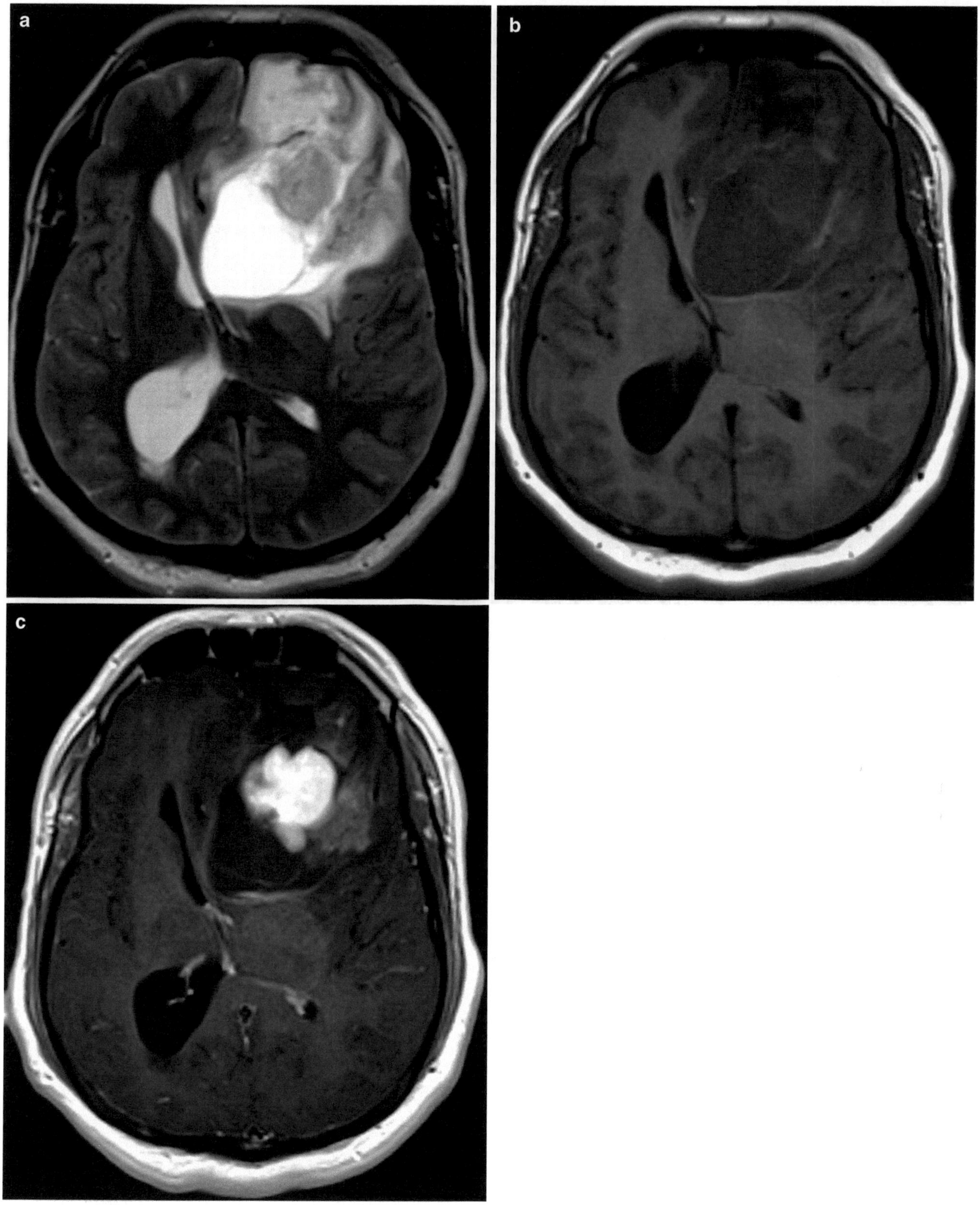

Fig. 1.33 Anaplastic oligodendroglioma. Axial T2-weighted (**a**), T1-weighted (**b**), and contrast T1-weighted (**c**) images of large left frontal anaplastic oligodendroglioma. Note the cystic-appearing component in the basal ganglia posteromedial to the enhancing component with a fluid-hemorrhage level. The tumor also extends to brain surface

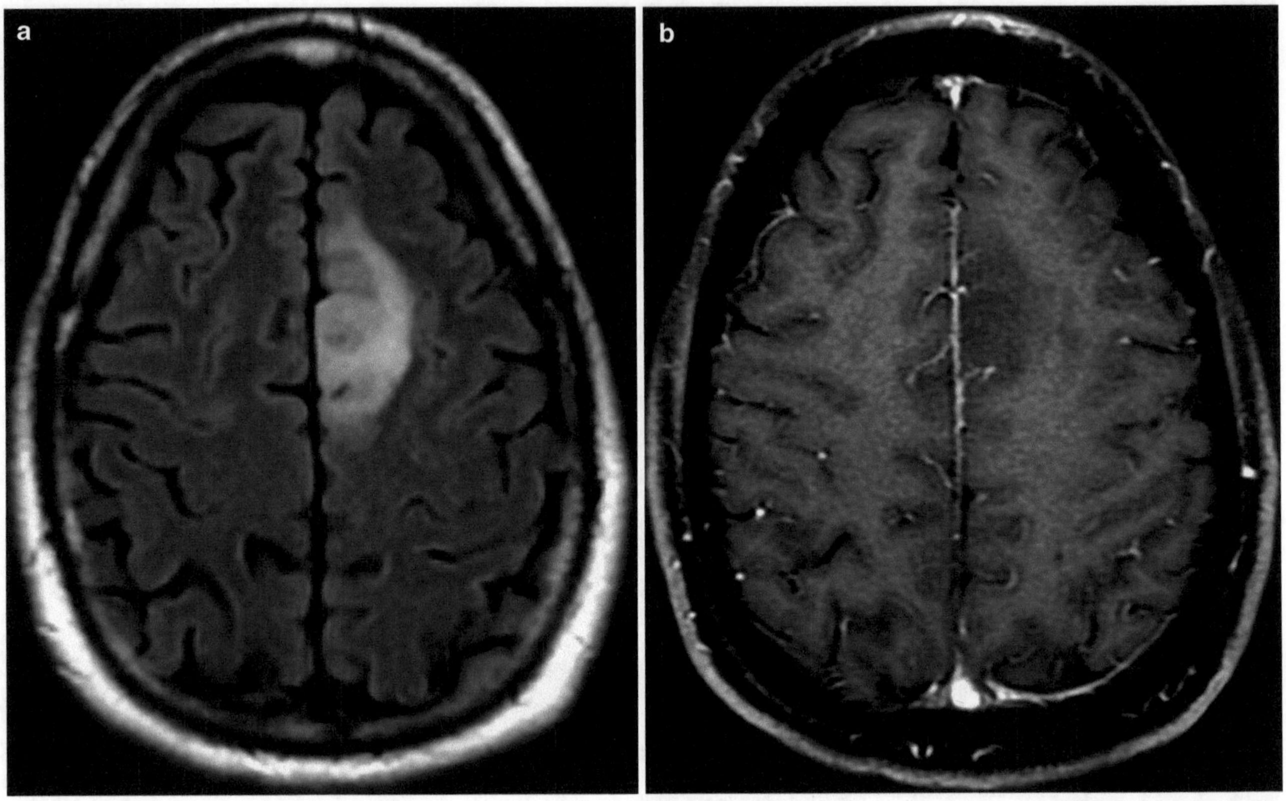

Fig. 1.34 Anaplastic oligodendroglioma. Axial FLAIR (**a**) and contrast T1-weighted (**b**) demonstrate a left paramedian nonenhancing tumor. Post-resection pathology revealed largely low-grade oligodendroglioma with focal region of high-grade (anaplastic) component. Enhancement is usually but not always associated with high-grade disease

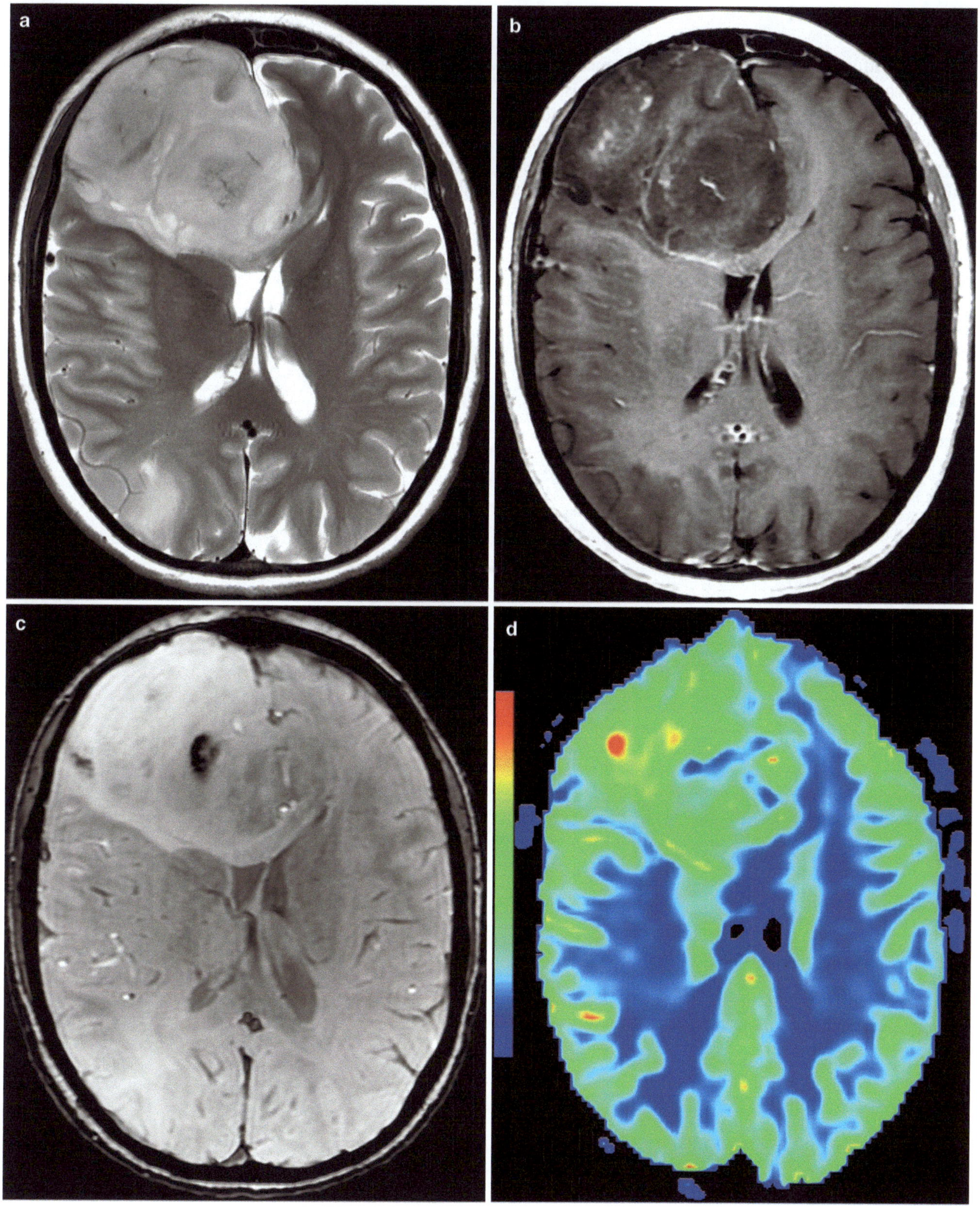

Fig. 1.35 Anaplastic oligodendroglioma. Axial T2-weighted (**a**), contrast T1-weighted (**b**), susceptibility-weighted angiography (SWAN) (**c**), and axial relative cerebral blood volume map (rCBV) (**d**) images. Large, expansile, predominantly nonenhancing, right frontal lobe tumor with bony remodeling of the right frontal bone (**a** and **c**). The tumor is hyperperfused with a focal region of marked hyperperfusion (*red area* on the rCBV map). Focal marked hypointensity is suggestive of calcification on the SWAN image (**c**). Note discontinuous nonenhancing tumor within the right parietal lobe (**a**)

Gliomatosis Cerebri

This rare, diffusely infiltrating, glial brain tumor involves more than one lobe of the brain [20, 21]. Gliomatosis cerebri can occur at any age but typically has a peak incidence between the fifth and sixth decade of life [20]. This tumor has no gender predominance [20, 22]. Patients diagnosed with gliomatosis cerebri have a poor prognosis with 50 % mortality at 1 year [20]. Gliomatosis cerebri typically involves more than two lobes and has hemispheric white matter involvement [20, 22]. This tumor is more infiltrative than histological features may suggest [20].

Imaging features. Gliomatosis cerebri appears as a poorly marginated, hyperintense mass with enlargement of affected structures on T2-weighted imaging sequences [21]. A majority of these tumors do not enhance or show only minimal enhancement [21].

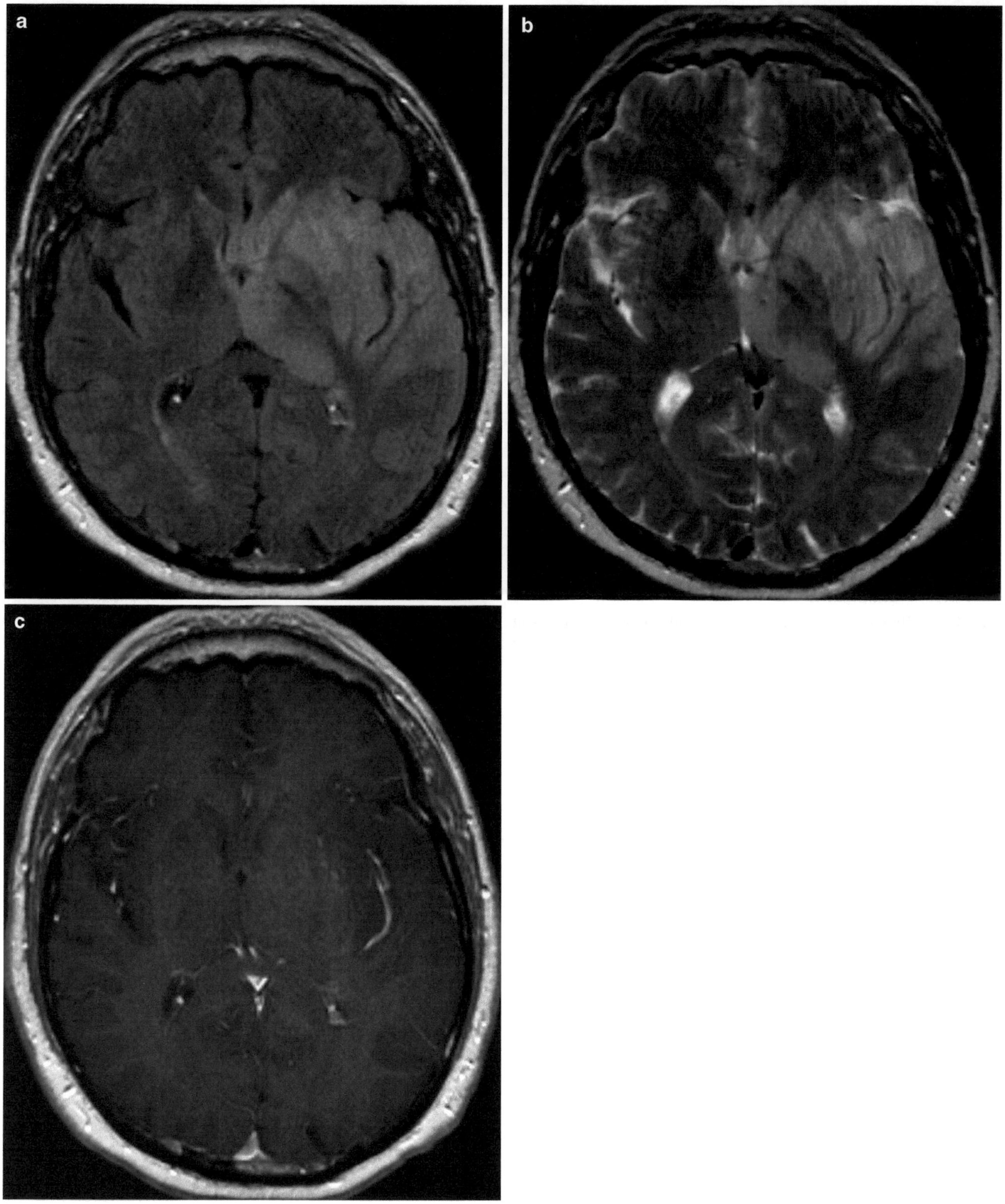

Fig. 1.36 Gliomatosis cerebri. Axial FLAIR (**a**), T2-weighted (**b**), and contrast T1-weighted (**c**) images demonstrate a mildly expansile left hemispheric infiltrative nonenhancing tumor involving the temporal lobe, frontal lobe, insula, subinsula, basal ganglia, thalamus and septum pellucidum

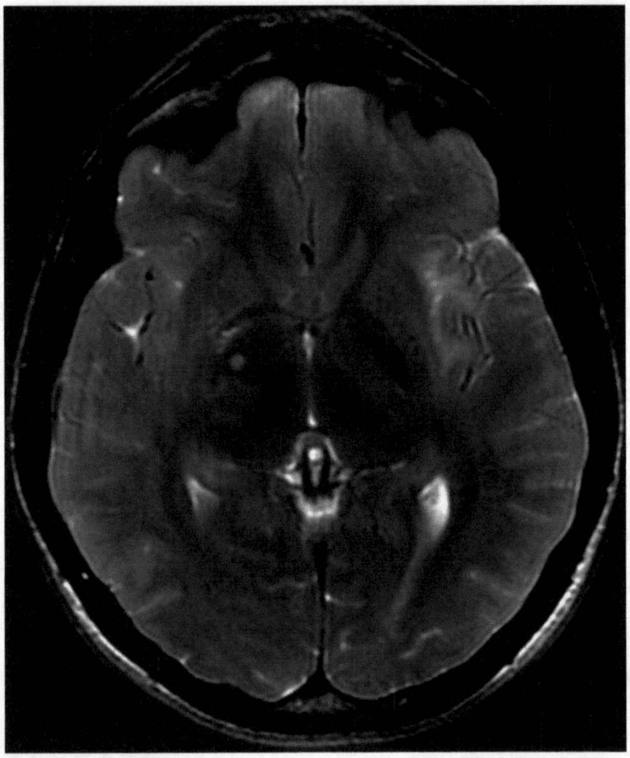

Fig. 1.37 Gliomatosis cerebri. Axial T2-weighted image of a patient with left insular and peri-insular hyperintensity consistent with the diagnosis of gliomatosis cerebri

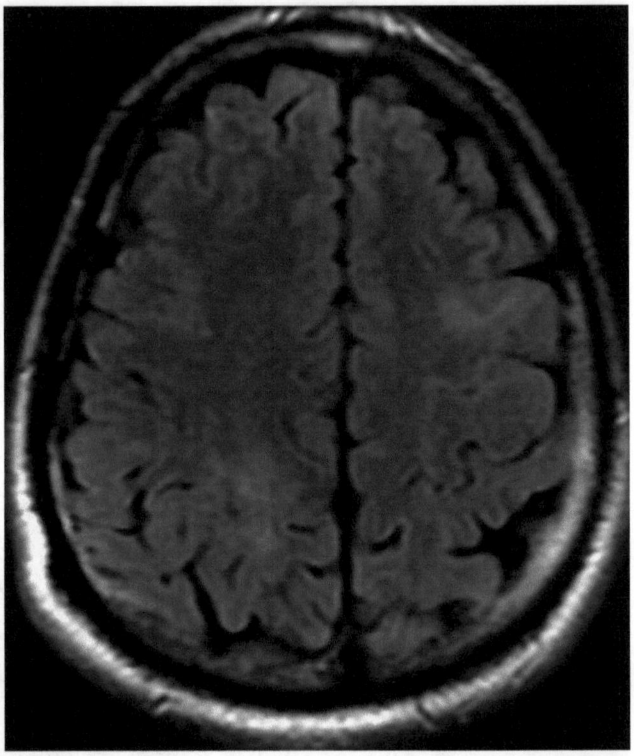

Fig. 1.38 Gliomatosis cerebri. Axial FLAIR image of a patient with biopsy-proven gliomatosis cerebri demonstrates subtle multifocal left frontal and right parietal lobe infiltrative hyperintense tumor

Primary CNS Lymphoma

This is a primary CNS malignancy that is usually B-cell, non-Hodgkin lymphoma (NHL) [23]. Primary CNS lymphoma (PCNSL) accounts for 1–7 % of all primary brain tumors and around 1 % of all lymphomas [24]. The incidence of this tumor in both immunocompetent and immunocompromised patients has risen in recent years [23, 24]. PCNSL is an AIDS-defining condition and is present in up to 6 % of patients with an AIDS diagnosis. This tumor type can occur at any age but tends to have an earlier age of onset in immunocompromised patients and later age of onset in immunocompetent patients. As there is no benefit with gross tumor resection, unlike metastases and malignant gliomas, standard treatment consists of biopsy followed by radiation therapy and chemotherapy [24]. Patients may require whole brain radiation therapy because this is a diffuse disease, unlike patients with malignant gliomas who receive partial brain radiation therapy [24]. Recurrence may occur months or years after treatment, at the original site or in a different part of the brain [24]. Patients generally have a poor prognosis with a median survival of 17–45 months [23, 24].

Imaging features. A large majority of PCNSL are well-circumscribed enhancing lesions found supratentorially within the basal ganglia or within white matter surrounding the ventricles [24]. The frontal and parietal lobes are the most common lobes of involvement [24]. These tumors often involve the corpus callosum and/or deep gray nuclei [23, 24]. PCNSL can appear as either a solitary mass or as multiple lesions [23, 24]. Tumor imaging and prognosis can vary with status of patient immunocompetence [23]. PCNSL are homogenous in immunocompetent patients and heterogenous in immunocompromised patients [24]. Tumors in immunocompromised patients are more likely to contain hemorrhage, calcium, and/or necrosis [24].

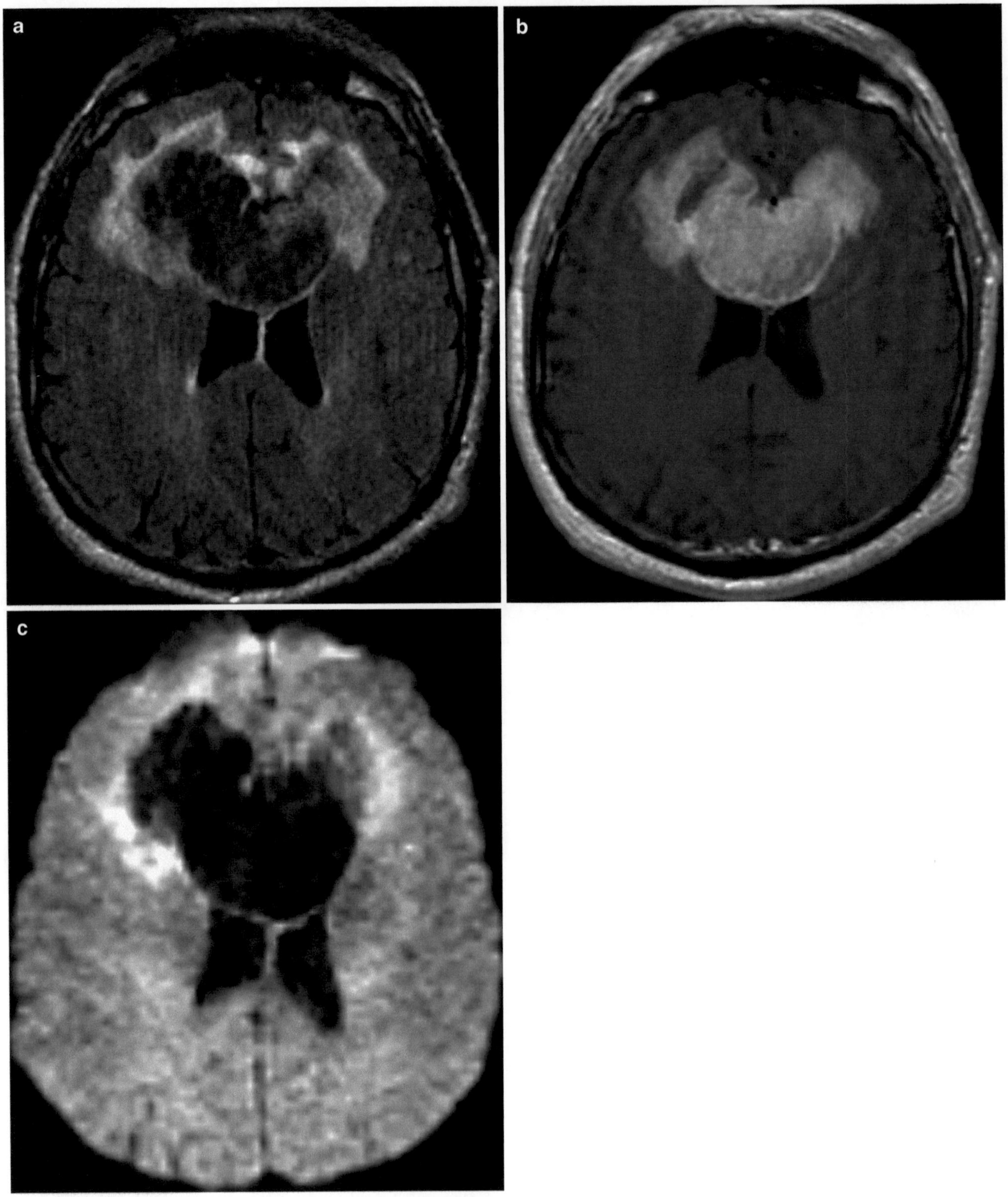

Fig. 1.39 Primary CNS lymphoma. Axial FLAIR (**a**), contrast T1-weighted (**b**), and diffusion-weighted (**c**) images of a butterfly lymphoma. There is peripheral diffusion restriction (**c**) rather than the usual homogenous restriction. The central diffusion-weighted imaging (DWI) and FLAIR hypointensity is due to acute blood products

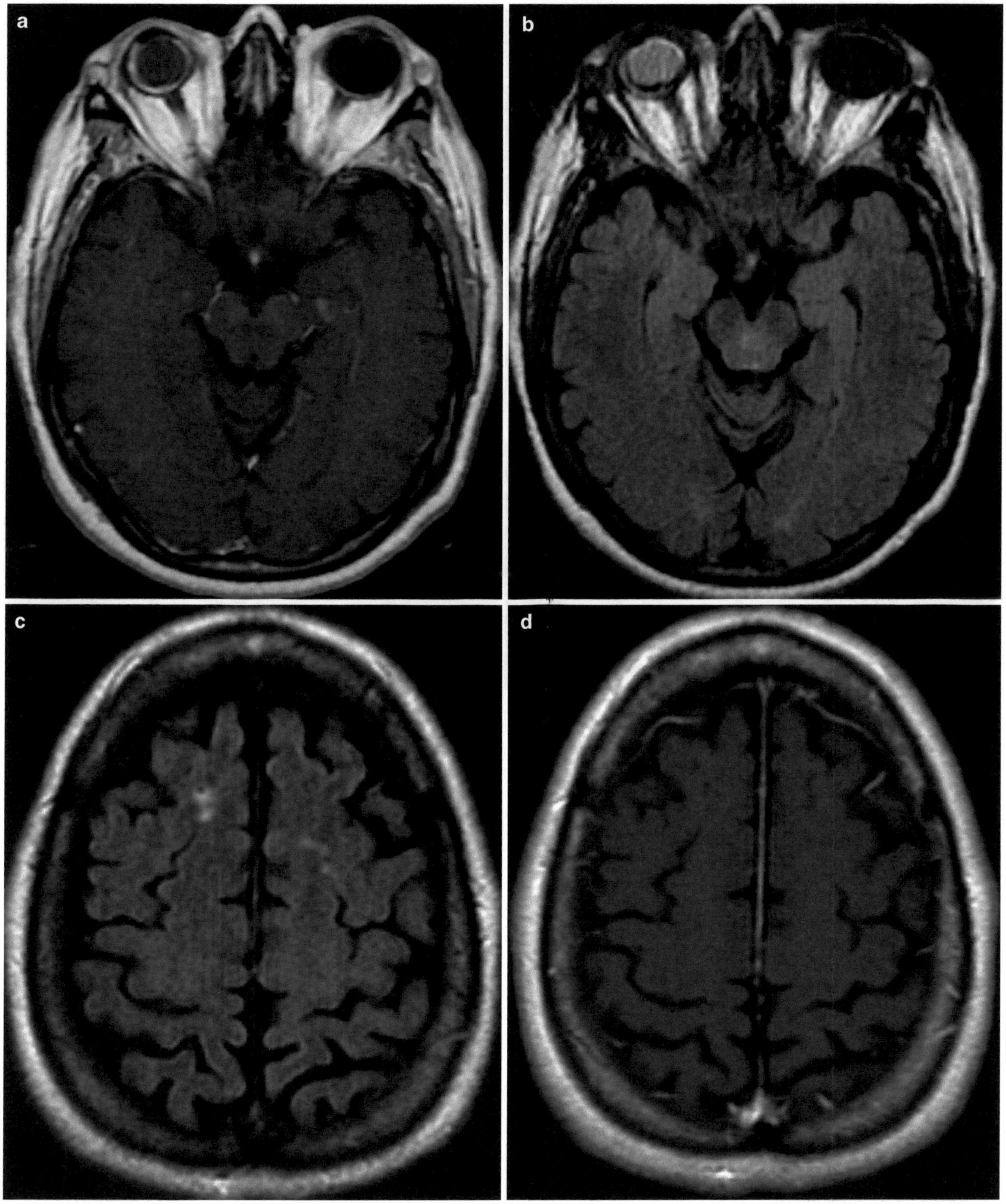

Fig. 1.40 Primary CNS lymphoma. Axial contrast T1-weighted (**a** and **d**) and FLAIR (**b** and **c**) images demonstrate subtle nonenhancing abnormal signal within mesial right temporal lobe and in high right frontal lobe. Diffusion-weighted images (**e** and **f**) show corresponding restriction

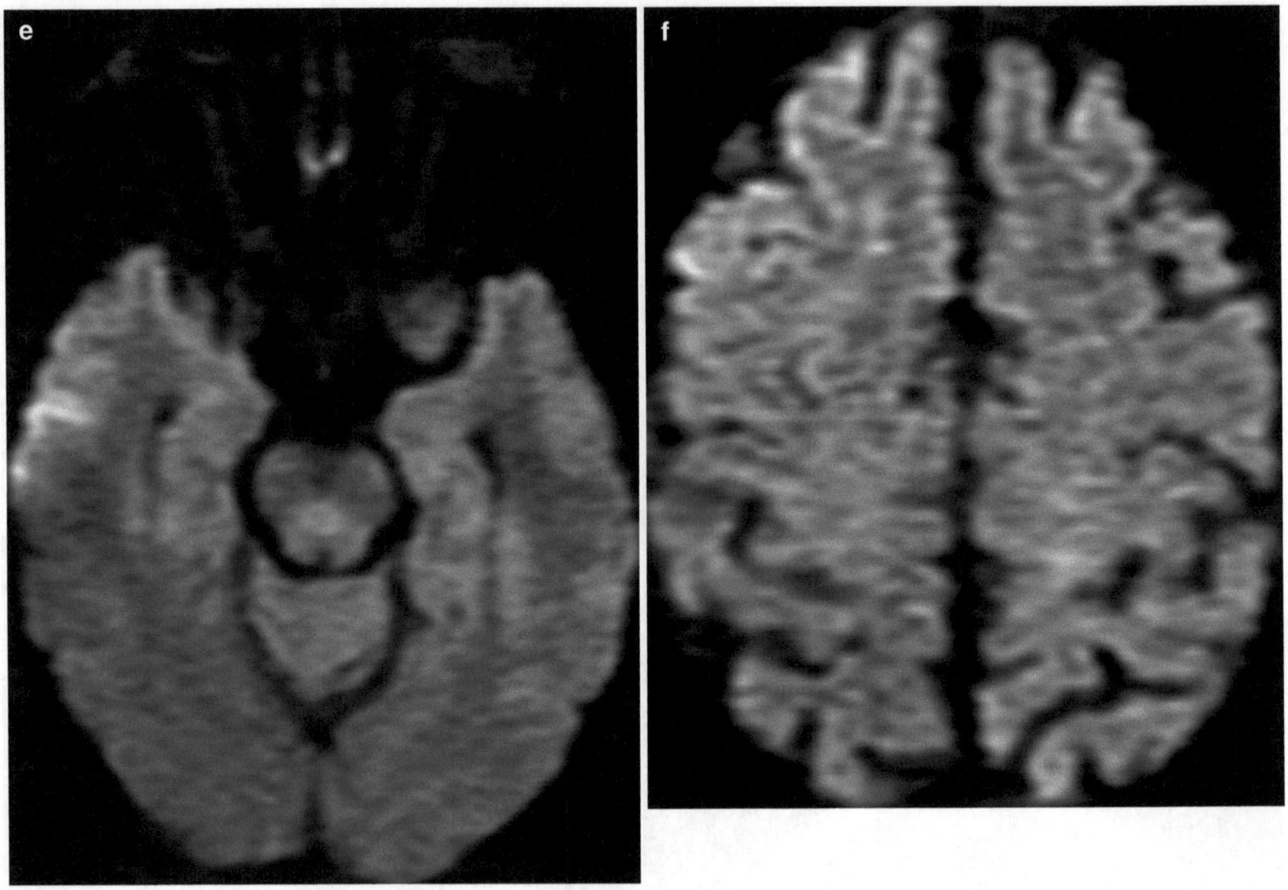

Fig. 1.40 (continued)

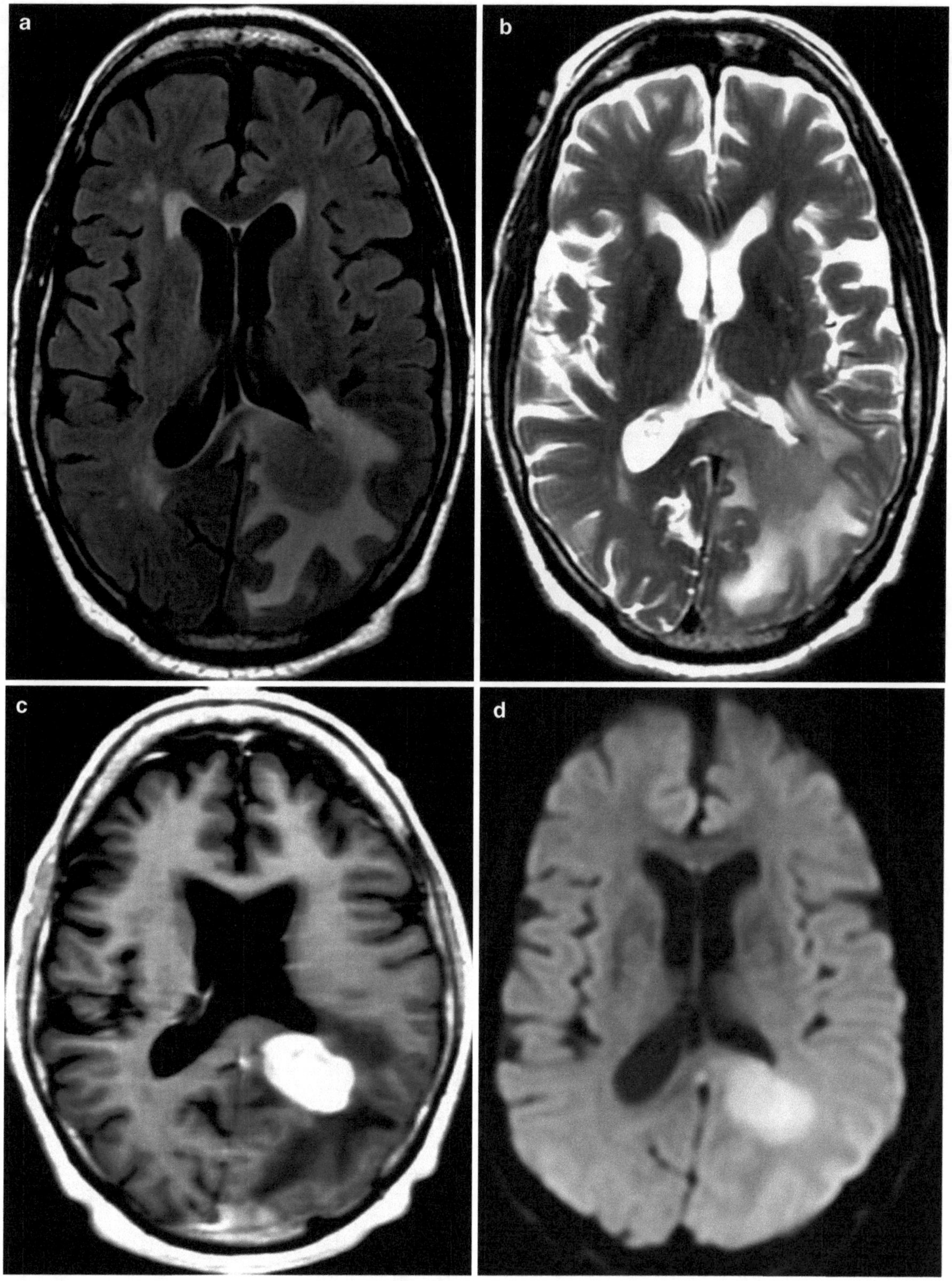

Fig. 1.41 Primary CNS lymphoma. Axial FLAIR (**a**), T2-weighted (**b**), and contrast T1-weighted (**c**) images demonstrate a homogeneously and intensely enhancing "cloud-like" tumor in left periventricular white matter extending into the corpus callosum. Note that the tumor is isointense on the long TR (time to repetition) images (**a** and **b**) and restricted on the diffusion-weighted image (**d**)

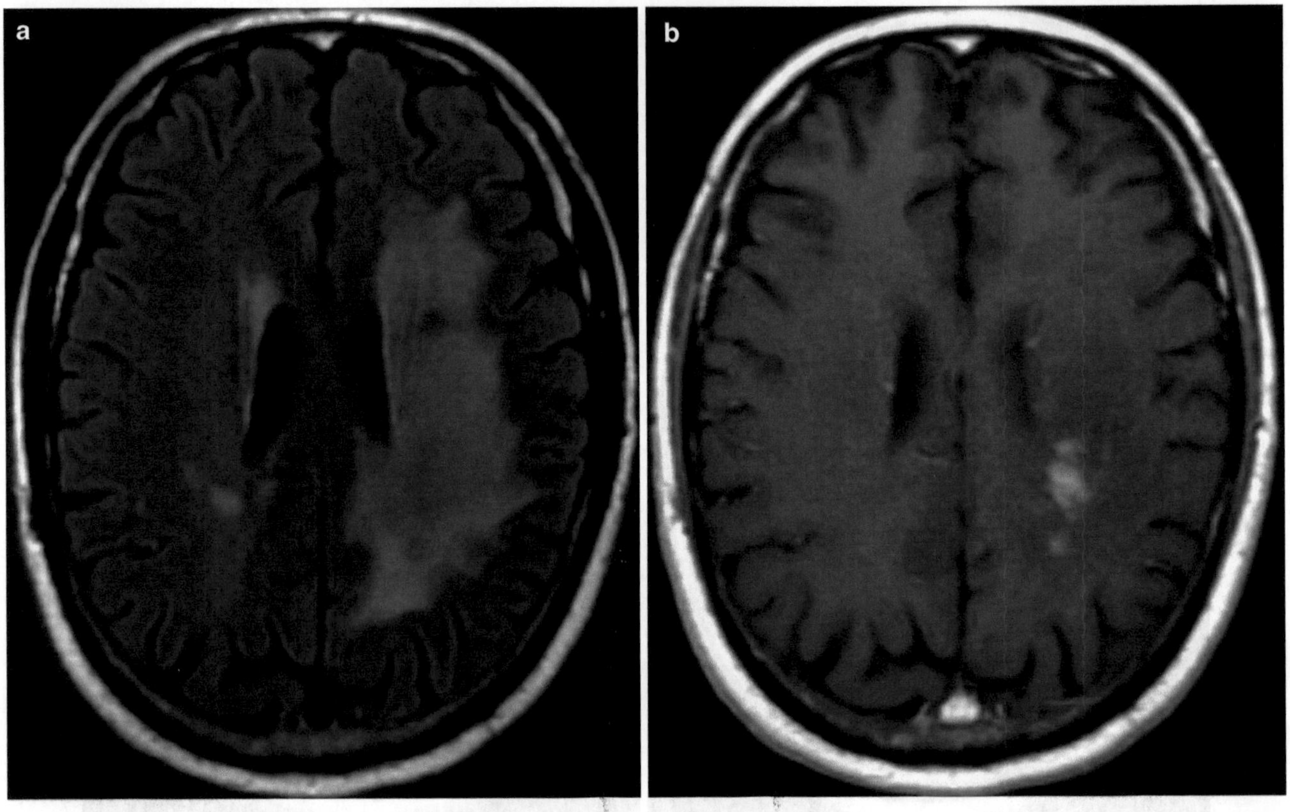

Fig. 1.42 Primary CNS lymphoma. Axial FLAIR (**a**) and contrast T1-weighted (**b**) images of primary CNS lymphoma. Large region of deep and periventricular white matter T2 hyperintensity (**a**) within the left frontal and parietal lobes extending into the corpus callosum containing patchy enhancement (**b**). The FLAIR hyperintensity represents a combination of nonenhancing tumor and edema

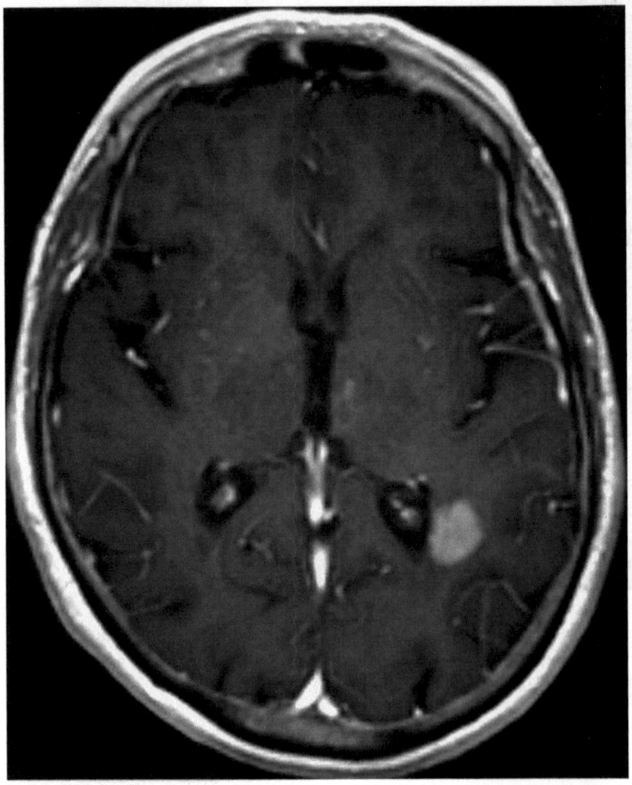

Fig. 1.43 Primary CNS lymphoma. Axial contrast T1-weighted image shows left periatrial homogeneous-enhancing nodule. Additional small foci of enhancing tumor are evident within the left basal ganglia and thalamus

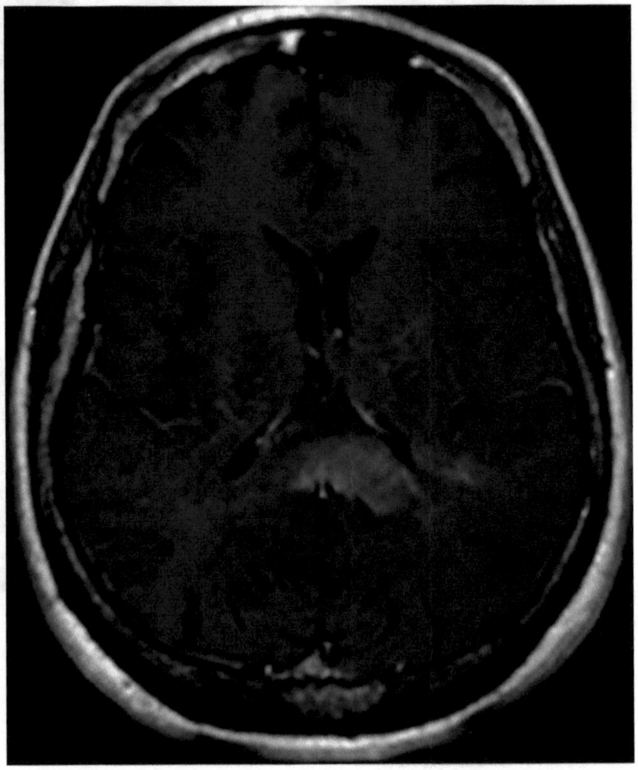

Fig. 1.44 Primary CNS lymphoma. Axial contrast T1-weighted image of butterfly lymphoma of the splenium of the corpus callosum

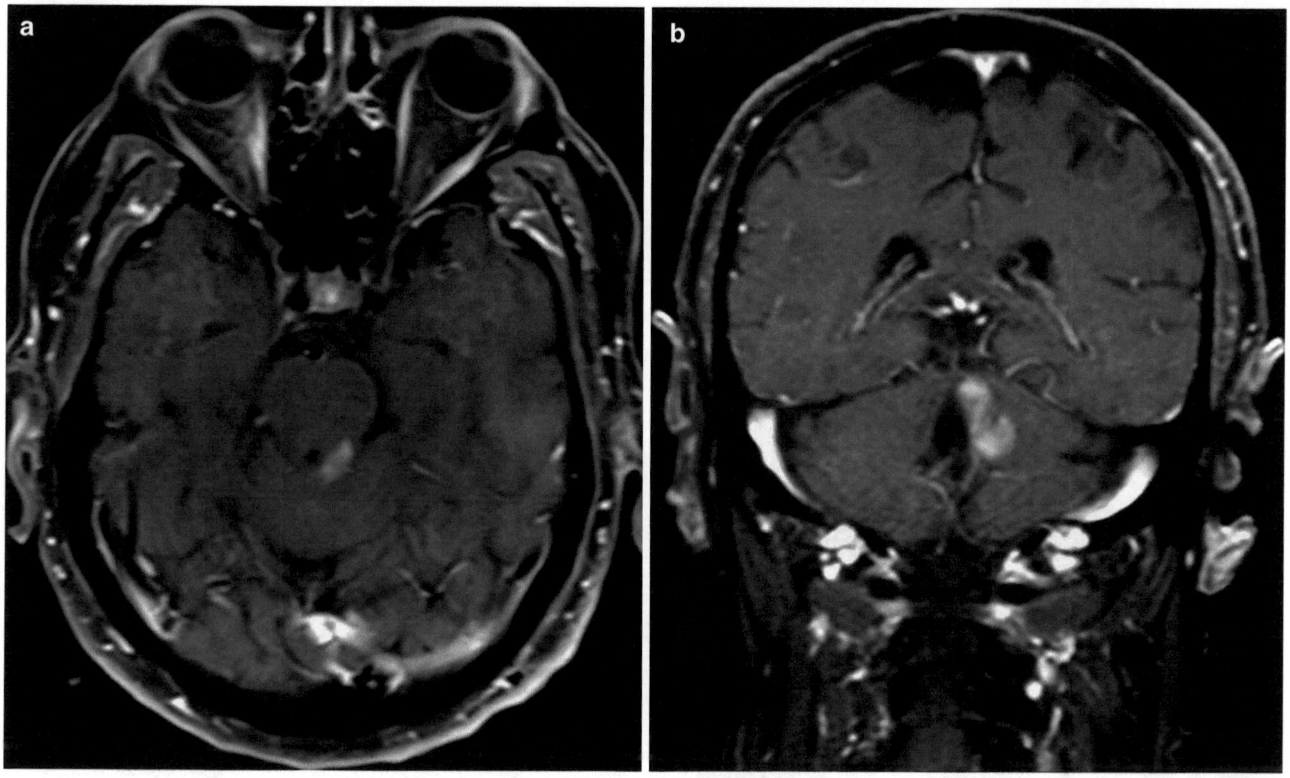

Fig. 1.45 Primary CNS lymphoma. Axial (**a**) and coronal (**b**) contrast T1-weighted images with fat suppression show an enhancing mass extending from the tectum to the cerebellum

Adult Ependymoma

This is a rare grade II or III glial brain tumor made of ependymal cells [25]. Ependymomas are responsible for up to 5 % of all adult intracranial glial brain tumors [25, 26]. This tumor type tends to peak at 35 years old and has a slight predominance in men [25]. Adult ependymomas have a fair prognosis with a 5-year overall survival rate of 76 % [25, 27]. Gross total resection with chemotherapy and radiation therapy may improve overall prognosis [25, 27].

Imaging features. The majority of adult ependymomas are large, heterogeneously enhancing, supratentorial masses located in the brain parenchyma and less often in the ventricles [25, 28]. This contrasts with pediatric ependymomas, which are usually located in the infratentorial compartment within the fourth ventricle [28]. This tumor type may contain calcium, cysts, and/or hemorrhage [25, 28]. CSF dissemination can occur in up to 15 % of patients with ependymoma [25]. Spinal imaging may be useful for identification of drop leptomeningeal metastases.

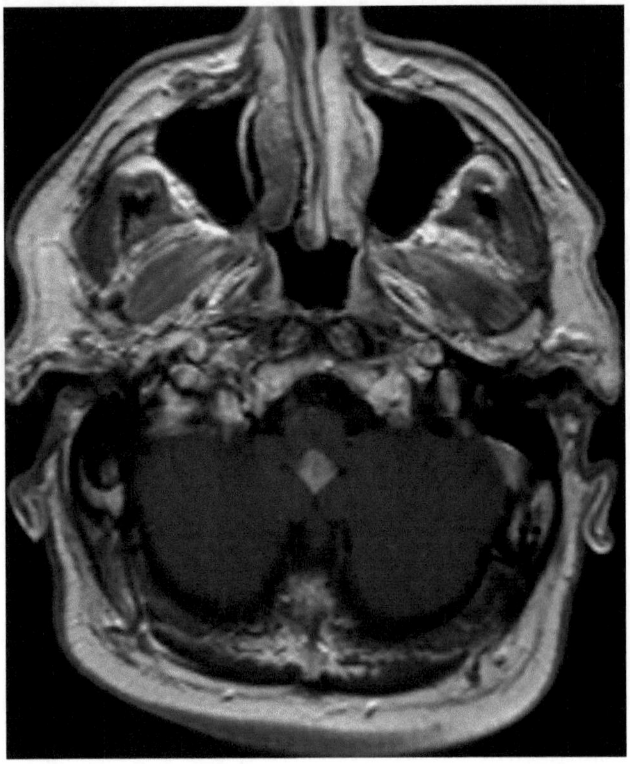

Fig. 1.46 Adult ependymoma. Axial contrast T1-weighted image of a typical posterior fossa ependymoma in an adult extending from the inferior fourth ventricle down into the foramen of Magendie

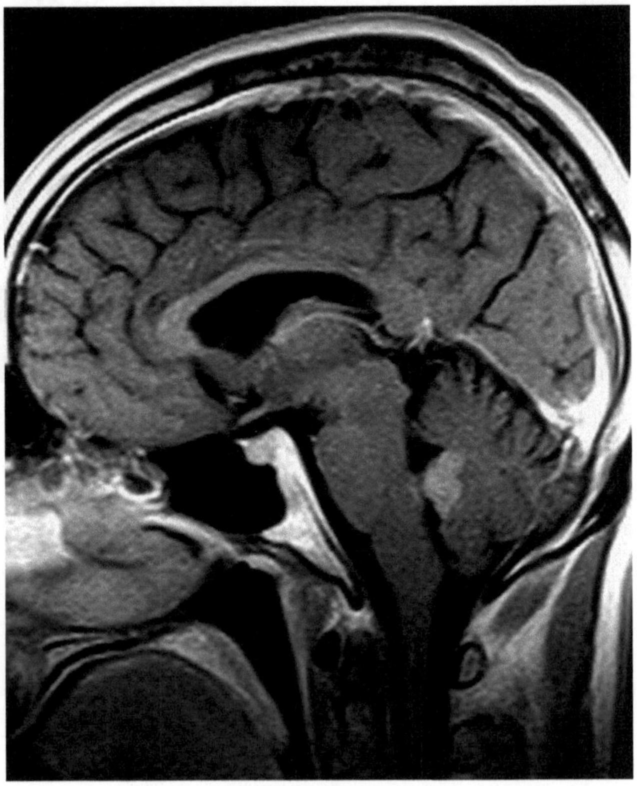

Fig. 1.47 Adult ependymoma. Sagittal contrast T1-weighted image of a different patient from Fig. 1.46 demonstrates another typical posterior fossa ependymoma extending from inferior fourth ventricle into the foramen of Magendie

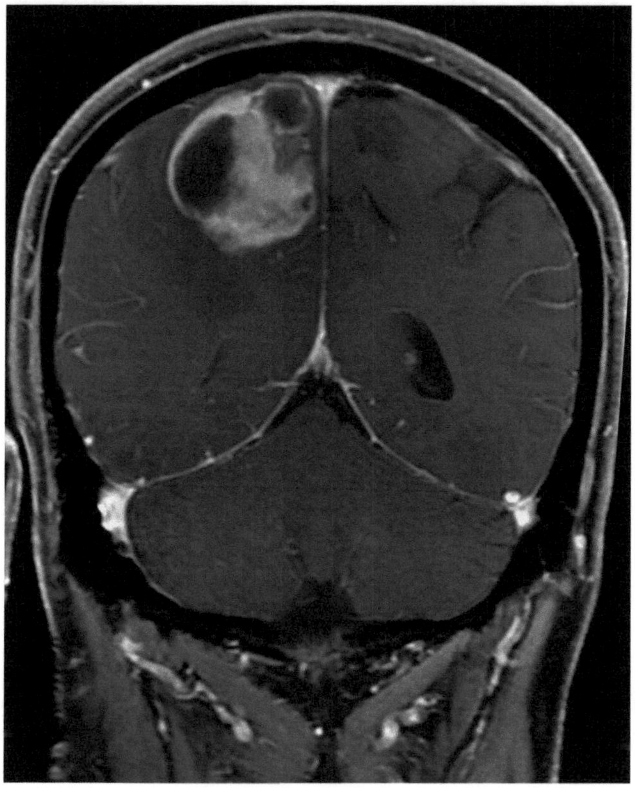

Fig. 1.48 Adult ependymoma. Coronal contrast T1-weighted image of an adult with supratentorial ependymoma shows a heterogeneously enhancing mass in the right parietal lobe with solid and cystic/necrotic components

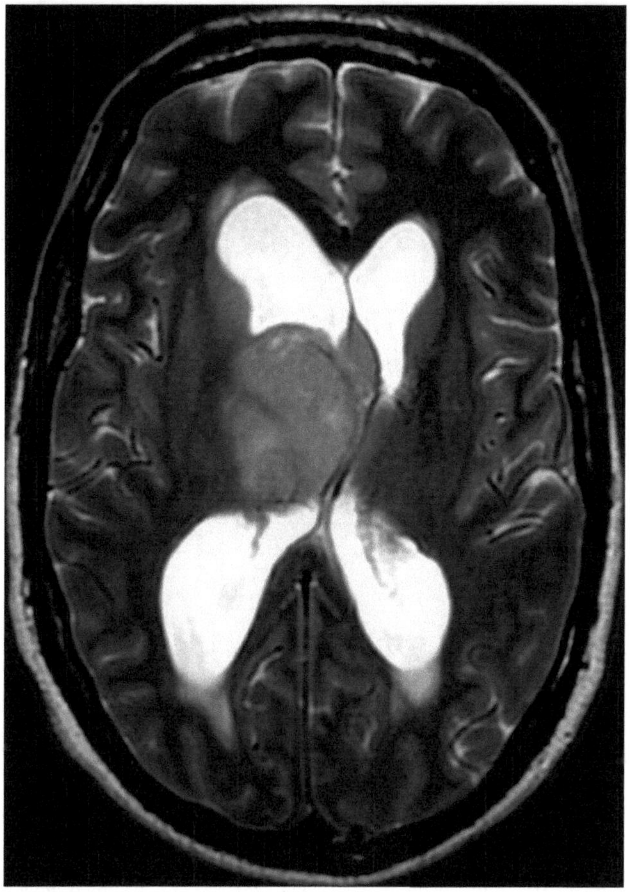

Fig. 1.49 Adult ependymoma. Axial T2-weighted image shows an expansile right thalamic tumor protruding in the lateral ventricle and bowing the septum pellucidum with obstructive hydrocephalus

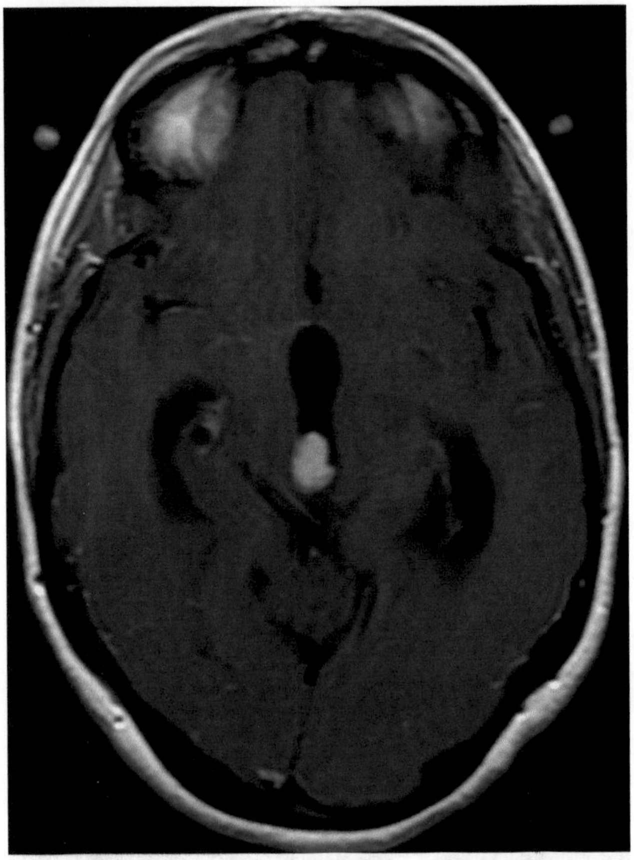

Fig. 1.50 Adult ependymoma. Axial contrast T1-weighted image shows an enhancing tumor in the posterior third ventricle

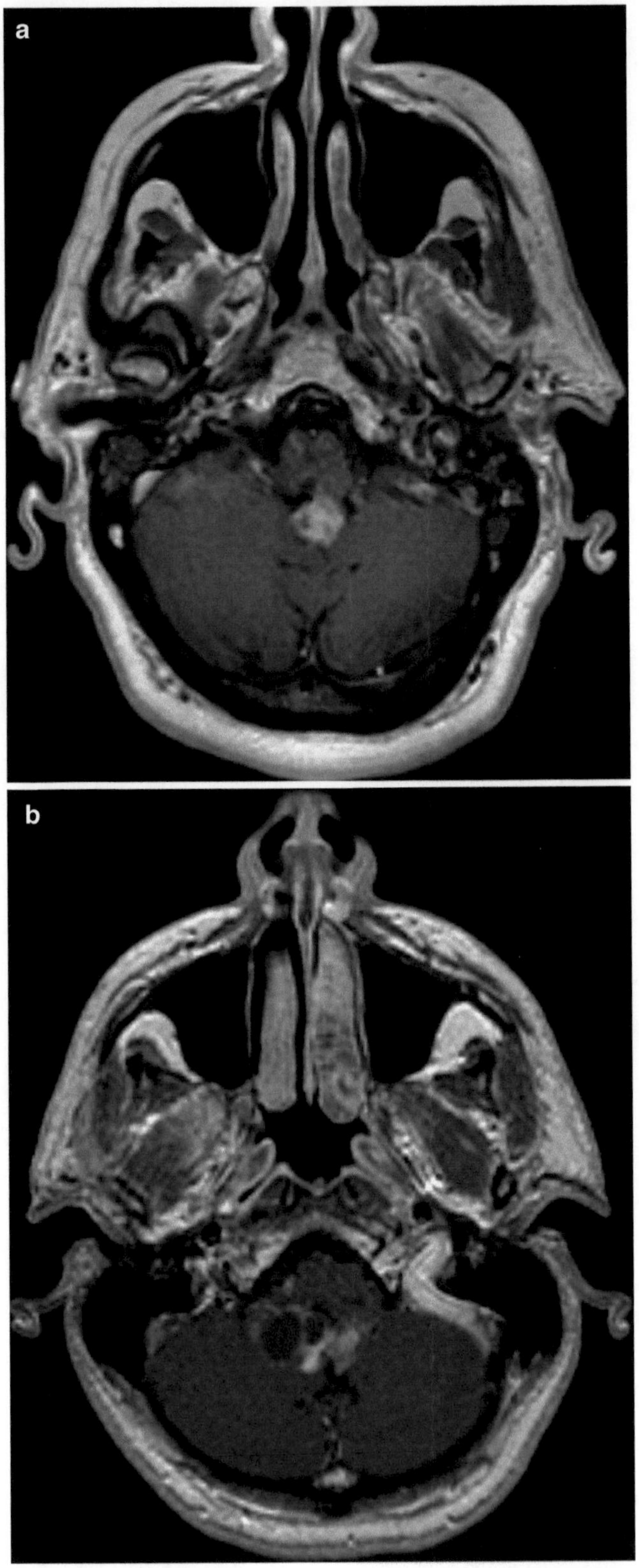

Fig. 1.51 Adult ependymoma. Axial contrast T1-weighted images (**a** and **b**) demonstrate a heterogeneously enhancing mass in the fourth ventricular outlet foramina

Infratentorial

Hemangioblastoma

A hemangioblastoma is a grade I vascular meningeal tumor of uncertain histogenesis [29]. These tumors account for 1–2 % of all intracranial tumors and for up to 10 % of posterior fossa tumors [29]. Up to 40 % of patients with hemangioblastoma have underlying Von Hippel-Lindau syndrome [29]. These patients show younger age of onset than the sporadic tumors that are most common in the third and fourth decades of life [29, 30]. Hemangioblastomas are slow growing and have a fair prognosis with a 10-year survival of 85 %. In familial forms, screening of the entire neuraxis is recommended as new hemangioblastomas may occur on average every 2 years [29, 30].

Imaging features. Hemangioblastomas classically present as superficial intra-axial masses in the cerebellum with cysts that contain an enhancing mural nodule and contact a pial surface [29]. Up to 90 % of these tumors are located within the posterior fossa [29, 30]. Supratentorial location, specifically near the optic pathway, usually occur in patients with Von Hippel-Lindau syndrome [30]. Blood products and prominent flow voids may be present within these highly vascular tumors [29, 30].

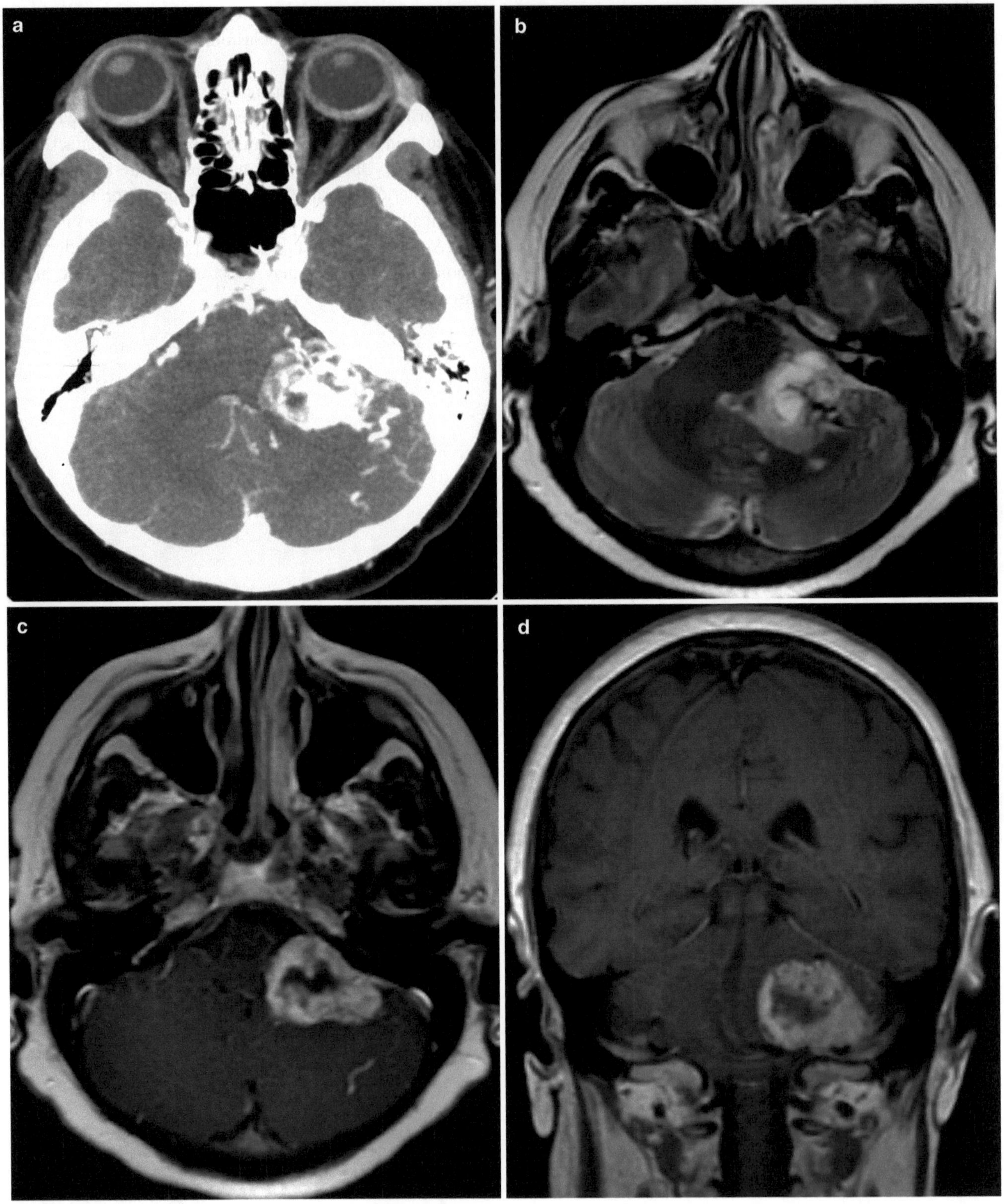

Fig. 1.52 Hemangioblastoma. Axial contrast CT (**a**) shows a tumor in the left brachium pontis with avid heterogeneous enhancement. The increased internal and adjacent vascularity manifests as flow voids on the T2-weighted image (**b**) and as curvilinear enhancement on axial (**c**) and coronal (**d**) contrast T1-weighted images

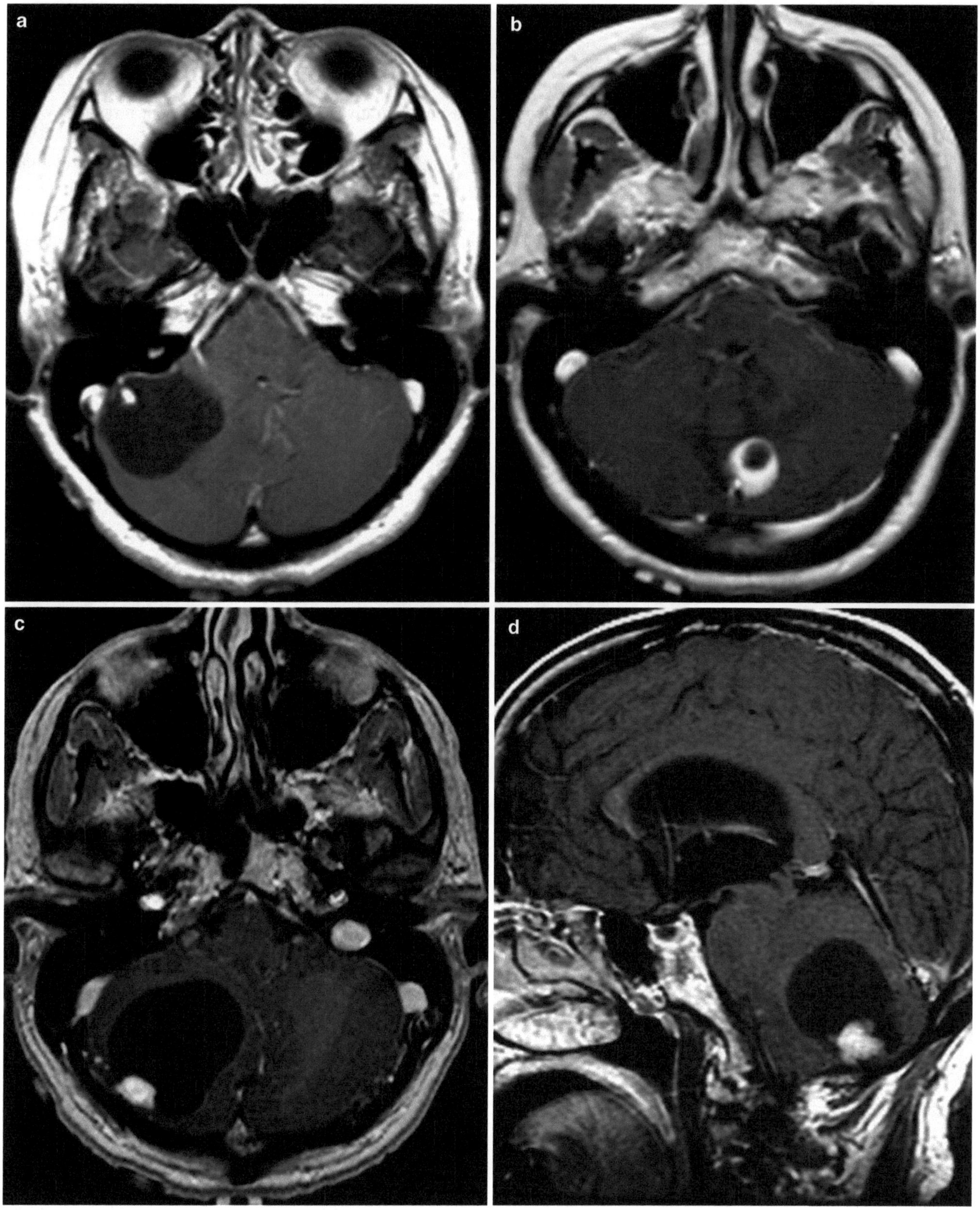

Fig. 1.53 Hemangioblastoma. Axial (**a–c**) and sagittal (**d**) contrast T1-weighted images in four different patients show similar cystic tumors in cerebellum with enhancing mural nodules. The superficial location and contact against a pial surface is typical for hemangioblastomas

Intraventricular

A location-based classification system is useful in formulating a differential diagnosis, which can then be narrowed down further using information gleaned from patient demographics and lesion-imaging characteristics. The ependymal cells of the choroid plexus produce cerebrospinal fluid (CSF), which flows from the lateral ventricles through the foramina of Monro into the third ventricle, then through the cerebral aqueduct into the fourth ventricle, and into the central canal of the spinal cord or through the foramina of Luschka and Magendie into the subarachnoid spaces. Tumors of the choroid plexus do not occur in the frontal horns of the lateral ventricles or in the cerebral aqueduct, as no choroid plexus is normally found in these locations.

Central Neurocytoma

A central neurocytoma is a grade II neuroepithelial brain tumor [31]. This tumor is responsible for less than 1 % of all intracranial tumors and has an incidence of 0.02 person-years [10]. This tumor represents around half of all intraventricular brain tumors in patients in their third through fifth decades of life [31]. Central neurocytomas have no gender predominance [31]. Surgical resection is the treatment of choice and is usually curative [32]. Patients have a fair prognosis with a 5-year survival rate of 81 % [31].

Imaging features. The majority of central neurocytomas are well-circumscribed lobulated lesions with a characteristic cystic and solid appearance [31, 32]. More than 50 % of these tumors are found in the lateral ventricle and attached to the septum pellucidum [31]. Hydrocephalus is common secondary to the obstruction of the foramen of Monro [31, 32]. Central neurocytomas commonly contain calcium and are rarely complicated by hemorrhage [31, 32].

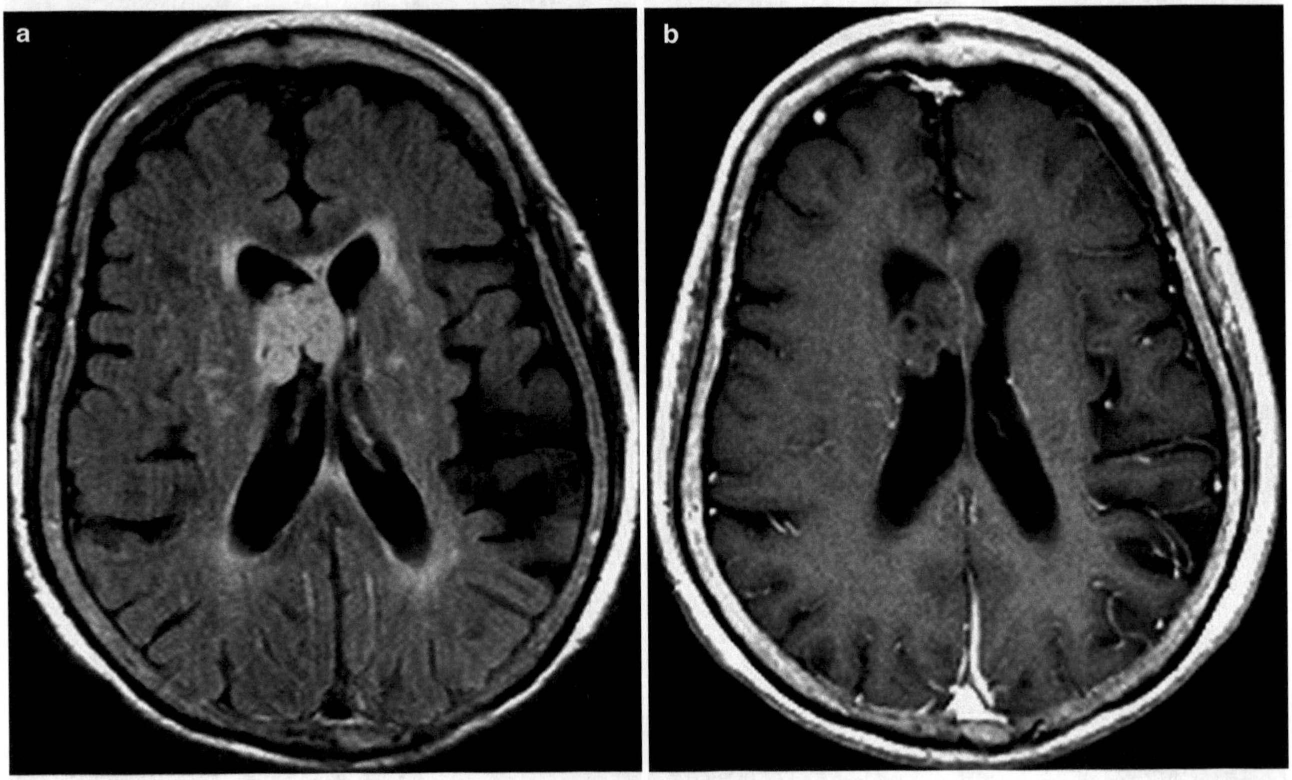

Fig. 1.54 Central neurocytoma. Axial FLAIR (**a**) and contrast T1-weighted (**b**) images show a lobulated nonenhancing tumor in the anterior body of the right lateral ventricle, closely apposed to the septum pellucidum that is bowed to the contralateral side

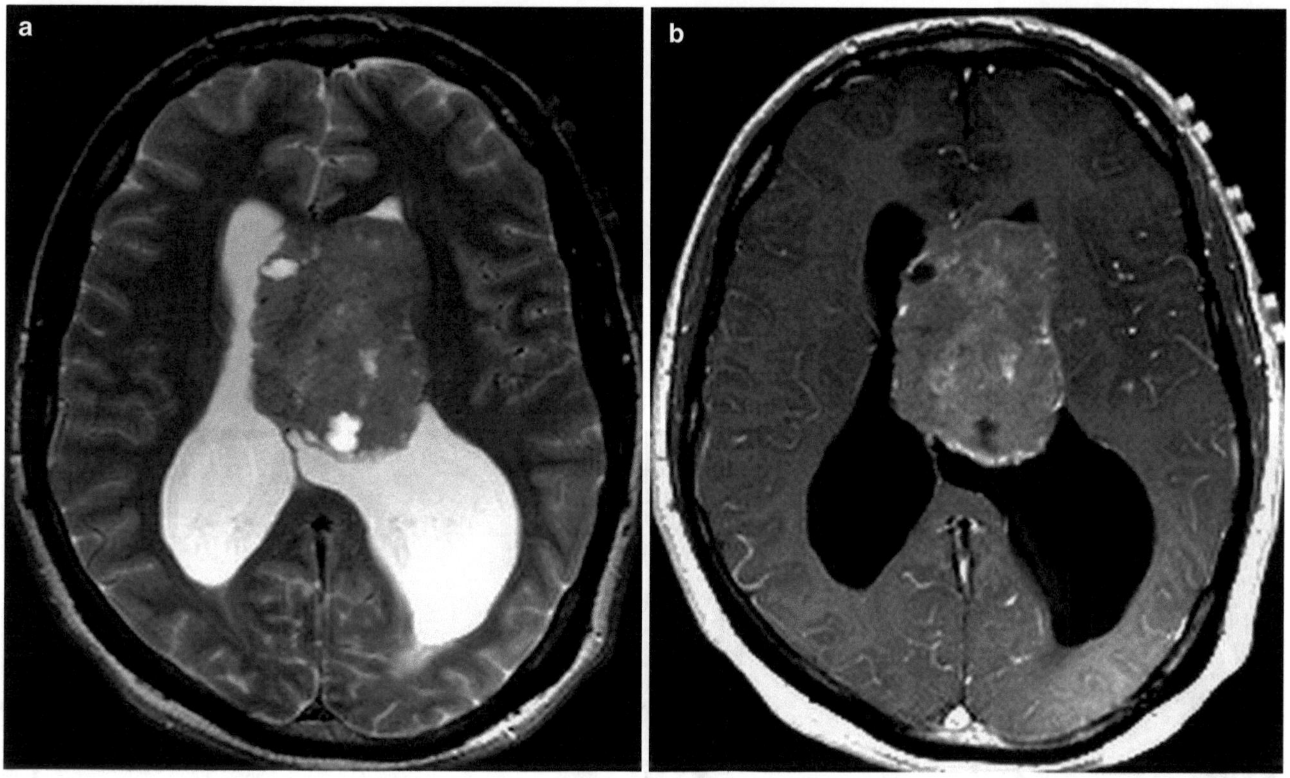

Fig. 1.55 Central neurocytoma. Axial T2- (**a**) and contrast T1-weighted (**b**) images show a solid tumor in the left lateral ventricle with small cystic components and mild heterogeneous enhancement. Mild hydrocephalus is due to obstruction of the foramen of Monro (*not shown*). The location and imaging appearance are both typical for central neurocytoma. An intraventricular oligodendroglioma and subependymoma may occasionally mimic this appearance

Subependymoma

A subependymoma is a grade I benign brain tumor comprised of well-differentiated ependymal cell lines [33]. This tumor is rare as it accounts for less than 0.1 % of all intracranial neoplasms and has an incidence of around one case per one million person-years [10, 33]. Subependymomas most commonly occur in the fifth and sixth decades of life and tend to have a predominance in men [32]. Supratentorial subependymomas have an excellent prognosis with low rate of recurrence after tumor resection [34].

Imaging features. Subependymomas are most commonly seen as small lobulated lesions with well-defined margins [33, 34]. These tumors are most commonly found in the inferior portion of the fourth ventricle but may also be found in the lateral ventricles, third ventricle, and spinal cord [33, 34]. Larger tumors may contain cysts, calcium, and/or hemorrhage [33, 34]. Subependymoma in particular are usually nonenhancing without associated edema in the adjacent brain parenchyma [34, 35].

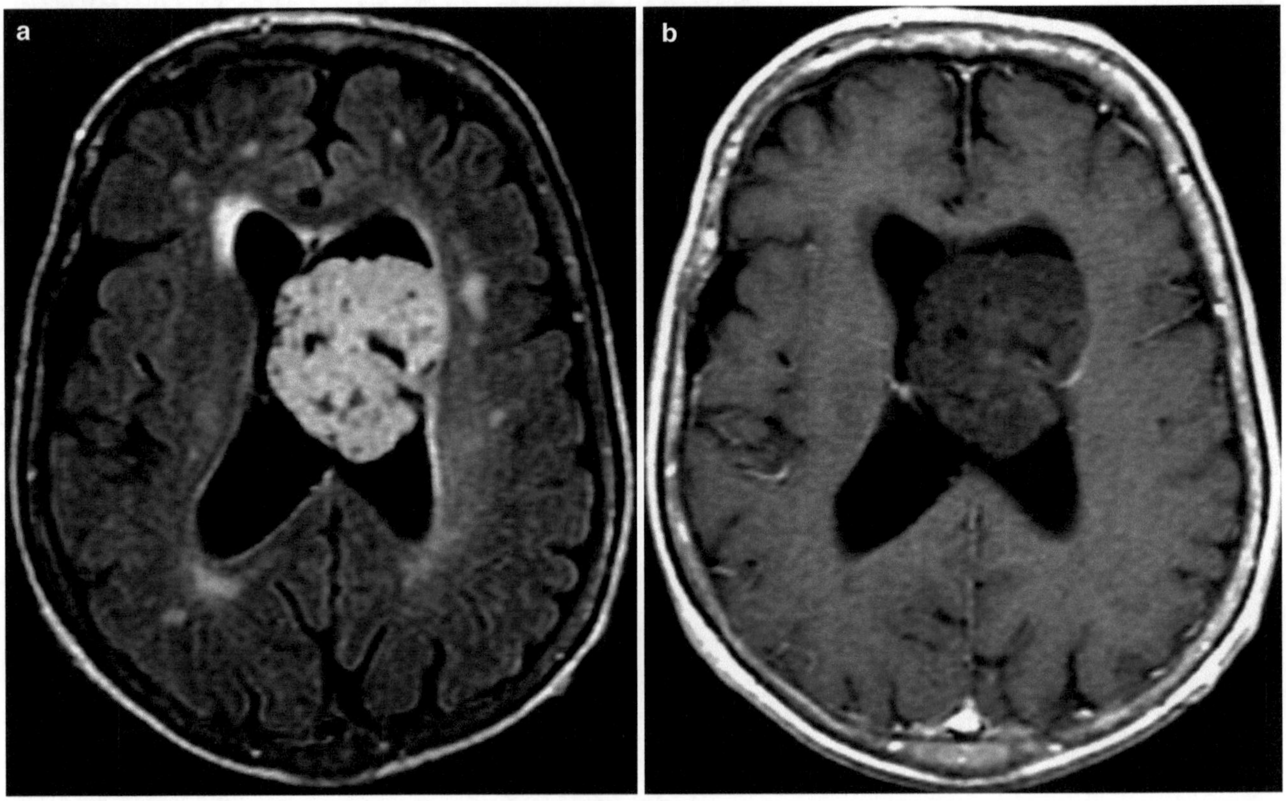

Fig. 1.56 Subependymoma. Axial FLAIR (**a**) and contrast T1-weighted (**b**) images show a solid and cystic nonenhancing tumor in the left lateral ventricle. Mass effect causes contralateral displacement of the septum pellucidum, mimicking a central neurocytoma (*see* Fig. 1.55) in a slightly younger patient

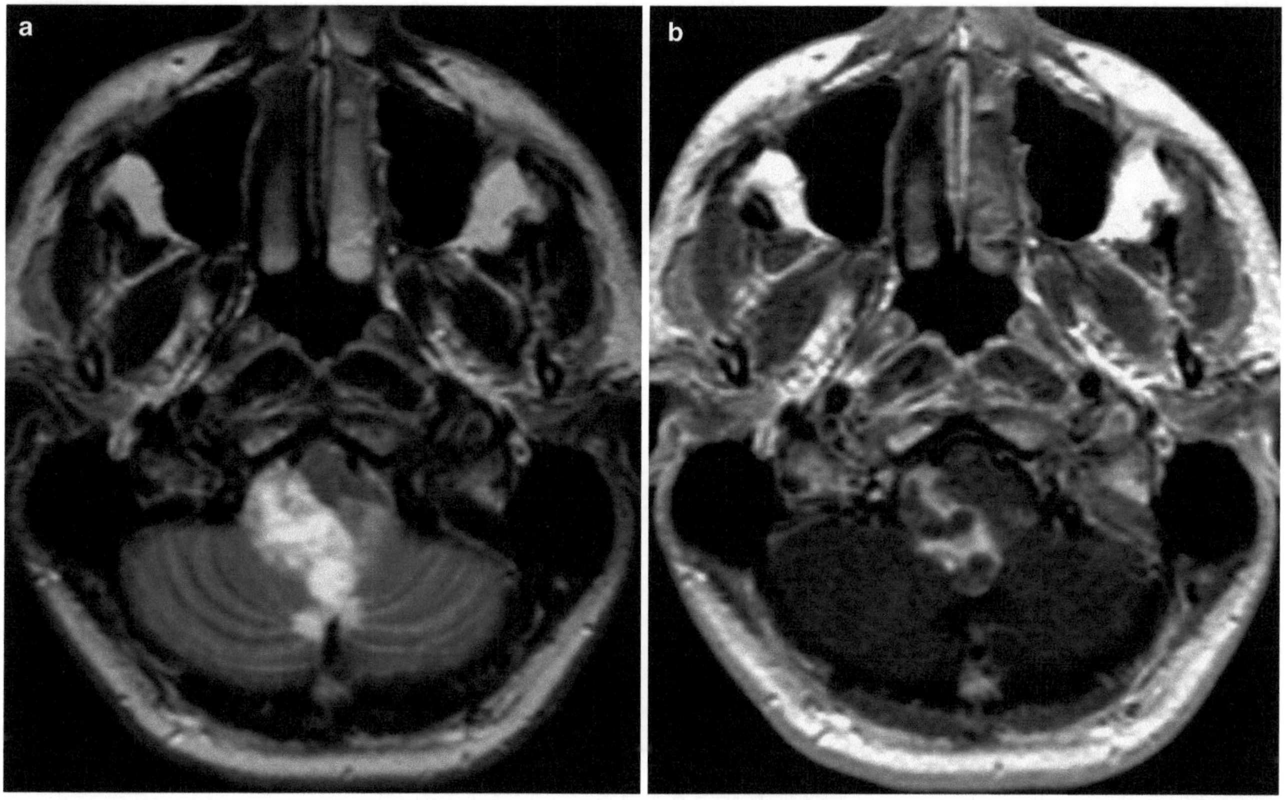

Fig. 1.57 Subependymoma. Axial FLAIR (**a**) and contrast T1-weighted (**b**) images reveal a heterogeneously enhancing cystic tumor in the fourth ventricle and right foramen of Luschka. In this location, the primary differential entity is an ependymoma (*see* Chap. 4)

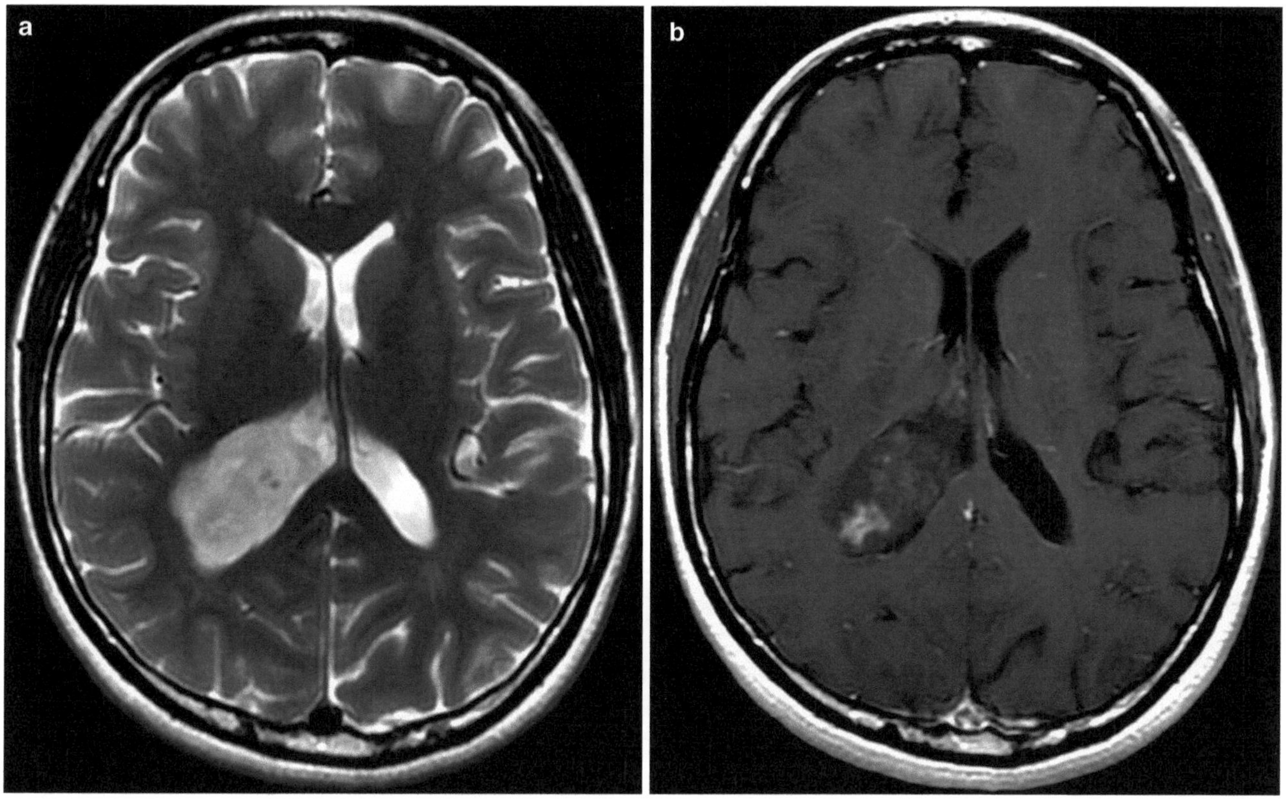

Fig. 1.58 Subependymoma. Axial T2- (**a**) and contrast T1-weighted (**b**) images demonstrate an expansile T2 hyperintense tumor in the right lateral ventricle with mild heterogeneous enhancement at its posterior margin. This appearance may also suggest an intraventricular oligodendroglioma or astrocytoma, but not central neurocytoma that should be attached to the septum pellucidum nor meningioma that should have avid homogeneous enhancement

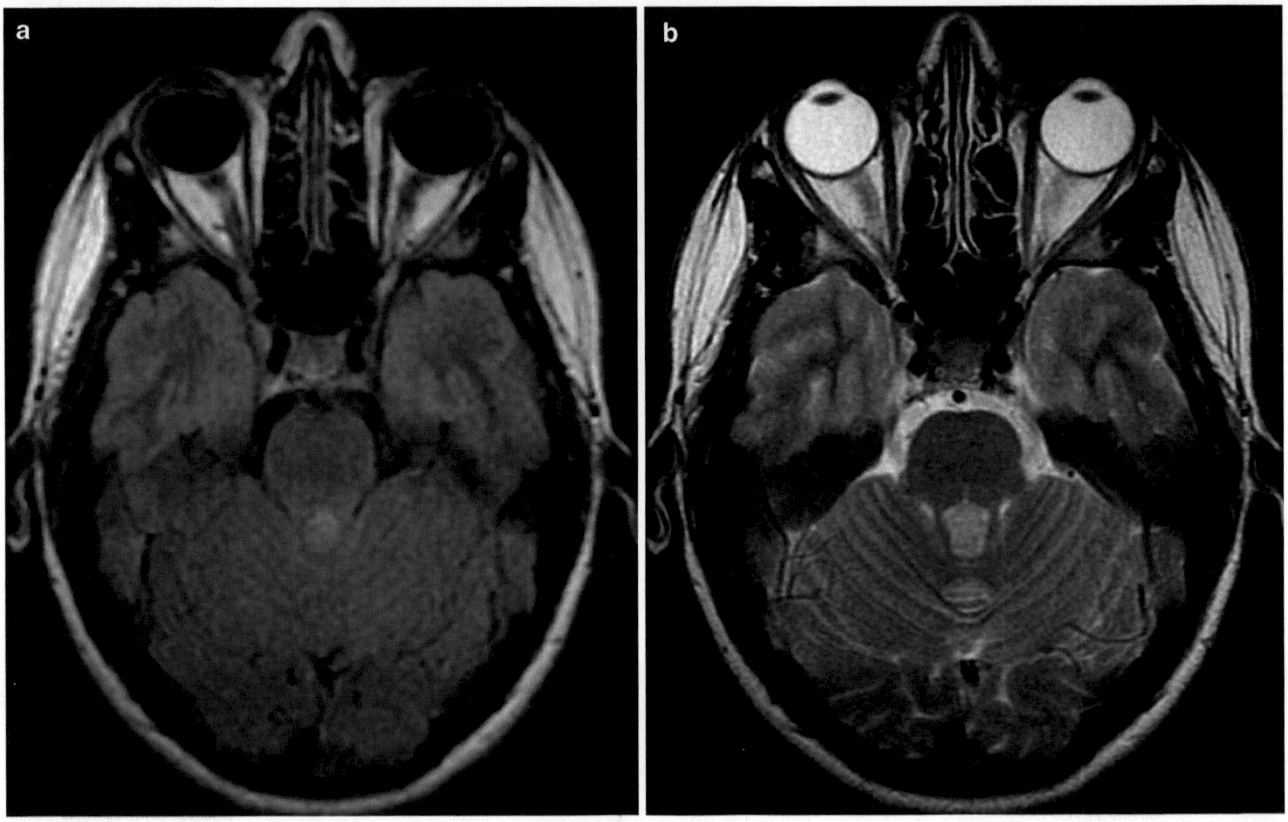

Fig. 1.59 Subependymoma. Axial FLAIR (**a**) and T2-weighted (**b**) images show an expansile hyperintense tumor filling the fourth ventricle. The lack of enhancement (*not shown*) would be unusual for other tumors that may occur in this location, such as ependymoma, choroid plexus tumor, or metastasis

Extra-axial

The term "extra-axial space" is used to define the space that is within the skull but outside of brain parenchyma. Tumors located within the extra-axial space are lesions that arise exterior to the pial membrane that covers the brain, spinal cord, and proximal nerve roots.

Meningioma

Meningiomas are tumors that arise from arachnoidal cap cells. Meningiomas are the most common primary intracranial neoplasm in adults [36]. Meningiomas have an incidence of around six cases per 100,000 person-years [10]. This tumor type peaks in the middle-aged population and has a slight predominance in women [36]. Meningiomas have a geographic predilection for the African subcontinent [36]. These are usually slow-growing grade I tumors in which gross total resection is curative [37]. Higher-grade atypical and anaplastic meningiomas are more likely to be difficult to completely resect, and to recur after resection [36, 38].

Imaging features. Meningiomas are dural-based lesions that show intense, homogeneous enhancement. Around 90 % of these lesions are supratentorial and 10 % are infratentorial [36, 39]. Meningiomas tend to be well-circumscribed lesions with a broad-based dural tail [36, 39]. Signs of extra-axial origin include cortical buckling of the subjacent brain and gray-white junction, which is separated by thin CSF clefts [39]. Calcium, hemorrhage, necrosis, and/or cysts may be present within the tumor [39]. Dense ossification usually indicates a burnt-out meningioma without potential for future growth [36, 39]. Larger tumors often show radial enhancement patterns that correspond to the appearance at digital subtraction angiography (DSA), which may also demonstrate a prolonged stain that "comes early and stays late" also known as the "mother-in-law" sign [36, 39]. This prolonged stain is visible on dynamic susceptibility contrast (DSC) T2-weighted magnetic resonance imaging (MRI) perfusion images with markedly increased permeability, where the contrast time-intensity curve shows rapid down slope (on T2-weighted perfusion) or rapid upslope (on T1-weighted perfusion) followed by delayed return to baseline [39]. Perfusion is very high as these lie outside the blood–brain barrier, and typically several times greater than the perfusion of high-grade gliomas and metastases [36, 39]. Hyperostosis of the overlying bone is pathognomonic [39].

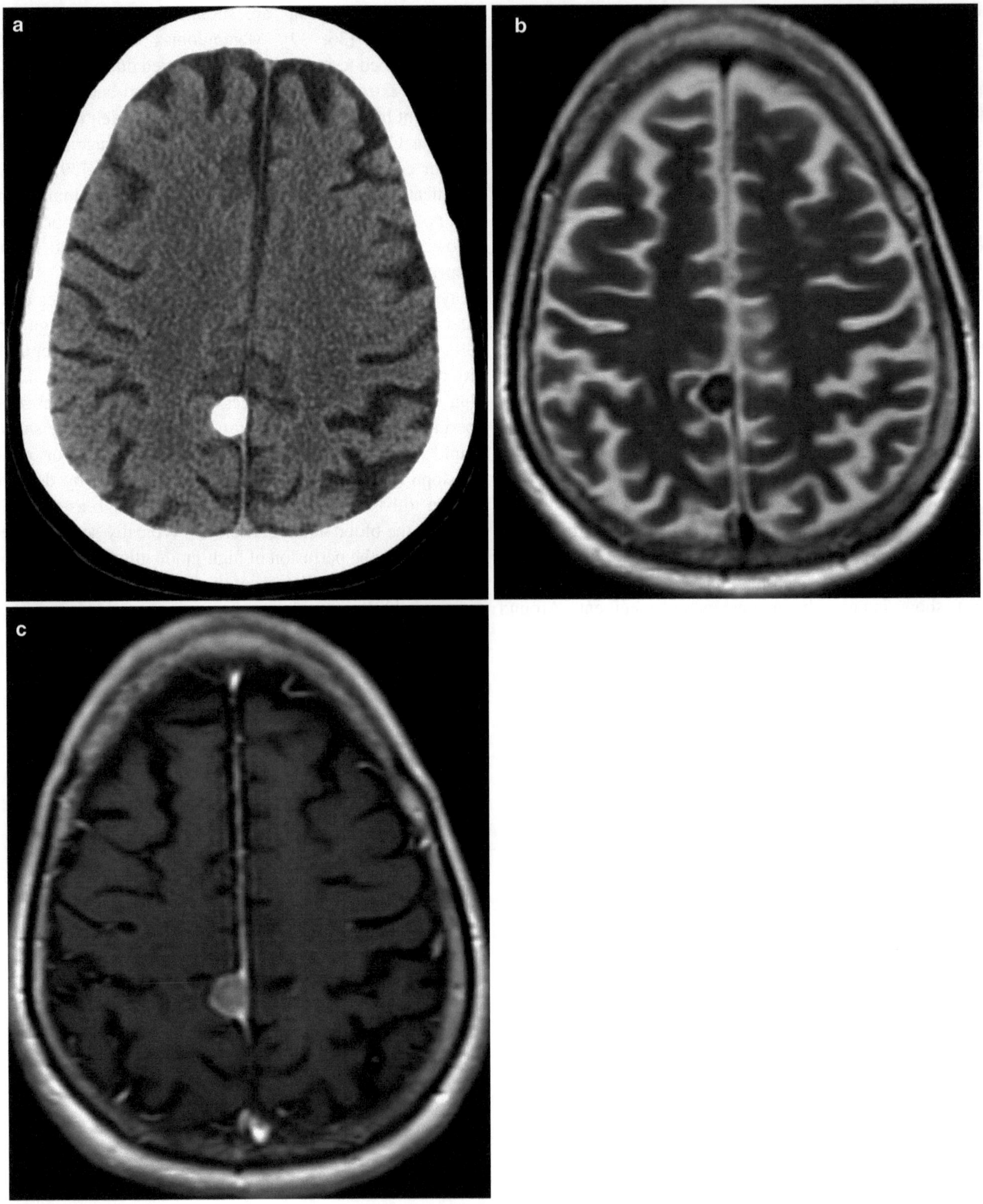

Fig. 1.60 Meningioma. Axial CT (**a**) shows a densely ossified posterior right parafalcine meningioma. The T2-weighted image (**b**) shows marked hypointensity. Despite enhancement on the contrast T1-weighted image (**c**), the dense ossification indicates a "burnt out" tumor with probably no future growth potential

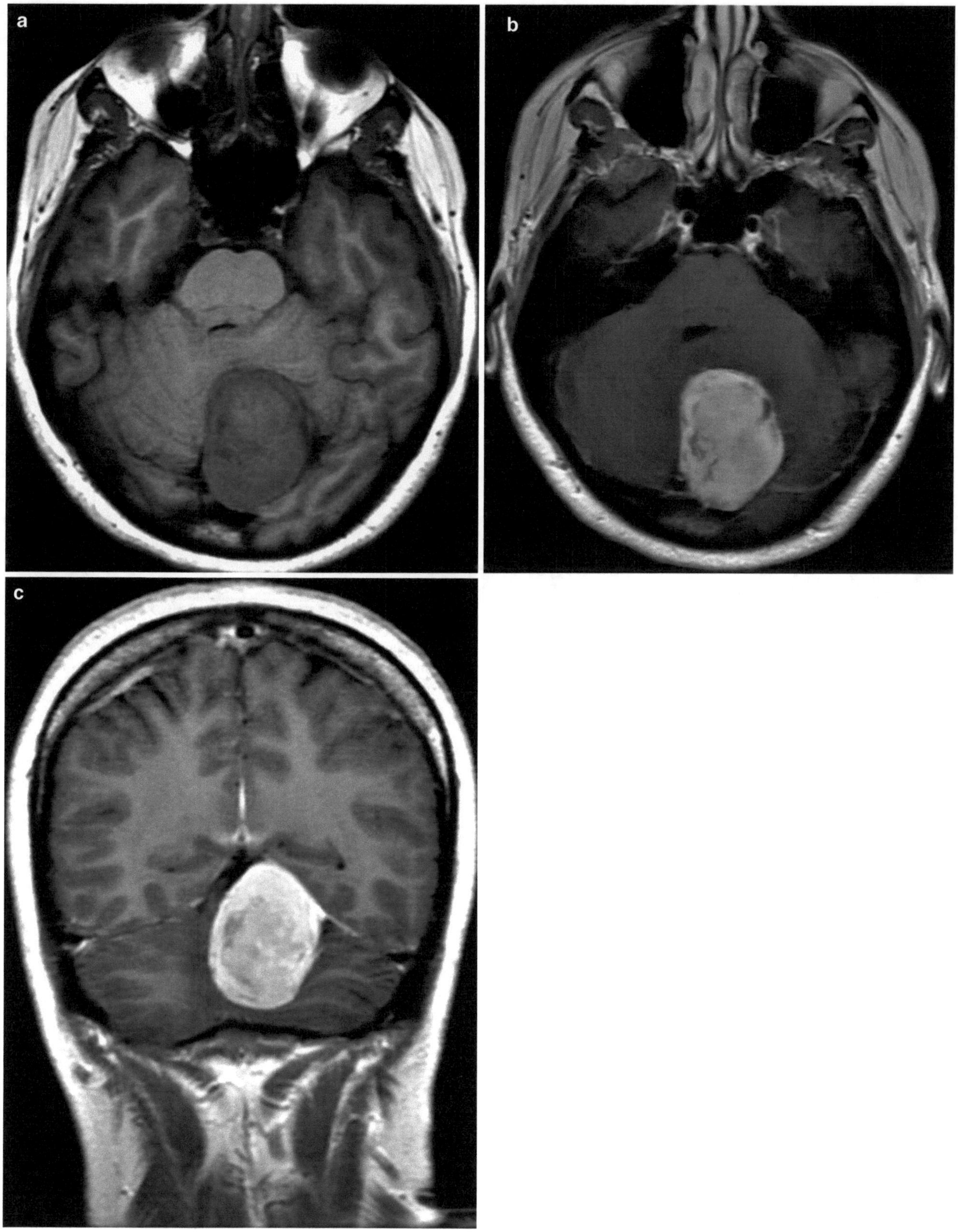

Fig. 1.61 Meningioma. Axial T1-weighted (**a**) and axial (**b**) and coronal (**c**) contrast T1-weighted images show a homogeneously enhancing tumor projecting from the tentorium down into the posterior fossa

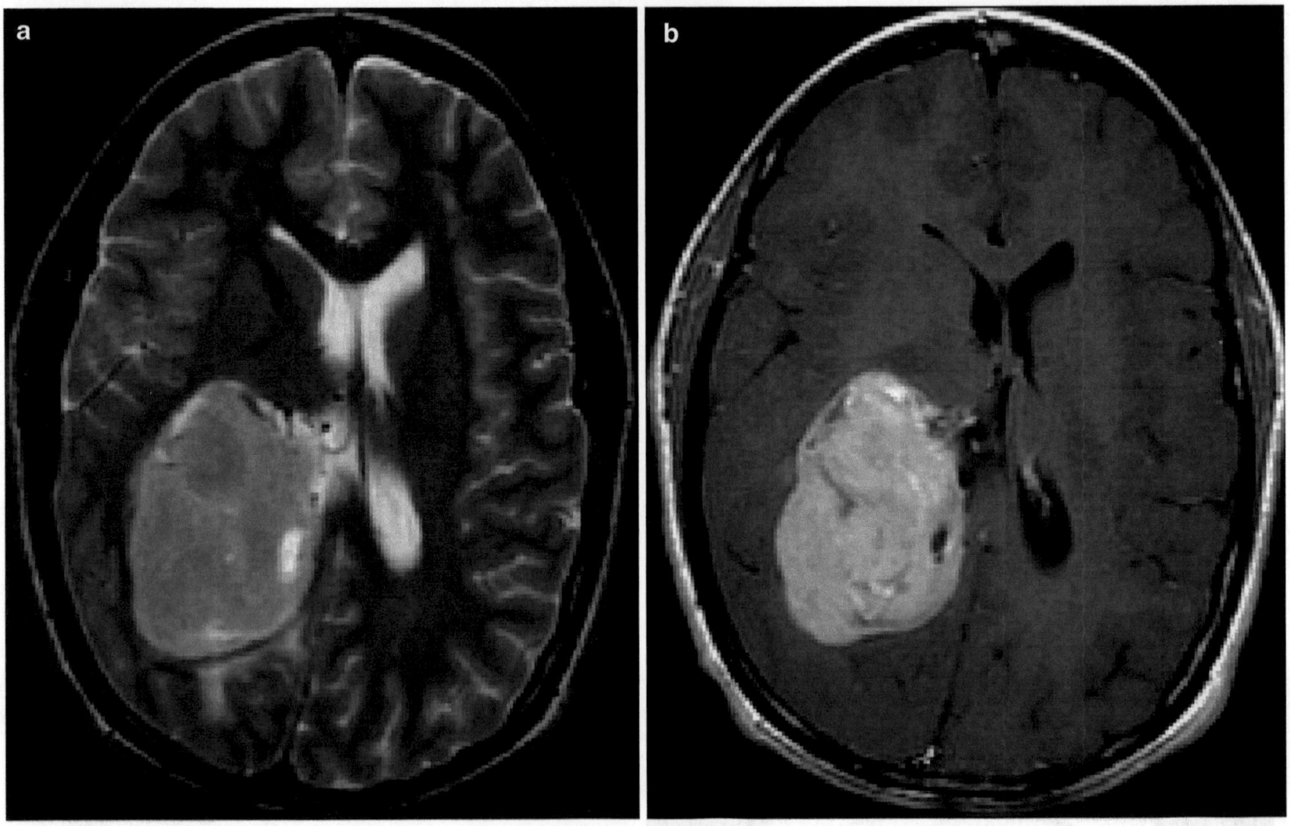

Fig. 1.62 Meningioma. Axial T2-weighted (**a**) and contrast T1-weighted (**b**) images show an expansile, avidly enhancing tumor in the atrium of the right lateral ventricle. Although the small cystic changes may mimic a subependymoma, the enhancement is otherwise very intense, and the atrium is the most common location for meningiomas in adults

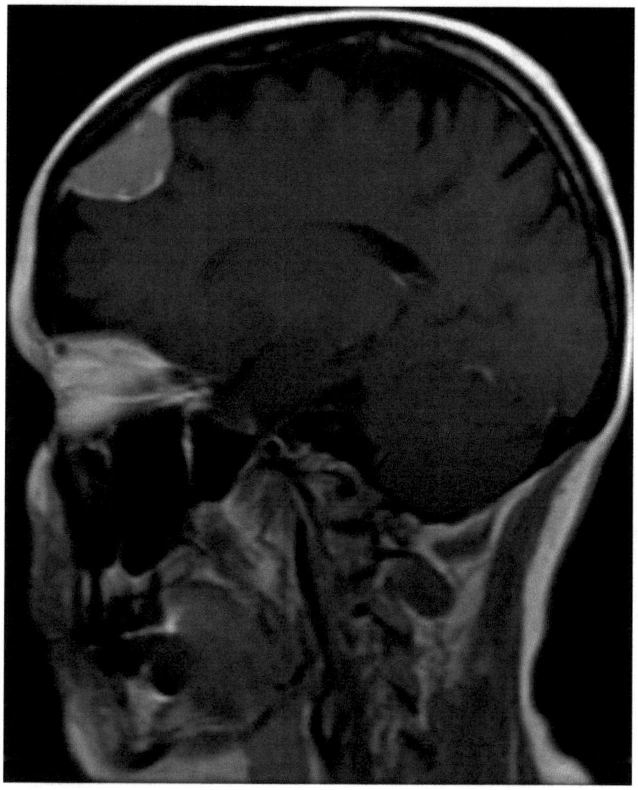

Fig. 1.63 Meningioma. Sagittal contrast T1-weighted image reveals a frontal convexity meningioma with enhancing dural tails and mild hyperostosis of the overlying frontal bone

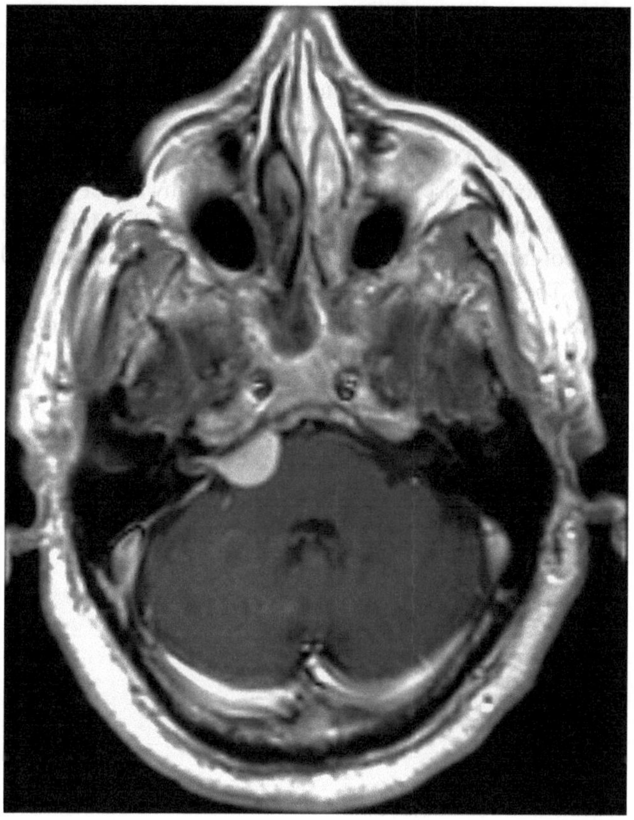

Fig. 1.64 Meningioma. Axial contrast T1-weighted image shows a meningioma in the right cerebellopontine angle cistern with an enhancing dural tail that extends posteriorly into the internal auditory canal. Contrast with vestibular schwannomas, which usually fill and expand the internal auditory canal and porus acousticus, and are more likely to show heterogeneous enhancement

Schwannoma

This is a grade I slow-growing nerve sheath tumor that consists of Schwann cells [40]. This tumor type is responsible for up to 8 % of all intracranial malignancies [40]. Almost all schwannomas arise from the myelinated Schwann cell nerve sheaths that surround cranial nerves [40, 41]. More than 50 % of intraparenchymal schwannomas occur before age 30 [40]. These tumors have a less than 10 % chance of recurrence after surgical resection [40, 41]. Radiation therapy is an option for some small tumors in patients who are poor surgical candidates [40, 42].

Imaging features. Around 90 % of these arise from the vestibular portion of cranial nerve VIII and 5 % occur in other cranial nerves such as V and VII [40, 41]. Cranial nerve schwannomas are commonly seen as solid, enhancing, noncalcified extra-axial masses [40, 42]. Heterogeneous enhancement is common. Rarely these tumors are intra-axial, located adjacent to the ventricle or superficially [40, 42]. Parenchymal schwannomas typically appear as well-demarcated cysts with a strongly enhancing nodule [40, 42].

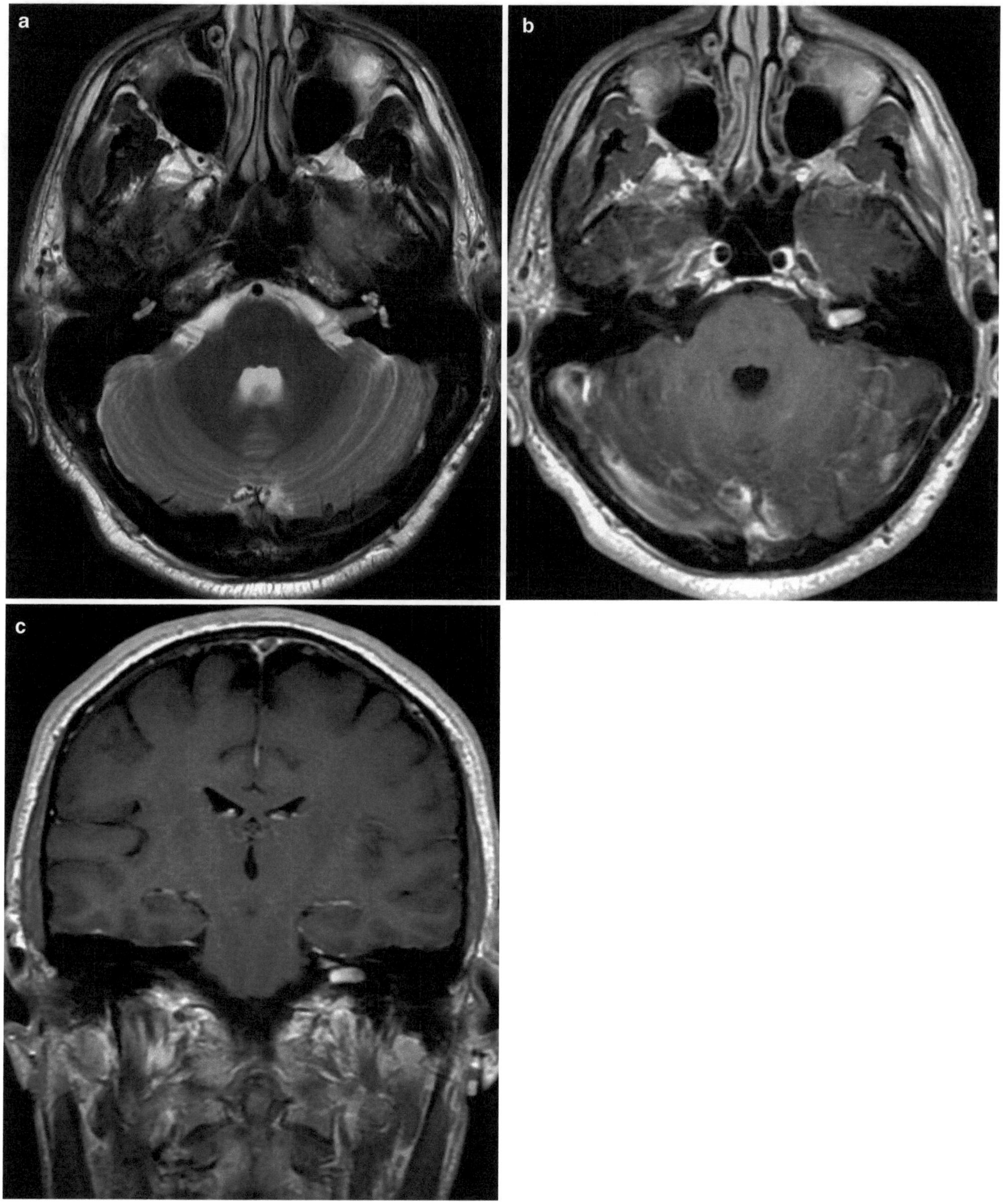

Fig. 1.65 Schwannoma. Axial T2-weighted (**a**) and axial (**b**) and coronal (**c**) contrast T1-weighted images reveal an enhancing intracanalicular tumor filling and confined to the left internal auditory canal

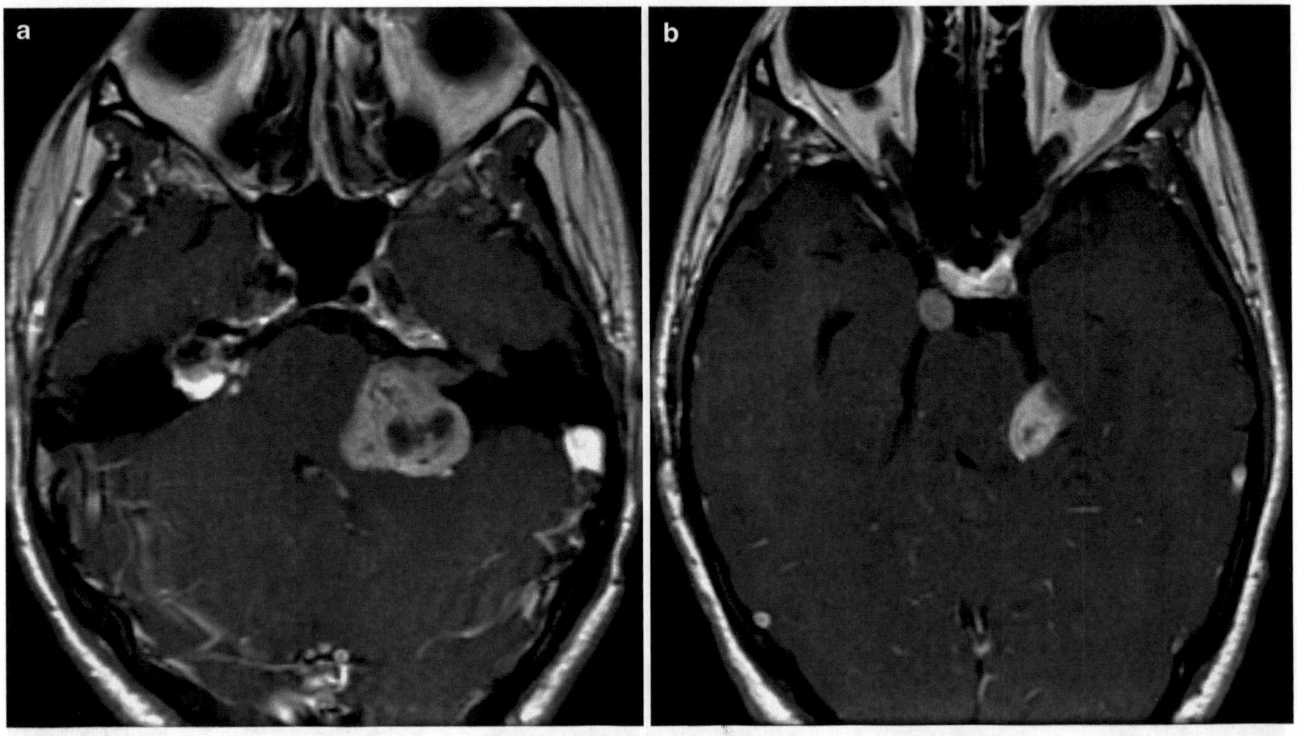

Fig. 1.66 Schwannoma. Axial contrast T1-weighted images (**a** and **b**) show a heterogeneously enhancing left vestibular schwannoma filling the internal auditory canal and widening the porus acousticus with a large component in the cerebellopontine angle cistern compressing the brachium pontis. Although the center of the tumor is outside the internal auditory canal, the complete filling and expansion of the canal are typical for a schwannoma. The presence of bilateral vestibular schwannomas (smaller one in right internal auditory canal in (**a**)) is diagnostic for neurofibromatosis type 2. Patient has additional schwannomas of the bilateral cranial nerves V in Meckel's caves in (**a**) and right cisternal cranial nerve III in (**b**). The enhancing lesion in the left ambient cistern represents the top of the dominant vestibular schwannoma

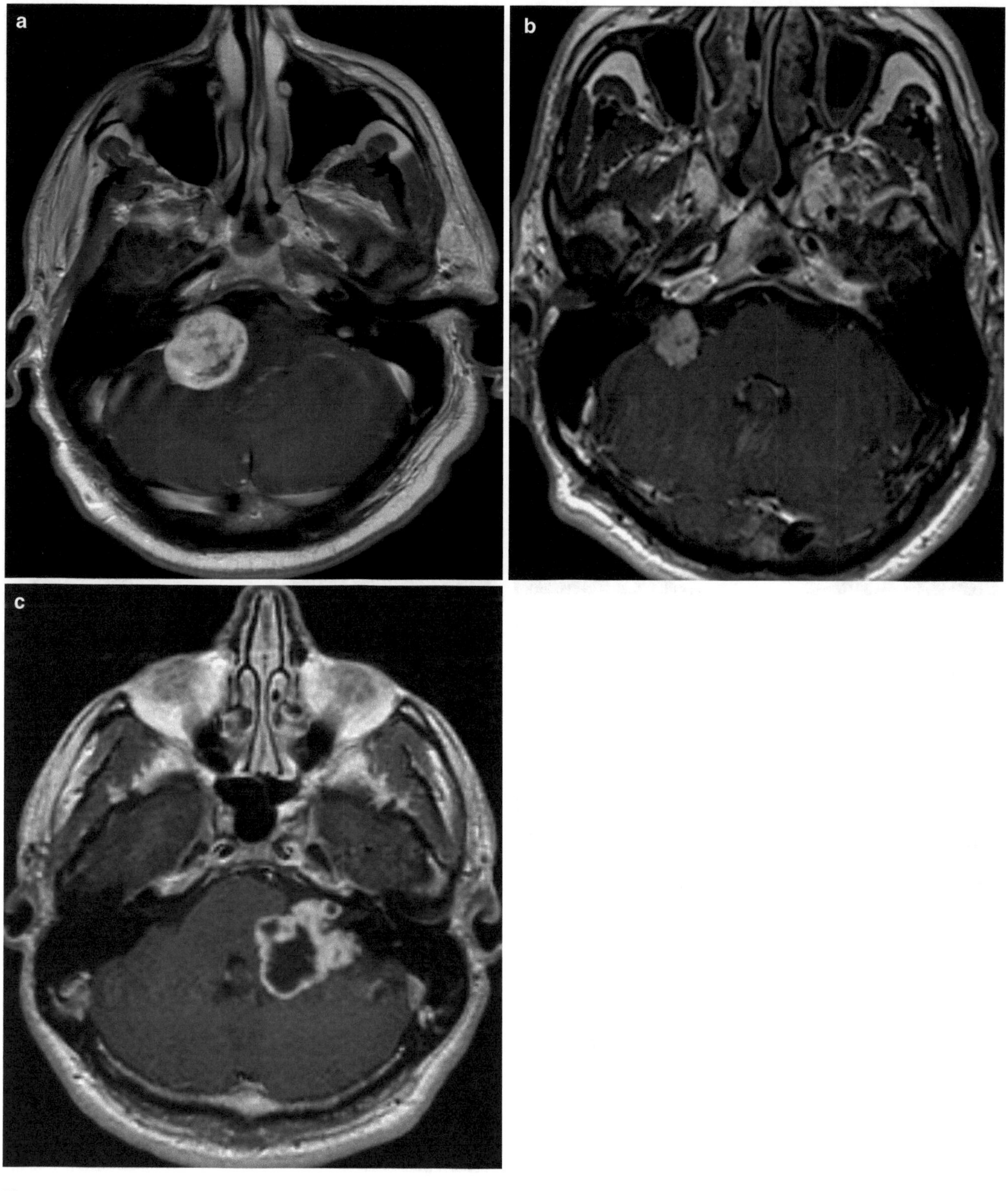

Fig. 1.67 Schwannoma. Axial contrast T1-weighted images (**a–c**) in three different patients show vestibular schwannomas involving the cisternal portion of the vestibular portions of cranial nerve VIII. Lack of involvement of the internal auditory canal is rare, and may dissuade correct identification as vestibular schwannomas. The heterogeneous enhancement would be unusual for untreated meningioma, which may show peritumoral arachnoid cysts without enhancing margins

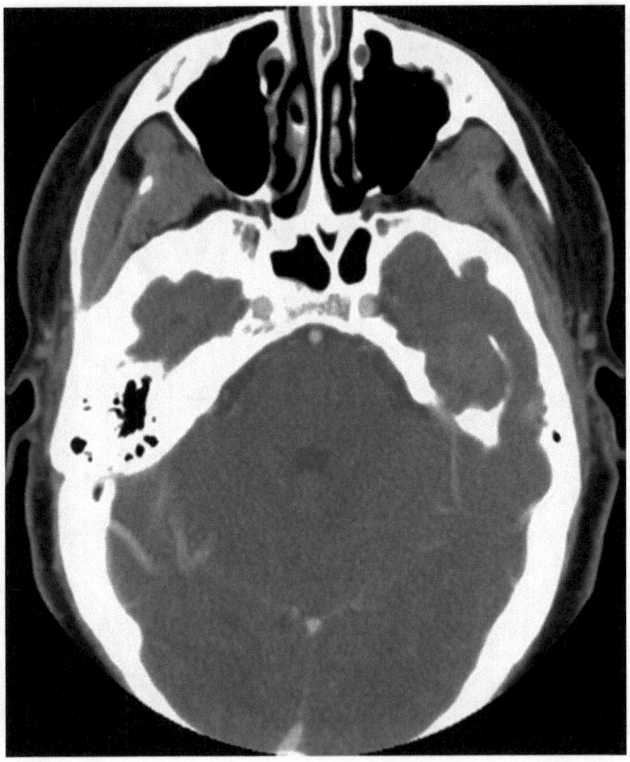

Fig. 1.68 Schwannoma. Axial contrast CT shows an expansile tumor in the region of the left geniculate ganglion in this patient with a schwannoma of cranial nerve VII. Smooth remodeling of the temporal bone is consistent with a slow-growing benign tumor

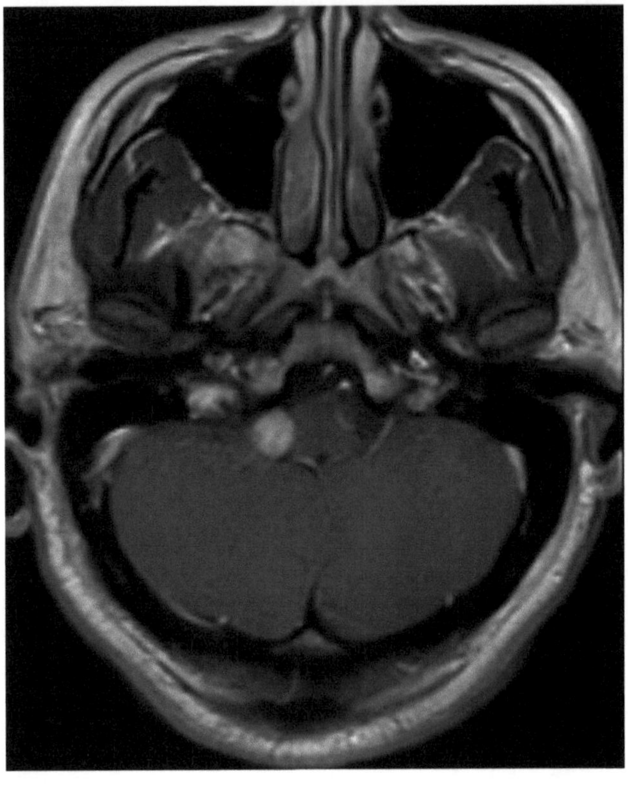

Fig. 1.69 Schwannoma. Axial contrast T1-weighted image reveals an enhancing tumor of the right cranial nerve XII

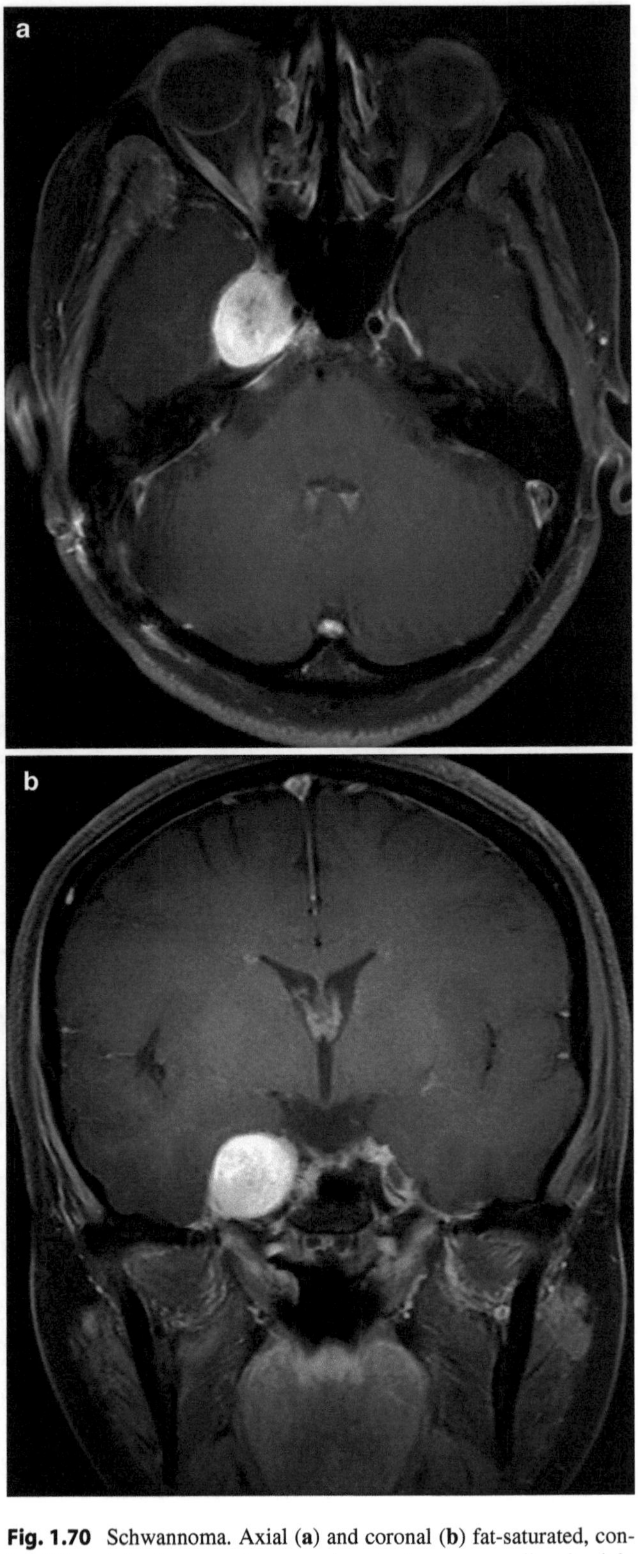

Fig. 1.70 Schwannoma. Axial (**a**) and coronal (**b**) fat-saturated, contrast T1-weighted images show an enhancing tumor expanding the right Meckel's cave, lateral to the cavernous sinus. This was a schwannoma of the trigeminal nerve or cranial nerve V

Hemangiopericytoma

This is an anaplastic sarcomatous mesenchymal tumor that involves the malignant transformation of pericytes found adjacent to capillaries within the body [43]. Hemangiopericytomas account for less than 1 % of all primary CNS lesions and around 2–4 % of meningeal tumors [43]. These tumors are most common in the fourth to sixth decades of life. Because local recurrence and extracranial metastases are common for patients with these tumors, careful follow-up is highly recommended [43]. Patients have a guarded prognosis with a 5-year survival rate of 5 % [43, 44].

Imaging features. Hemangiopericytomas are typically supratentorial and are most commonly found in the occipital region with involvement of the falx, tentorium, or dural sinuses [43, 45]. These often present as large heterogenous dural lesions with heterogeneous enhancement and areas of cystic and/or necrotic change [43, 45]. They may have broad or narrow dural bases, unlike meningiomas that usually have broad bases [43, 45]. Hemangiopericytomas can also be differentiated from meningiomas by their lack of calcium and hyperostosis as well as the presence of bone erosion and multiple flow voids [43].

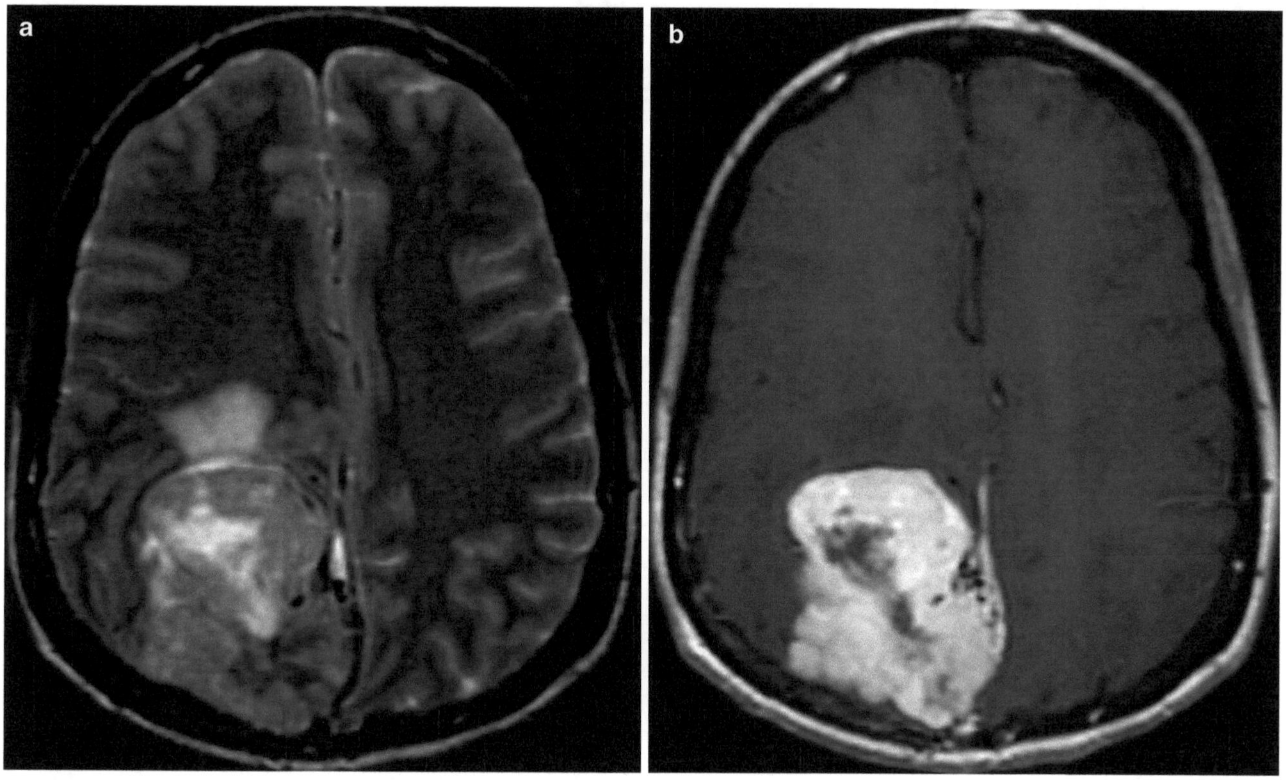

Fig. 1.71 Hemangiopericytoma. Axial T2-weighted (**a**) and contrast T1-weighted (**b**) images show a large heterogeneous enhancing tumor in the right occipital region with cystic/necrotic changes and mild adjacent brain edema. The tumor has broad dural bases against the posterior convexity and the posterior falx cerebri, which is bowed to the contralateral side

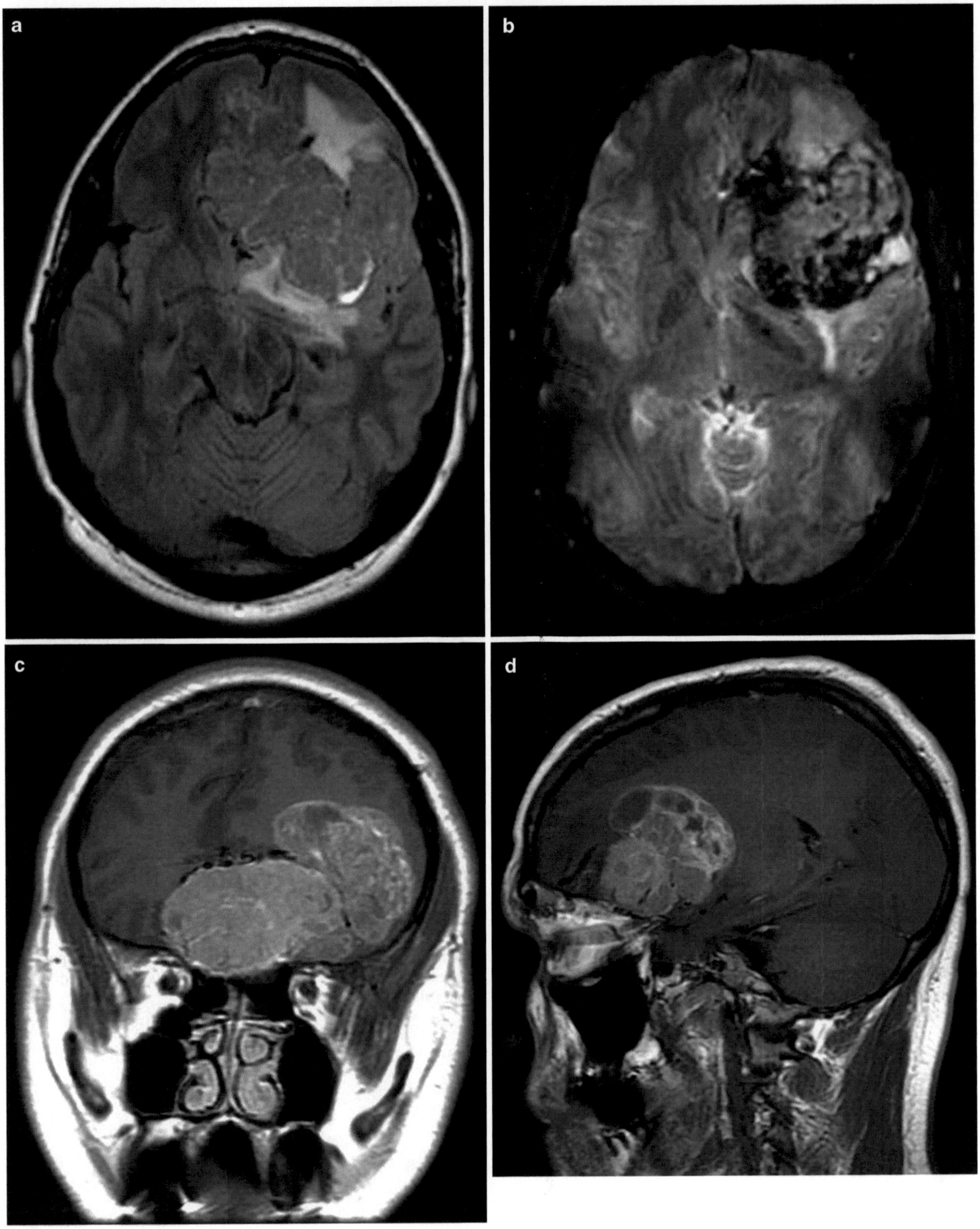

Fig. 1.72 Hemangiopericytoma. Axial FLAIR (**a**) and gradient-echo (**b**) images, as well as coronal (**c**) and sagittal (**d**) contrast T1-weighted images, show a large, heterogeneously enhancing tumor in the left frontal region with gradient hypointense flow voids and/or blood products. Calcifications have not been described in hemangiopericytomas

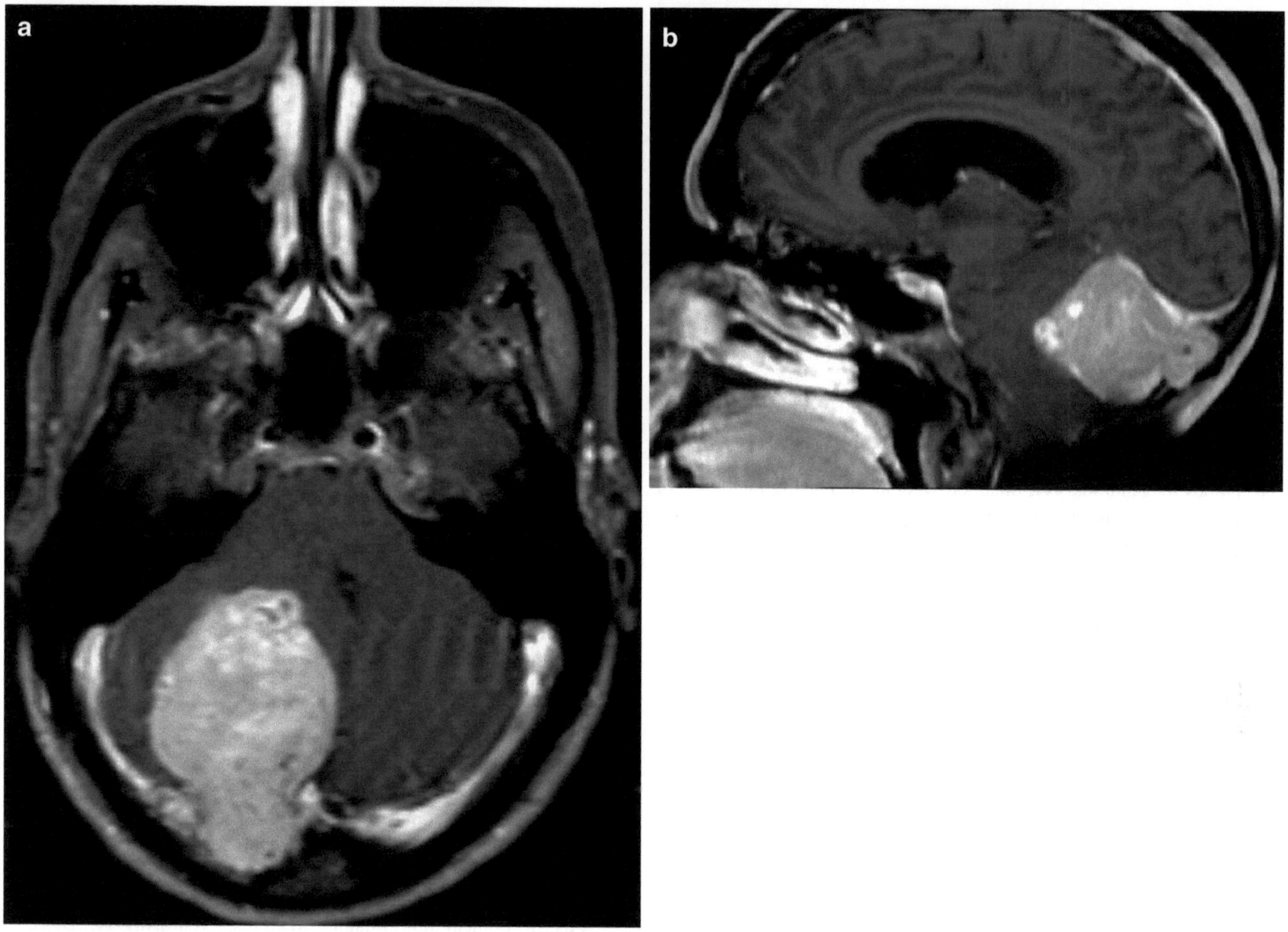

Fig. 1.73 Hemangiopericytoma. Axial (**a**) and sagittal (**b**) contrast T1-weighted images reveal a large enhancing tumor in the right posterior fossa. The homogeneous enhancement may mimic a more common meningioma, but the posterior erosion into the overlying occipital bone provides a clue that this is a hemangiopericytoma

References

1. Osborne AG. Neoplasms and tumorlike lesions. In: Mascarenaz AD, Dearth CL, Kaerli M, editors. Diagnostic imaging: brain. Salt Lake City: Amirsys; 2005. p. 140–2.
2. Nussbaum ES, Djalilian HR, Cho KH, Hall WA. Brain metastases. Histology, multiplicity, surgery, and survival. Cancer. 1996;78: 1781–8.
3. Lageraard FJ, Levendag PC, Nowak PJ, et al. Identification of prognostic factors in patients with brain metastases: a review of 1292 patients. Int J Radiat Oncol Biol Phys. 1999;43:795–803.
4. Osborne AG. Neoplasms and tumorlike lesions. In: Mascarenaz AD, Dearth CL, Kaerli M, editors. Diagnostic imaging: brain. Salt Lake City: Amirsys; 2005. p. 20–3.
5. Ohgaki H, Kleihues P. Population-based studies on incidence, survival rates, and genetic alterations in astrocytic and oligodendroglial gliomas. J Neuropathol Exp Neurol. 2005;64:479–89.
6. Dobes M, Khurana VG, Shadbolt B, et al. Increasing incidence of glioblastoma multiforme and meningioma and decreasing incidence of schwannoma (2000–2008): findings of a multicenter Australian study. Surg Neurol Int. 2011;2:176.
7. Lacroix M, Abi-Said D, Fourney DR, et al. A multivariate analysis of 416 patients with GBM: prognosis, extent of resection and survival. J Neurosurg. 2001;95:190–8.
8. Altman DA, Atkinson Jr DS, Brat DJ. Best cases from the AFIP: glioblastoma multiforme. Radiographics. 2007;27:883–8.
9. Osborne AG. Neoplasms and tumorlike lesions. In: Mascarenaz AD, Dearth CL, Kaerli M, editors. Diagnostic imaging: brain. Salt Lake City: Amirsys; 2005. p. 8–10.
10. Central Brain Tumor Registry of the United States. CBTRUS statistical report tables: primary brain and central nervous system tumors diagnosed in the United States in 2004–2008. Hinsdale: Central Brain Tumor Registry of the United States; 2012. Available at http://www.cbtrus.org/2007-2008/2007-20081.html. Accessed 12 May 2012.
11. Lote K, Egeland T, Hager B, et al. Survival, prognostic factors, and therapeutic efficacy in low-grade glioma: a retrospective study in 379 patients. J Clin Oncol. 1997;15:3129–40.
12. Recht LD, Bernstein M. Low-grade gliomas. Neurol Clin. 1995;13: 847–59.
13. Osborne AG. Neoplasms and tumorlike lesions. In: Mascarenaz AD, Dearth CL, Kaerli M, editors. Diagnostic imaging: brain. Salt Lake City: Amirsys; 2005. p. 42–4.
14. Celli P, Nofrone I, Palma L, et al. Cerebral oligodendroglioma: prognostic factors and life history. Neurosurgery. 1994;35:1018–34.
15. Jenkinson MD, du Plessis DG, Smith TS. Histological growth patterns and genotype in oligodendroglial tumours: correlation with MRI features. Brain. 2006;129:1884–91.
16. Tortosa A, Viñolas N, Villà S, et al. Prognostic implication of clinical, radiologic and pathologic features in patients with anaplastic gliomas. Cancer. 2003;97:1063–71.
17. Osborne AG. Neoplasms and tumorlike lesions. In: Mascarenaz AD, Dearth CL, Kaerli M, editors. Diagnostic imaging: brain. Salt Lake City: Amirsys; 2005. p. 16–8.
18. Engellard HH, Stelea A, Mundt A, et al. Oligodendroglioma and anaplastic oligodendroglioma: clinical features, treatment, prognosis. Surg Neurol. 2003;60:443–56.
19. Osborne AG. Neoplasms and tumorlike lesions. In: Mascarenaz AD, Dearth CL, Kaerli M, editors. Diagnostic imaging: brain. Salt Lake City: Amirsys; 2005. p. 46–8.
20. Osborne AG. Neoplasms and tumorlike lesions. In: Mascarenaz AD, Dearth CL, Kaerli M, editors. Diagnostic imaging: brain. Salt Lake City: Amirsys; 2005. p. 26–8.
21. Rust P, Ashkan K, Ball C, et al. Gliomatosis cerebri: pitfalls in diagnosis. J Clin Neurosci. 2001;8:361–3.
22. Kim DG, Yang HJ, Park IA, et al. Gliomatosis cerebri: clinical features, treatment and prognosis. Acta Neurochir (Wien). 1998;140: 755–62.
23. Abrey LE, DeAngelis LM, Yahalom J. Long-term survival in primary CNS lymphoma. J Clin Oncol. 1998;16:859.
24. Osborne AG. Neoplasms and tumorlike lesions. In: Mascarenaz AD, Dearth CL, Kaerli M, editors. Diagnostic imaging: brain. Salt Lake City: Amirsys; 2005. p. 122–4.
25. Osborne AG. Neoplasms and tumorlike lesions. In: Mascarenaz AD, Dearth CL, Kaerli M, editors. Diagnostic imaging: brain. Salt Lake City: Amirsys; 2005. p. 52–4.
26. Schwartz TH, Kim S, Glick RS, et al. Supratentorial ependymomas in adult patients. Neurosurgery. 1999;44:721–31.
27. Applegate GL, Marymont MH. Intracranial ependymomas: a review. Cancer Invest. 1998;16:588–93.
28. Koeller KK, Sanberg GD. From the archives of the AFIP: cerebral intraventricular neoplasms: radiologic-pathologic correlation. Radiographics. 2002;22:1473–505.
29. Osborne AG. Neoplasms and tumorlike lesions. In: Mascarenaz AD, Dearth CL, Kaerli M, editors. Diagnostic imaging: brain. Salt Lake City: Amirsys; 2005. p. 114–6.
30. Neumann HP, Eggert HR, Weigel K, et al. Hemangioblastomas of the central nervous system. A 10-year study with special reference to von Hippel-Lindau syndrome. J Neurosurg. 1989;70:24–30.
31. Osborne AG. Neoplasms and tumorlike lesions. In: Mascarenaz AD, Dearth CL, Kaerli M, editors. Diagnostic imaging: brain. Salt Lake City: Amirsys; 2005. p. 80–2.
32. Chen C, Shen CC, Wang J, et al. Central neurocytoma: a clinical, radiological and pathological study of nine cases. Clin Neurol Neurosurg. 2008;110:129–36.
33. Osborne AG. Neoplasms and tumorlike lesions. In: Mascarenaz AD, Dearth CL, Kaerli M, editors. Diagnostic imaging: brain. Salt Lake City: Amirsys; 2005. p. 56–8.
34. Ragel BT, Osborn AG, Whang K, et al. Subependymomas: an analysis of clinical and imaging features. Neurosurgery. 2006;58: 881–90.
35. Koral K, Kedzierski RM, Gimi B, et al. Subependymoma of the cerebellopontine angle and prepontine cistern in a 15-year-old adolescent boy. AJNR Am J Neuroradiol. 2008;29:190–1.
36. Osborne AG. Skull, scalp and meninges. In: Mascarenaz AD, Dearth CL, Kaerli M, editors. Diagnostic imaging: brain. Salt Lake City: Amirsys; 2005. p. 56–8.
37. Palma L, Celli P, Franco C, et al. Long-term prognosis for atypical and malignant meningiomas: a study of 71 surgical cases. J Neurosurg. 1997;86:793–800.
38. Ko KW, Nam DH, Kong DS, et al. Relationship between malignant subtypes of meningioma and clinical outcome. J Clin Neurosci. 2007;14:747–53.
39. Buetow MP, Buetow PC, Smirniotopoulos JG. Typical, atypical and misleading features in meningioma. Radiographics. 1991;11: 1087–106.
40. Osborne AG. Neoplasms and tumorlike lesions. In: Mascarenaz AD, Dearth CL, Kaerli M, editors. Diagnostic imaging: brain. Salt Lake City: Amirsys; 2005. p. 108–10.
41. Colreavy MP, Lacy PD, Hughes J, et al. Head and neck schwannomas – a 10 year review. J Laryngol Otol. 2000;114:119–24.
42. Chung SY, Kim DI, Lee BH, et al. Facial nerve schwannomas: CT and MR findings. Yonsei Med J. 1998;39:148–53.
43. Osborne AG. Neoplasms and tumorlike lesions. In: Mascarenaz AD, Dearth CL, Kaerli M, editors. Diagnostic imaging: brain. Salt Lake City: Amirsys; 2005. p. 118–20.
44. Espat NJ, Lewis JJ, Leung D, et al. Conventional hemangiopericytoma: modern analysis of outcome. Cancer. 2002;95:1746–51.
45. Chiechi MV, Smirniotopoulos JG, Mena H. Intracranial hemangiopericytomas: MR and CT features. AJNR Am J Neuroradiol. 1996;17:1365–71.

Pediatric Brain Tumors

2

Gitanjali V. Patel, Robert J. Young, and Sasan Karimi

Intra-axial

Supratentorial

Dysembryonic neuroepithelial tumor. A dysembryonic neuroepithelial tumor (DNET) is a grade 1, slow-growing lesion that is located within the cortex of the brain. This tumor accounts for up to 2 % of all intracranial brain tumors in patients younger than 20 years old [1]. DNETs most commonly occur in children and young adults and have no gender predominance [2]. Uncontrollable epilepsy is a common clinical finding in patients with DNET [3].

Imaging features. This is a benign, wedge-shaped mass that is usually multi-cystic appearing and is most commonly located within the temporal lobe [2, 3]. DNETs have minimal or no mass effect and lack any surrounding edema [2]. These tumors can vary in size but typically do not enhance. These tumors may contain calcium and are rarely complicated by hemorrhage [2].

Ganglioglioma. A ganglioglioma is a grade I or II, tumor comprised of glial and ganglion cells [4]. Ganglioglioma is the most frequent cause of chronic epilepsy originating in the temporal lobe, representing up to 4 % of all pediatric intracranial neoplasms [5]. Gangliogliomas most commonly occur in patients younger than 30 years old with a slight male predominance [5]. Patients have an excellent prognosis following curative complete surgical resection.

Imaging features. The majority of Gangliogliomas are most commonly seen as well-circumscribed cystic-appearing lesions with mural nodules that extend from the cortex [4]. Gangliogliomas in younger patients tend to be larger and more cystic than gangliogliomas in adults. These tumors can occur anywhere within the brain but are often found within the temporal lobe or within the superficial cerebral hemispheres [4, 5]. Ganglioglioma have a variable enhancement pattern and may contain calcium [4].

G.V. Patel
Department of Radiology,
Memorial Sloan-Kettering Cancer Center,
1275 York Avenue, MRI-1156, New York,
NY 10065, USA
e-mail: gita.patel@gmail.com

R.J. Young • S. Karimi (✉)
Department of Radiology,
New York Presbyterian Hospital/Weill Cornell Medical College,
New York, NY, USA

Neuroradiology Service, Department of Radiology,
Memorial Sloan-Kettering Cancer Center,
1275 York Avenue, MRI-1156, New York, NY 10065, USA
e-mail: youngr@mskcc.org; karimis@mskcc.org

S. Karimi (ed.), *Atlas of Brain and Spine Oncology Imaging*, Atlas of Oncology Imaging,
DOI 10.1007/978-1-4614-5653-7_2, © Springer Science+Business Media New York 2013

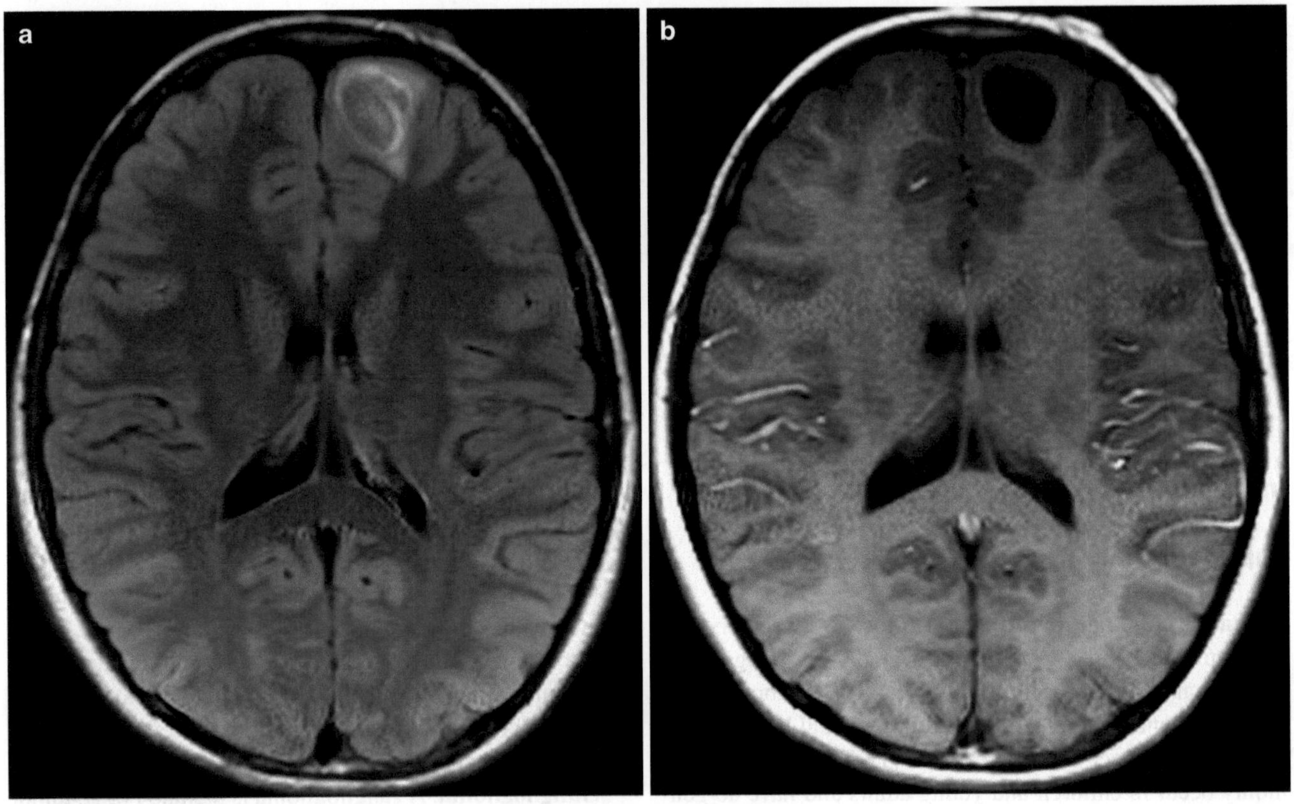

Fig. 2.1 Dysembryonic neuroepithelial tumor. Axial fluid attenuated inversion recovery (FLAIR) (**a**) and contrast T1-weighted (**b**) images show a heterogeneously FLAIR hyperintense cystic-appearing tumor in the anterior left frontal lobe with no enhancement and minor adjacent peritumoral FLAIR hyperintense changes

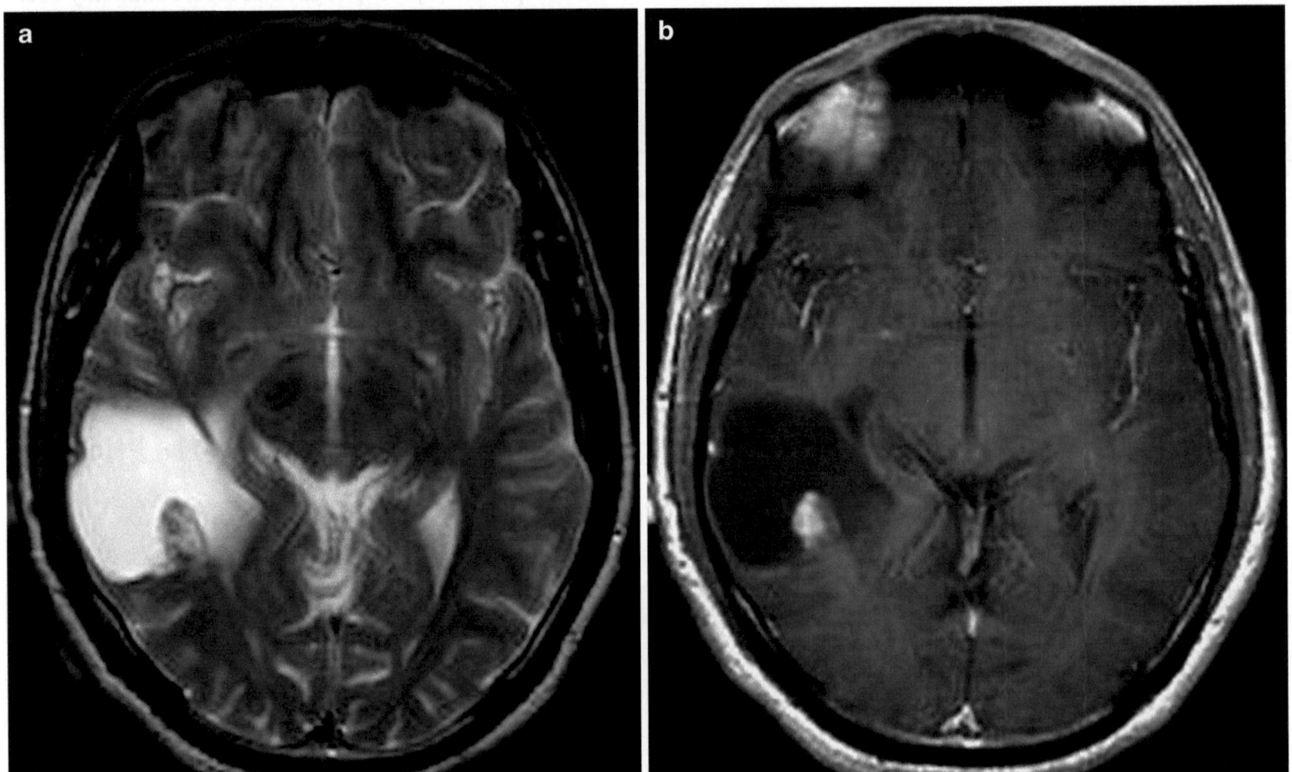

Fig. 2.2 Dysembryonic neuroepithelial tumor. Axial T2-weighted (**a**) and contrast T1-weighted (**b**) images show a cystic cortical/subcortical tumor in the right temporal lobe with a posterior enhancing nodule

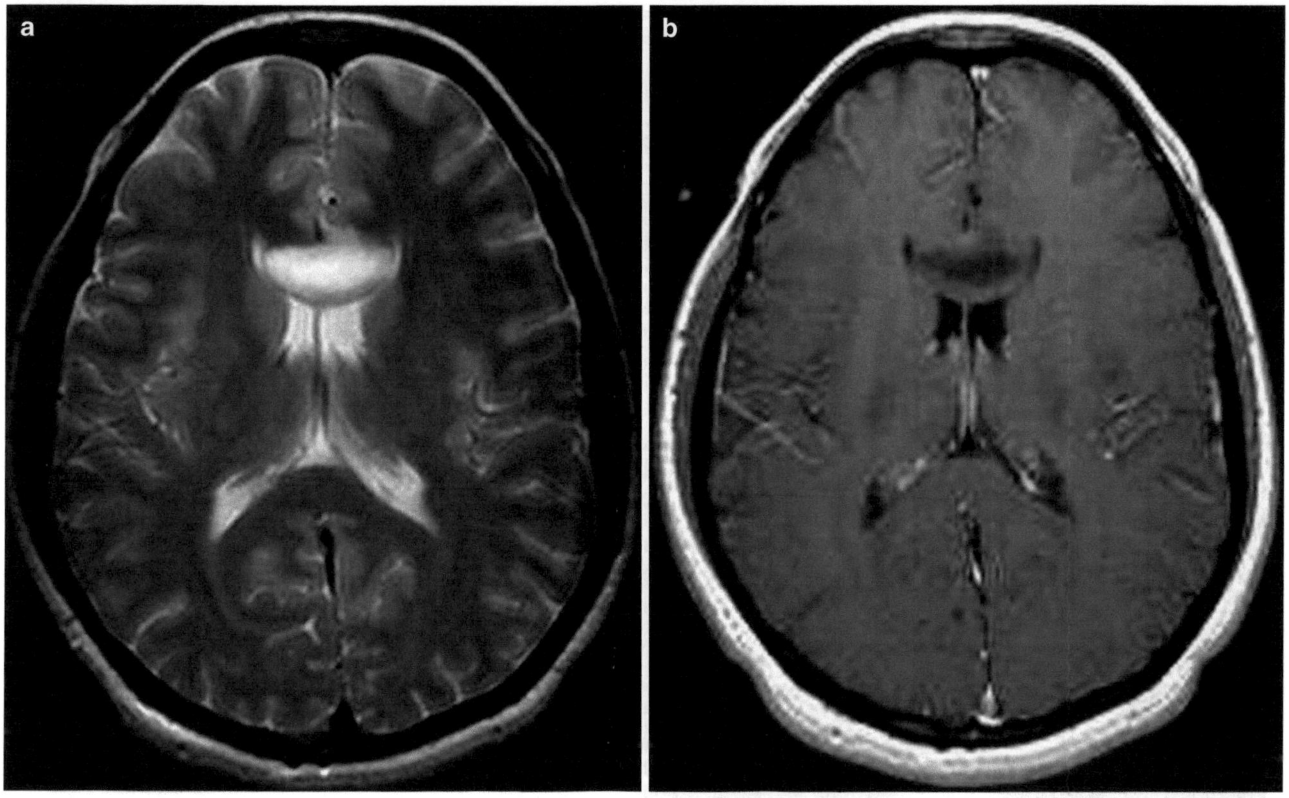

Fig. 2.3 Dysembryonic neuroepithelial tumor. Axial T2-weighted (**a**) and contrast T1-weighted (**b**) images demonstrate an expansile cystic-appearing nonenhancing tumor in the genu of the corpus callosum. Despite the unusual location, a biopsy confirmed the diagnosis of DNET

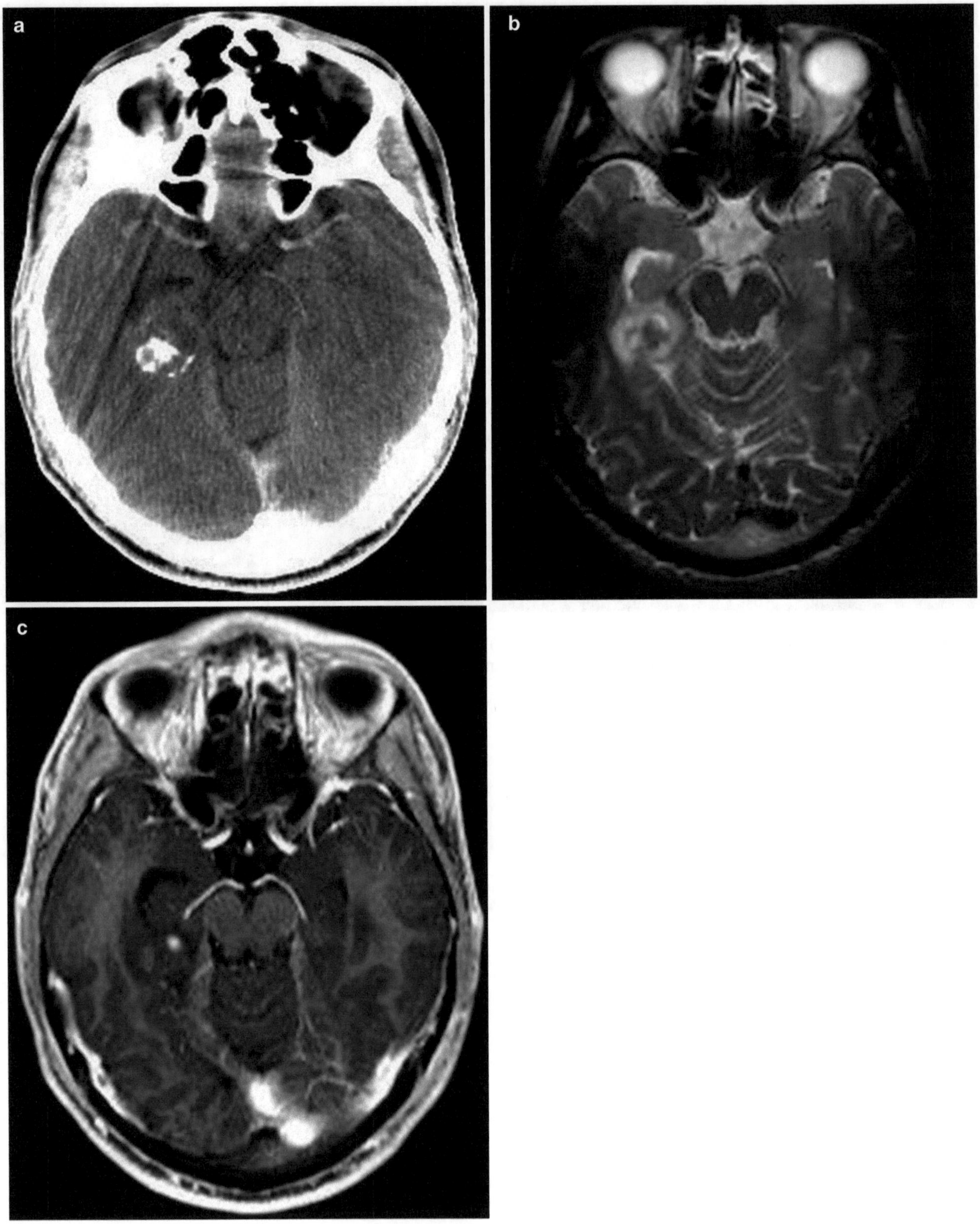

Fig. 2.4 Ganglioglioma. Axial noncontrast CT (**a**), T2-weighted (**b**), and contrast T1-weighted (**c**) images show a heterogeneous, partially calcified tumor in the right mesial temporal lobe with focal nodular enhancement. The temporal lobe location in a young patient presenting with seizures is characteristic

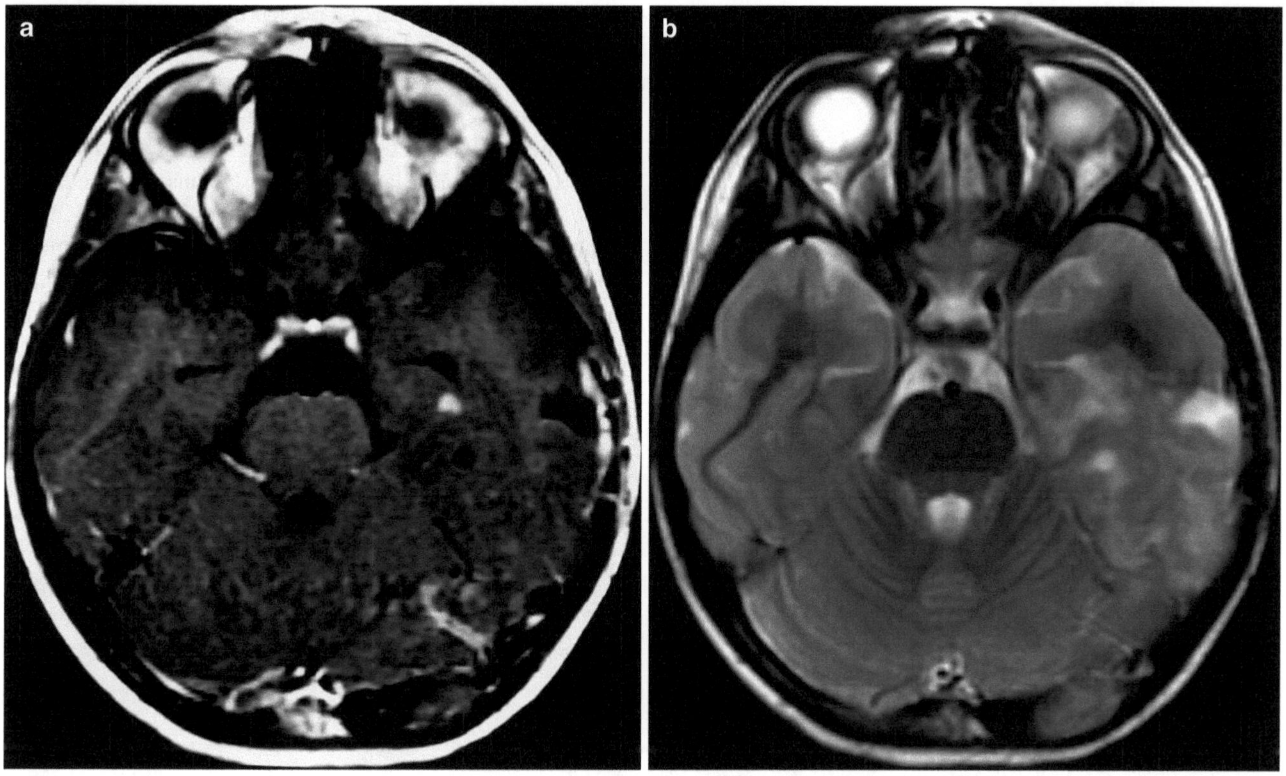

Fig. 2.5 Ganglioglioma. Axial contrast T1-weighted (**a**) and T2-weighted (**b**) images in a 6-year-old male reveal an enhancing nodule in the left mesial temporal lobe, and more diffuse expansile T2 hyperintense abnormality involving most of the visualized temporal lobe (while sparing the anterior temporal pole)

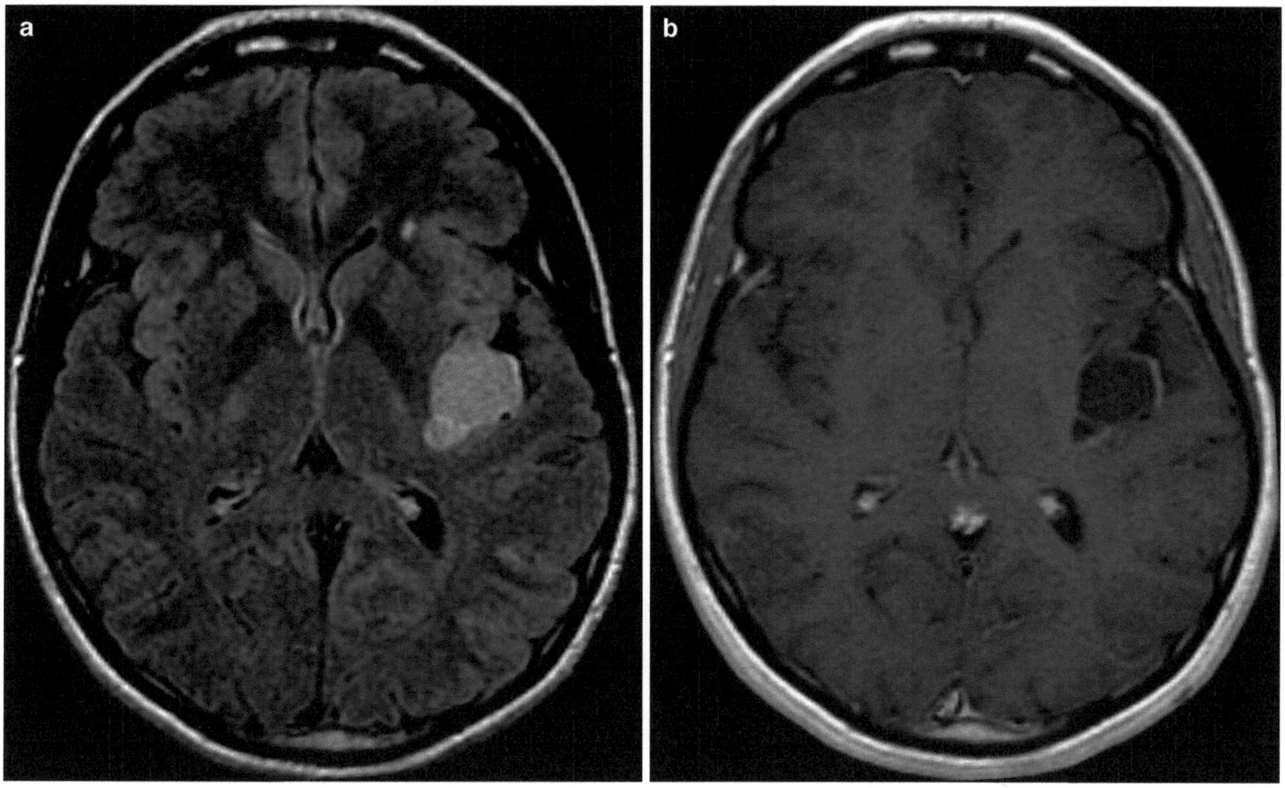

Fig. 2.6 Ganglioglioma. Axial FLAIR (**a**) and contrast T1-weighted (**b**) images in a 22 year old show a FLAIR hyperintense tumor with thin curvilinear peripheral enhancement in the posterior left insula and subinsula

Intratentorial

Atypical Teratoid Rhabdoid Tumor

Atypical teratoid rhabdoid tumor (ATRT) is a rare, grade IV, malignant brain tumor [6]. This tumor accounts for up to 3 % of all pediatric brain tumors and 20 % of central nervous system (CNS) malignancies in children under the age of 3 [6, 7]. Around 15–20 % of patients with ATRT present with a disseminated lesion [6]. This tumor type is the primary consideration for a malignant-appearing brain lesion in a newborn or infant [7]. ATRTs carry a poor prognosis, with a median survival of 6 months [6, 7].

Imaging features. Around half of ATRTs are large tumors that are located infratentorially within the cerebellopontine angle, cerebellum, and/or brainstem [7]. These tumors are typically large irregular lesions with heterogeneous enhancement [7]. ATRT commonly contain cysts, hemorrhage, and/or calcium. Large tumors commonly compress the fourth ventricle and cause hydrocephalus. Imaging of the entire CNS is recommended to search for disseminated tumor.

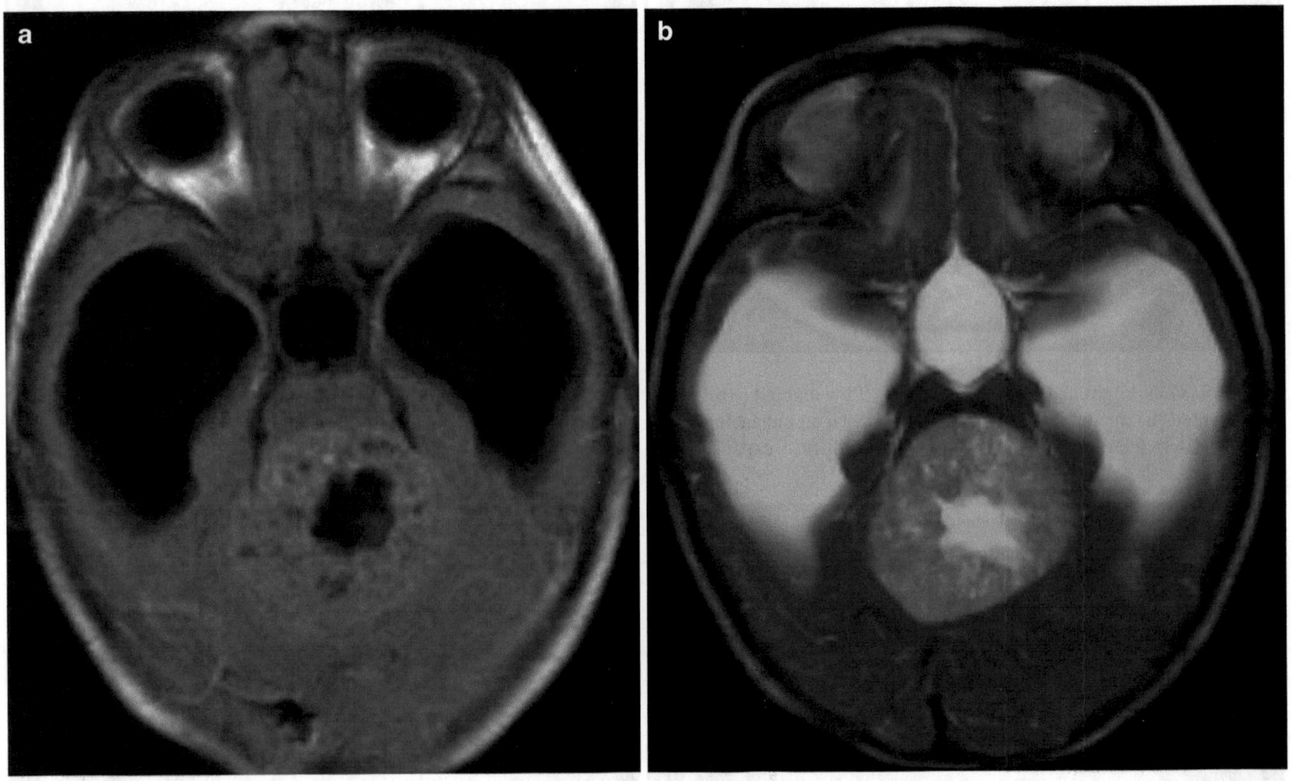

Fig. 2.7 Atypical teratoid rhabdoid tumor. Axial FLAIR (**a**), T2-weighted (**b**), and contrast axial (**c**) and sagittal (**d**) T1-weighted images in a 4 month old show an expansile tumor centered in the superior cerebellar cistern with central cystic/necrotic change and mild heterogeneous enhancement causing severe obstructive hydrocephalus due to compression of the cerebral aqueduct and fourth ventricle, with markedly dilated lateral and third ventricles. This appearance in a neonate is typical for ATRT. The patient also had a rhabdoid left renal tumor (**e**). Brain and kidney tumors share a common deletion of the INI1/hSNF5 tumor suppressor gene in chromosome 22

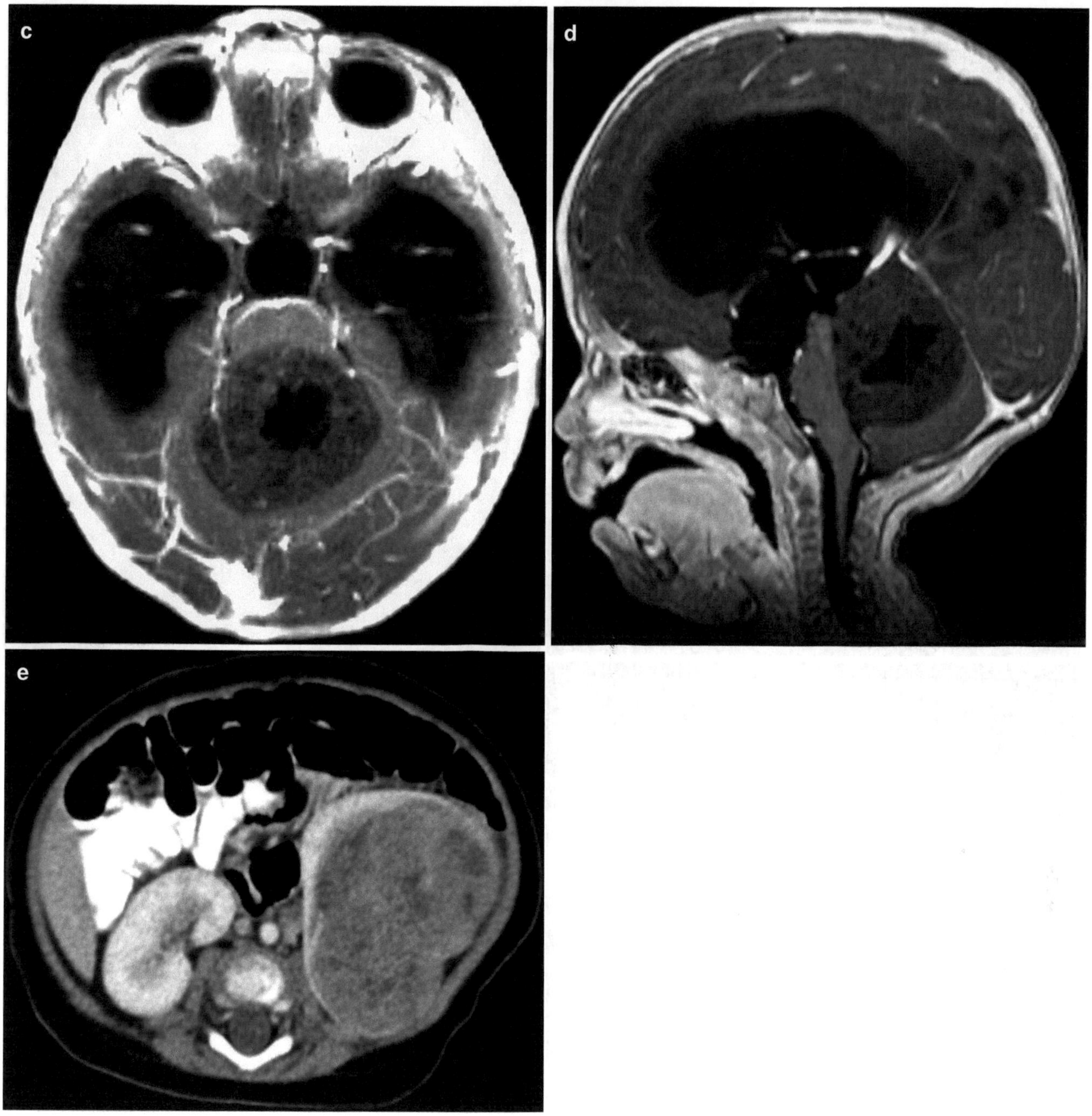

Fig. 2.7 (continued)

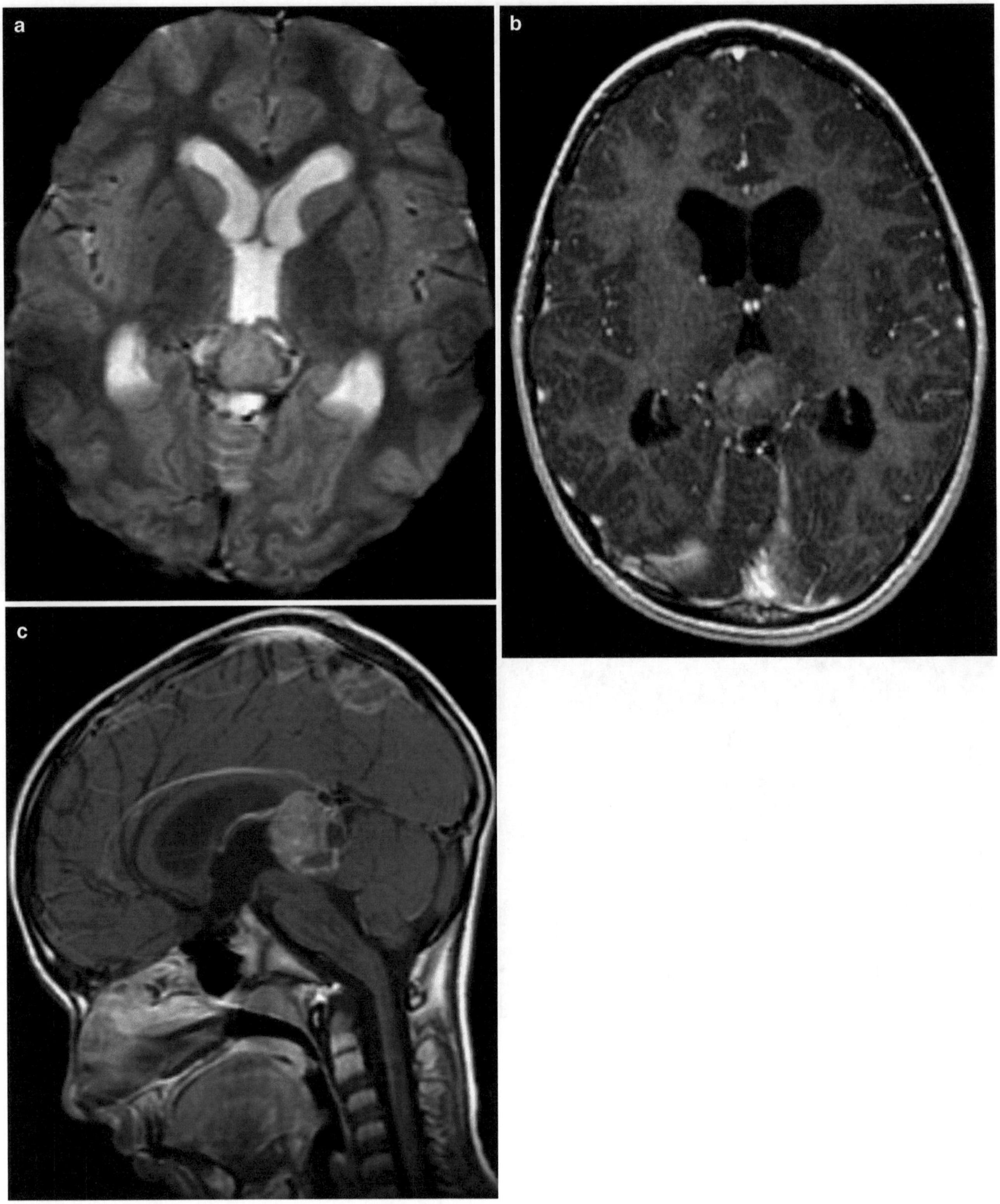

Fig. 2.8 Atypical teratoid rhabdoid tumor. Axial T2-weighted (**a**) and contrast axial (**b**) and sagittal (**c**) T1-weighted images in a 6 year old reveal a heterogeneously enhancing tumor in the pineal region with effacement of the posterior third ventricle and cerebral aqueduct causing mild obstructive hydrocephalus

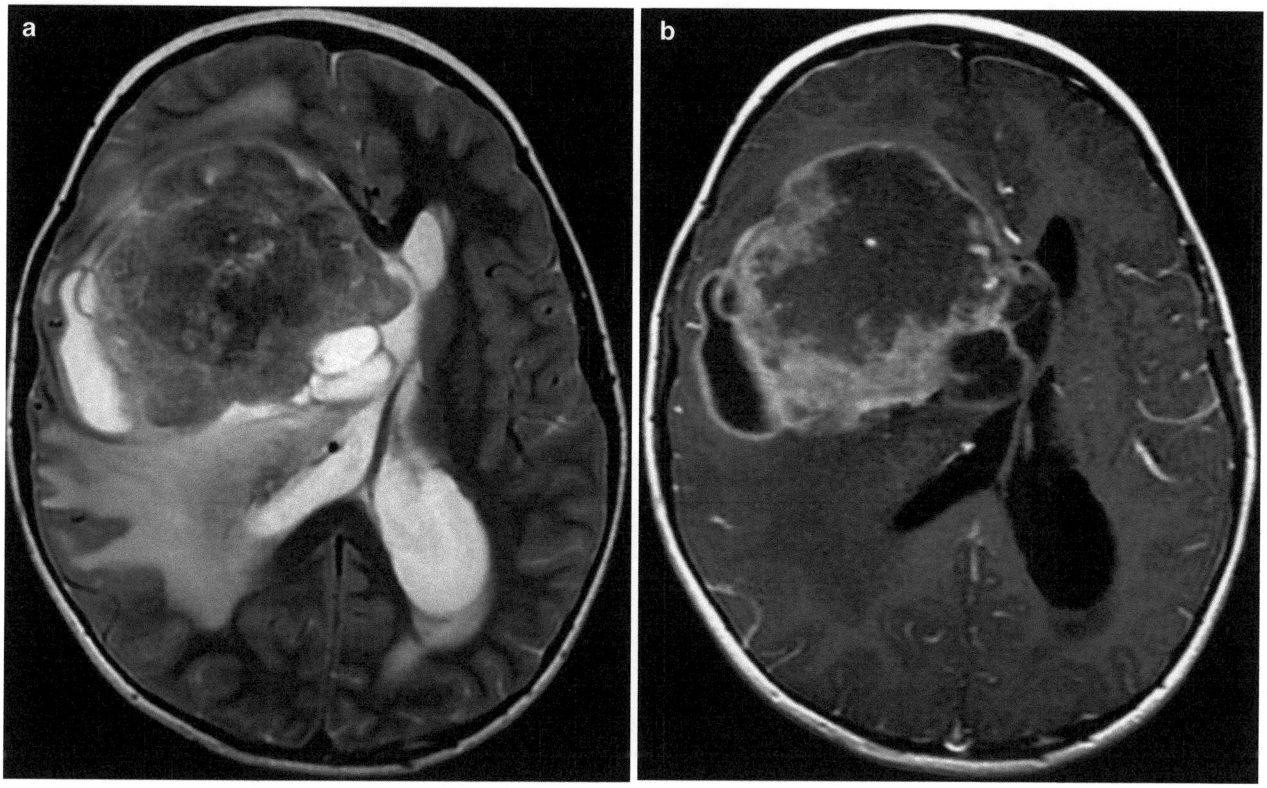

Fig. 2.9 Atypical teratoid rhabdoid tumor. Axial T2-weighted (**a**) and contrast T1-weighted (**b**) images in a 9-year-old female demonstrate a large heterogeneously enhancing tumor in the right frontal lobe and basal ganglia with prominent cystic/necrotic components and marked surrounding T2 hyperintense edema-type changes. Mass effect causes contralateral midline shift. Despite compression of the lateral ventricles, mild obstructive hydrocephalus at the level of the foramen of Monro (*not shown*) and mild interstitial edema from transependymal cerebrospinal fluid (CSF) flow

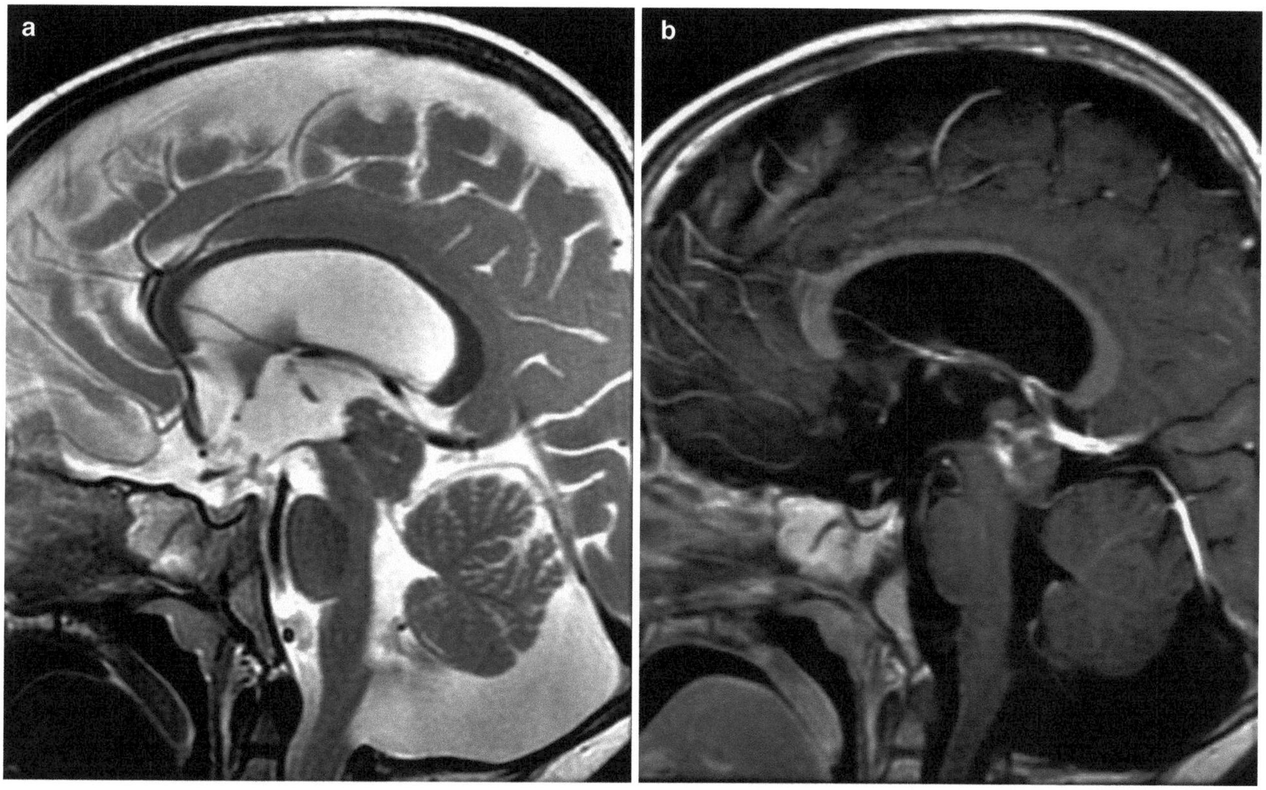

Fig. 2.10 Atypical teratoid rhabdoid tumor. Sagittal T2- (**a**) and contrast T1-weighted (**b**) images in 19-month-old male demonstrate a heterogeneously enhancing tumor in the tectum, located inferior to the internal cerebral veins and straight sinus. The cerebral aqueduct is compressed and its normal CSF flow void is missing on the sagittal T2-weighted image, indicating the level of the mild obstructive hydrocephalus (note mildly dilated lateral and third ventricles)

Brainstem Glioma

A brainstem glioma is a diffuse or focal gliomatous brain tumor that involves the midbrain, pons, and/or medulla [8]. This tumor type is responsible for around 10–20 % of all pediatric brain tumors [8]. Brainstem gliomas are found at a mean age of 7 years and have no gender predilection [9]. The grade of brainstem glioma varies by histologic type: pilocytic tumors are considered to be grade I tumors whereas fibrillary tumors can range from grade II to IV [10]. In general, these tumors do not metastasize outside the CNS. The location and extent of involvement of the brainstem glioma are predictors of prognosis [9, 10].

Imaging features. Appearance of brainstem glioma depends upon tumor type and location [9, 10]. Tectal gliomas are usually pilocytic, focal, have a variable enhancement pattern, and usually contain calcium [8, 9]. Focal tegmental mesencephalic gliomas usually contain a cystic and a nodular component [8]. Diffuse pontine gliomas are fibrillary, diffuse tumors that do not enhance [8]. All brainstem gliomas are variably hyperintense on T2-weighted imaging sequences [8].

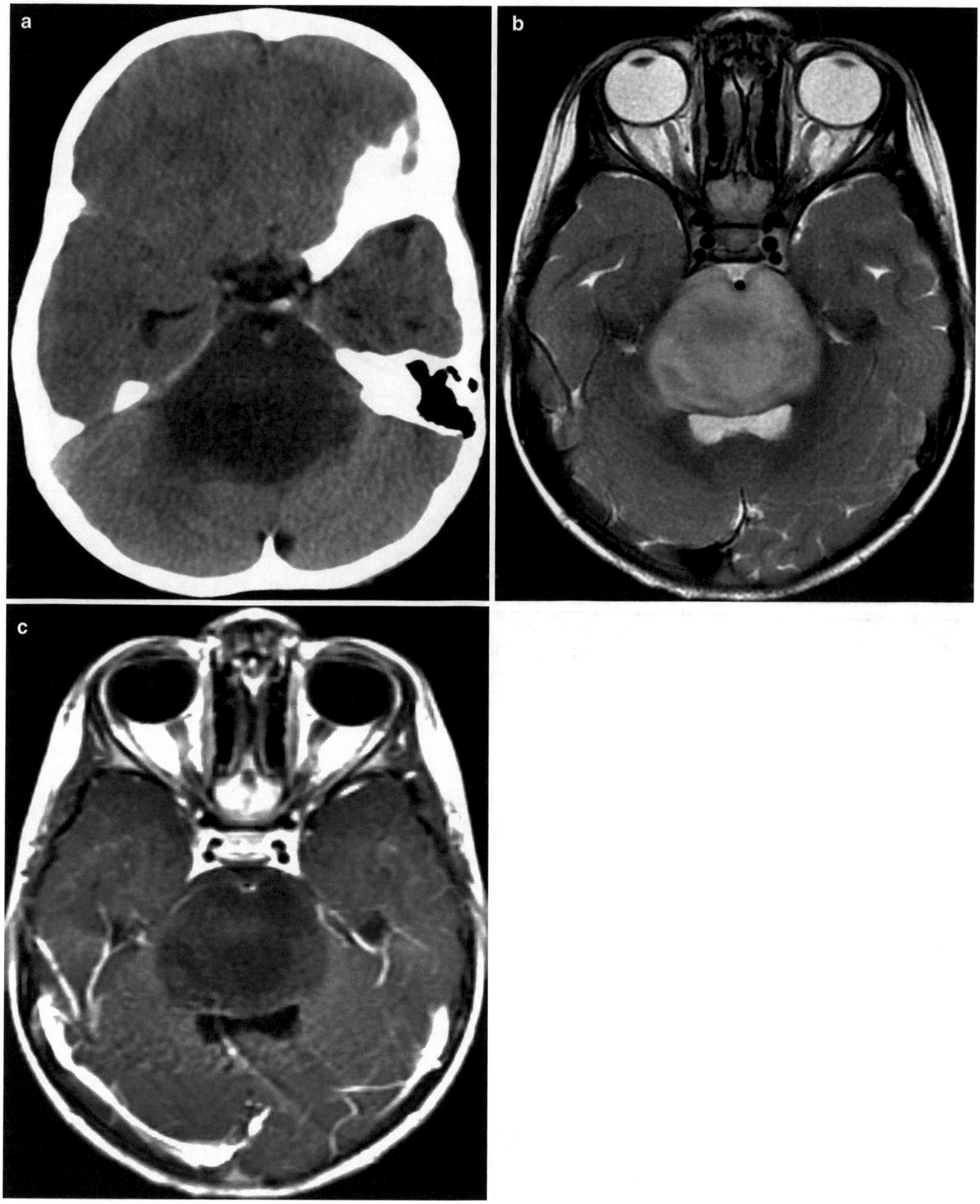

Fig. 2.11 Brainstem glioma. Axial noncontrast CT (**a**), T2-weighted (**b**), and contrast T1-weighted (**c**) images in a 3 year old reveal a hypodense, T2 hyperintense tumor expanding the pons with anterior filling of the prepontine cistern and partial encasement of the basilar artery. There is no discernible enhancement

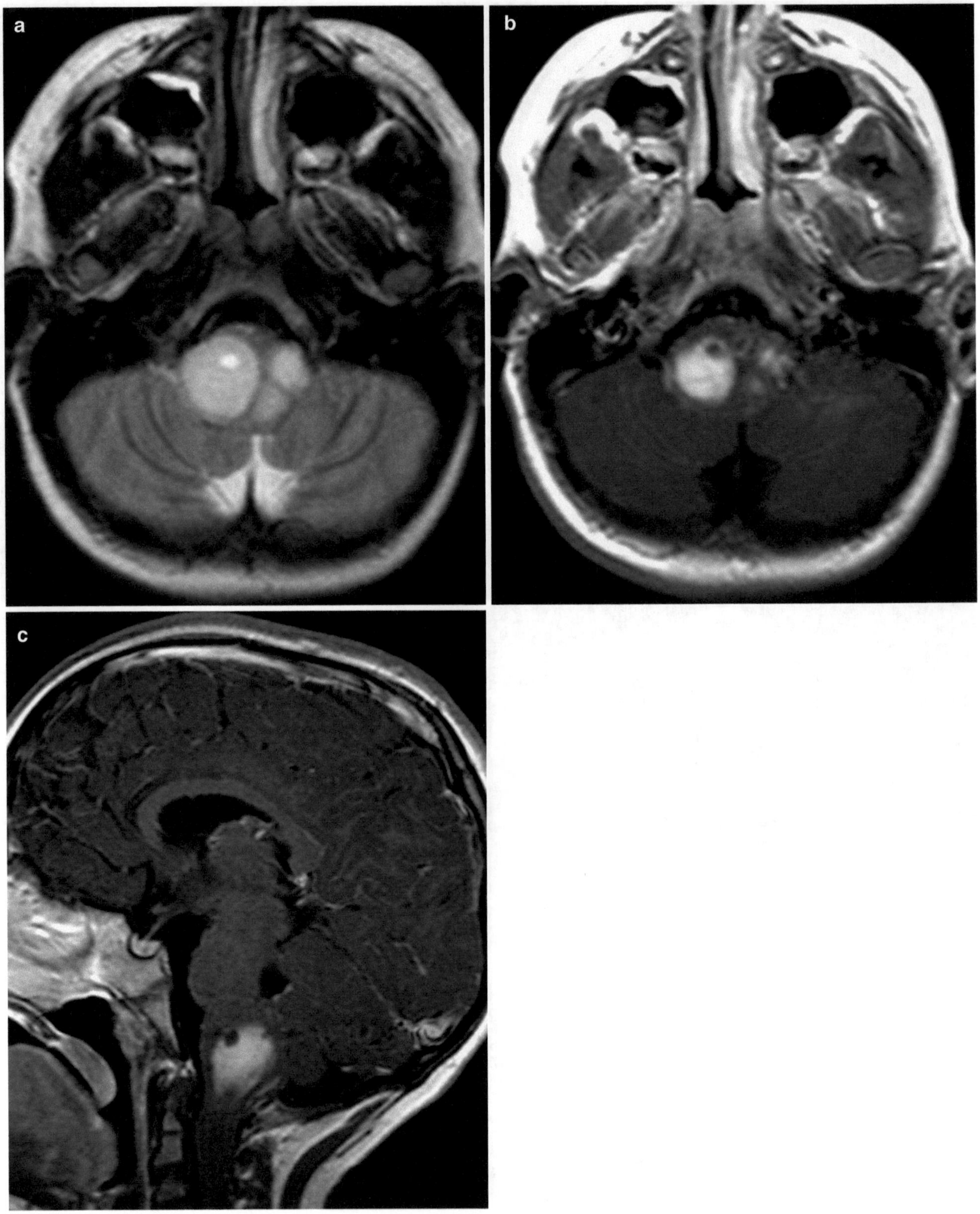

Fig. 2.12 Brainstem glioma. Axial T2-weighted (**a**) and contrast axial (**b**) and sagittal (**c**) T1-weighted images in a 5-year-old male demonstrate a multiloculated expansile tumor in the medulla with multiple heterogeneously enhancing components

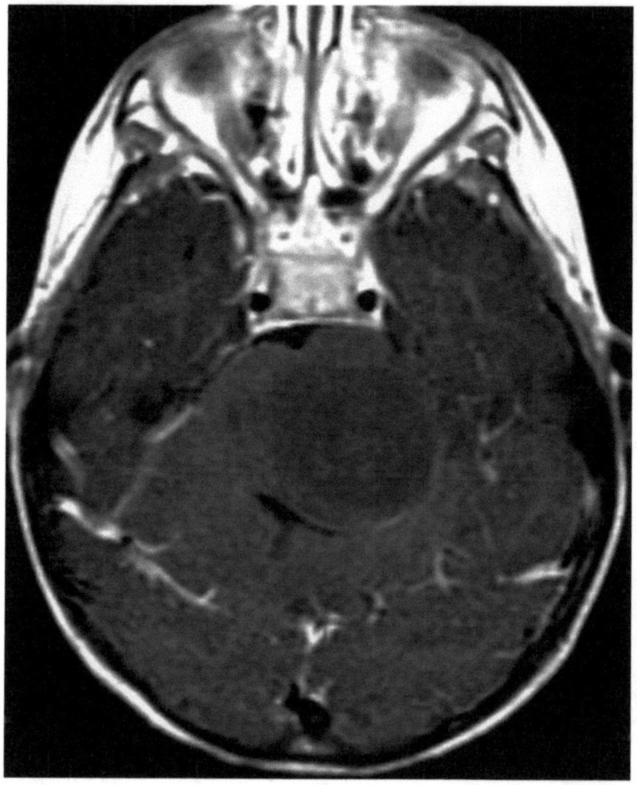

Fig. 2.13 Brainstem glioma. Axial contrast T1-weighted image in a 4-year-old male reveals expansion of the pons, worse on the left, by this nonenhancing tumor

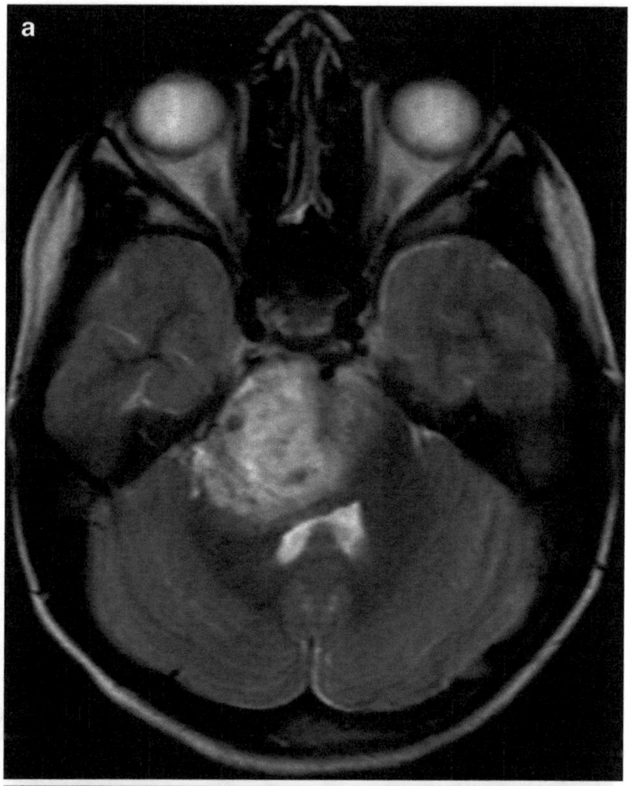

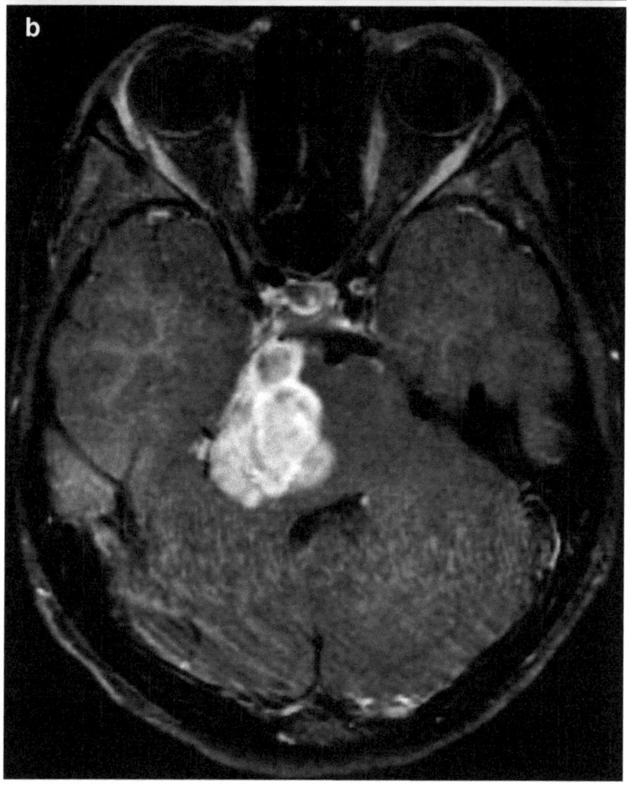

Fig. 2.14 Brainstem glioma. Axial T2-weighted (**a**) and contrast T1-weighted (**b**) images in a 6-year-old female show a heterogeneously enhancing tumor in the right pons with posterior extension into the brachium pontis

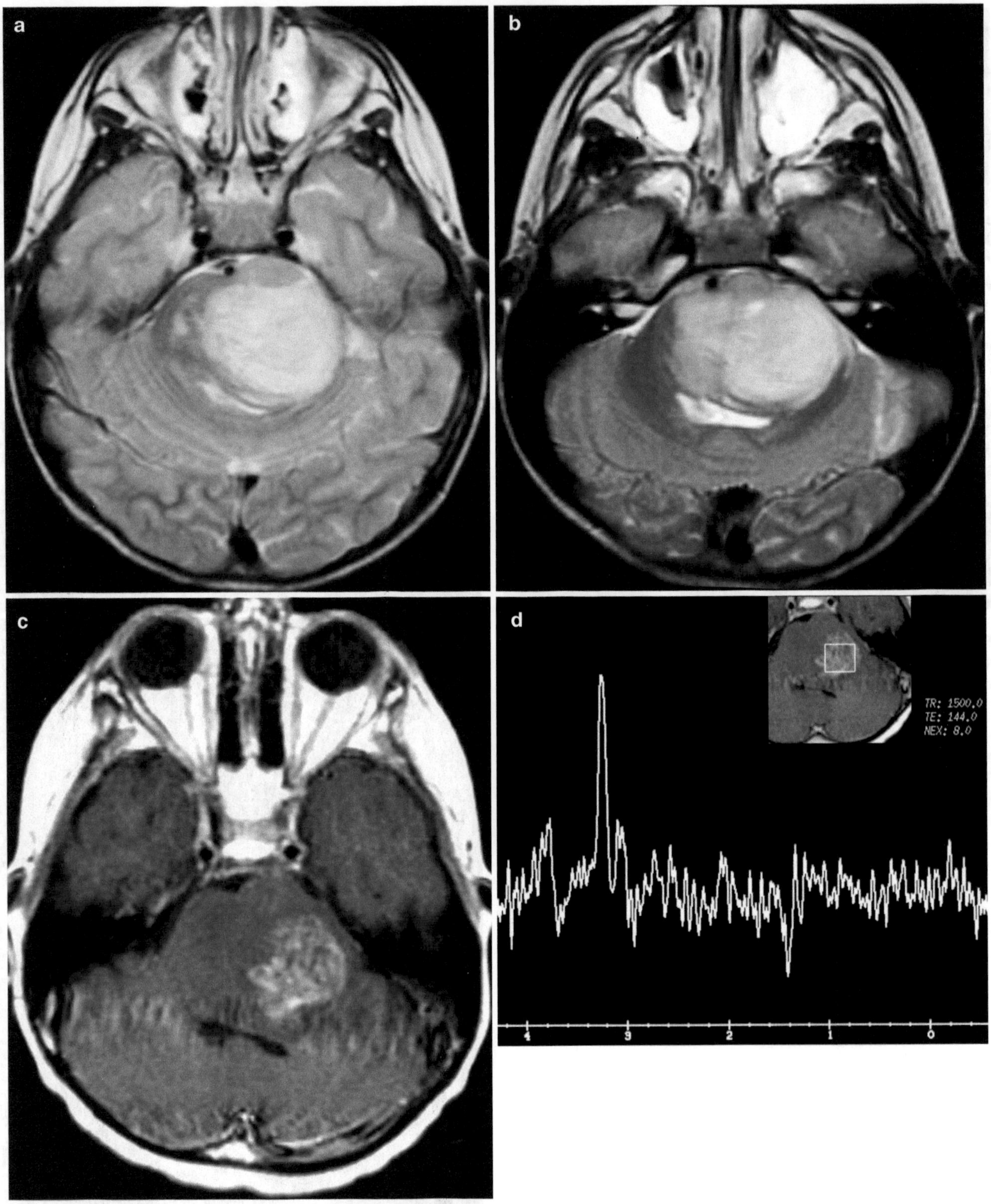

Fig. 2.15 Brainstem glioma. Axial T2-weighted (**a** and **b**) and contrast T1-weighted (**c**) images in a 4-year-old male demonstrate an expansile T2 hyperintense tumor in the pons that increases in (**b** and **c**) obtained 1 year after (**a**). Single voxel spectroscopy (**d**) at the time of (**b**) and (**c**) shows markedly reduced N-acetylaspartate (NAA) and elevated choline (Cho) with an inverted lipid/lactate peak due to anaerobic metabolism, consistent with high-grade tumor

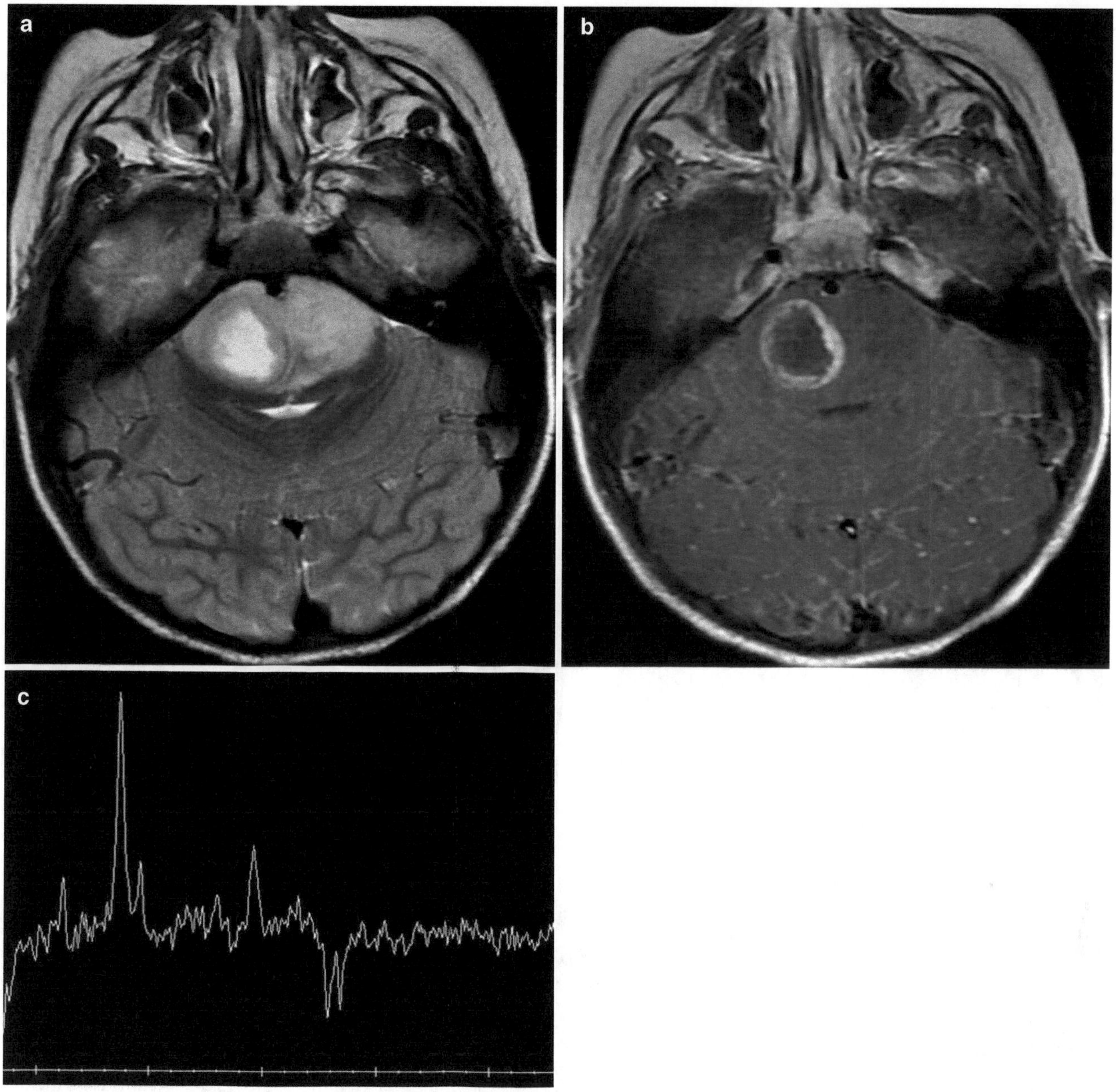

Fig. 2.16 Brainstem glioma. Axial T2-weighted (**a**) and contrast T1-weighted (**b**) images in a 3-year-old male show a heterogeneous tumor in the pons with a right component that has nodular peripheral enhancement and central cystic/necrotic change. Single voxel spectroscopy demonstrates malignant Cho/NAA ratio greater than 3 and inverted lipid/lactate peak (**c**)

Juvenile Pilocytic Astrocytoma

A juvenile pilocytic astrocytoma (JPA) is a benign brain tumor that often contains Rosenthal fibers and/or eosinophilic granules [11]. This tumor is associated with neurofibromatosis 1 (NF1); up to one third of patients with optic pathway JPA have NF1 [12]. JPAs occur equally in both genders [12]. A majority of patients with this brain tumor are between the ages of 5 and 15 years old upon diagnosis [12]. JPAs are slow-growing tumors that have a good prognosis, with a median survival rate of more than 70 % in 20 years [11]. Complete resection is usually curative.

Imaging features. JPAs are commonly seen as cystic lesions that contain an enhancing mural nodule [11]. JPAs are most commonly found within the cerebellum [11]. Less frequently this tumor can be found in the optic pathway, in areas adjacent to the third ventricle and in the brainstem [13]. Cerebellar JPAs are typically large whereas optic pathway JPAs are small. These lesions may contain calcium and rarely show signs of hemorrhage. Multiplanar or 3D volume post-contrast imaging can be useful in the evaluation of JPA specifically to determine the point-of-tumor origin and the degree of tumoral extension [12, 13].

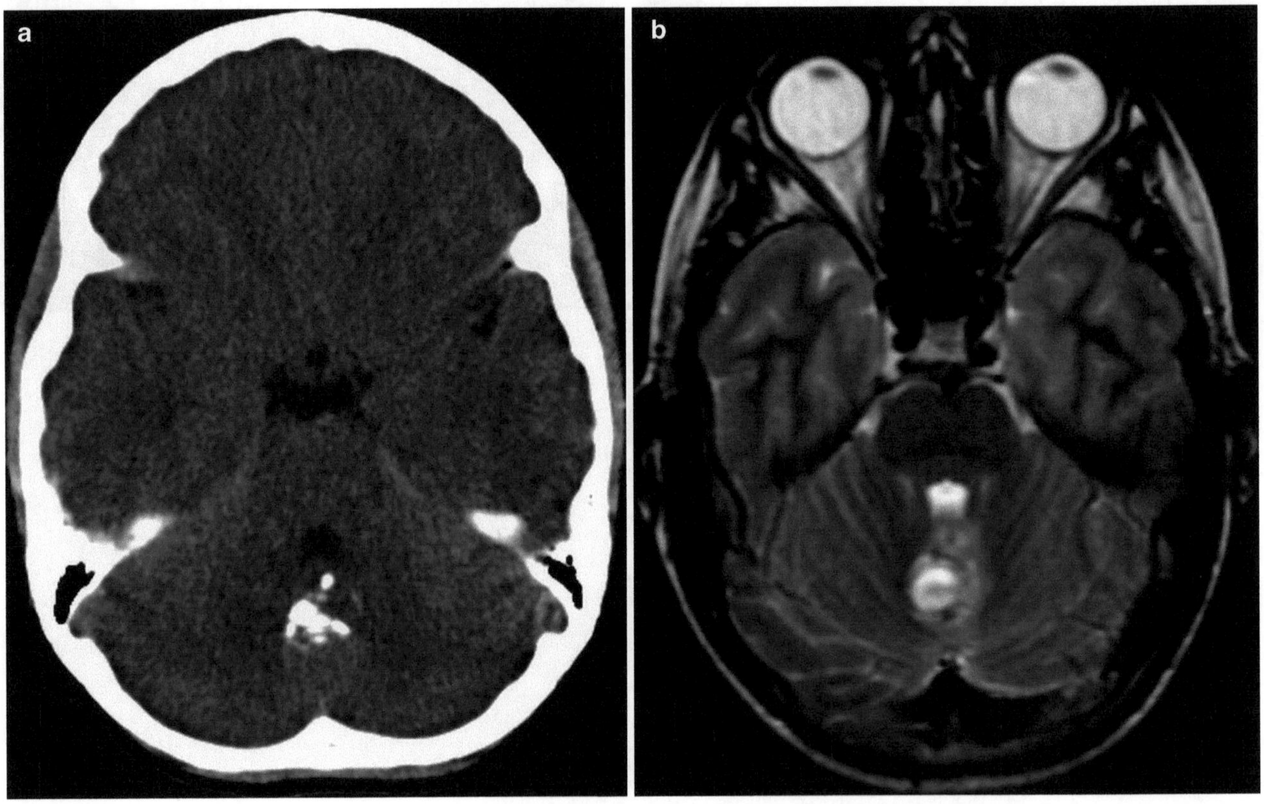

Fig. 2.17 Juvenile pilocytic astrocytoma. Axial CT (**a**) shows a partially calcified mass in the vermis in an 11-year-old male. Axial T2 (**b**), contrast axial (**c**), and sagittal (**d**) T1-weighted images reveal heterogeneous enhancement of this midline mass. Single voxel spectroscopy (**e**) demonstrate decreased NAA and increased Cho with Cho/Cr ratio of 2:8. Despite their benign course, JPAs often show malignant-appearing spectrum like this that may mimic that of a high-grade glioma. High perfusion may also mimic a high-grade glioma

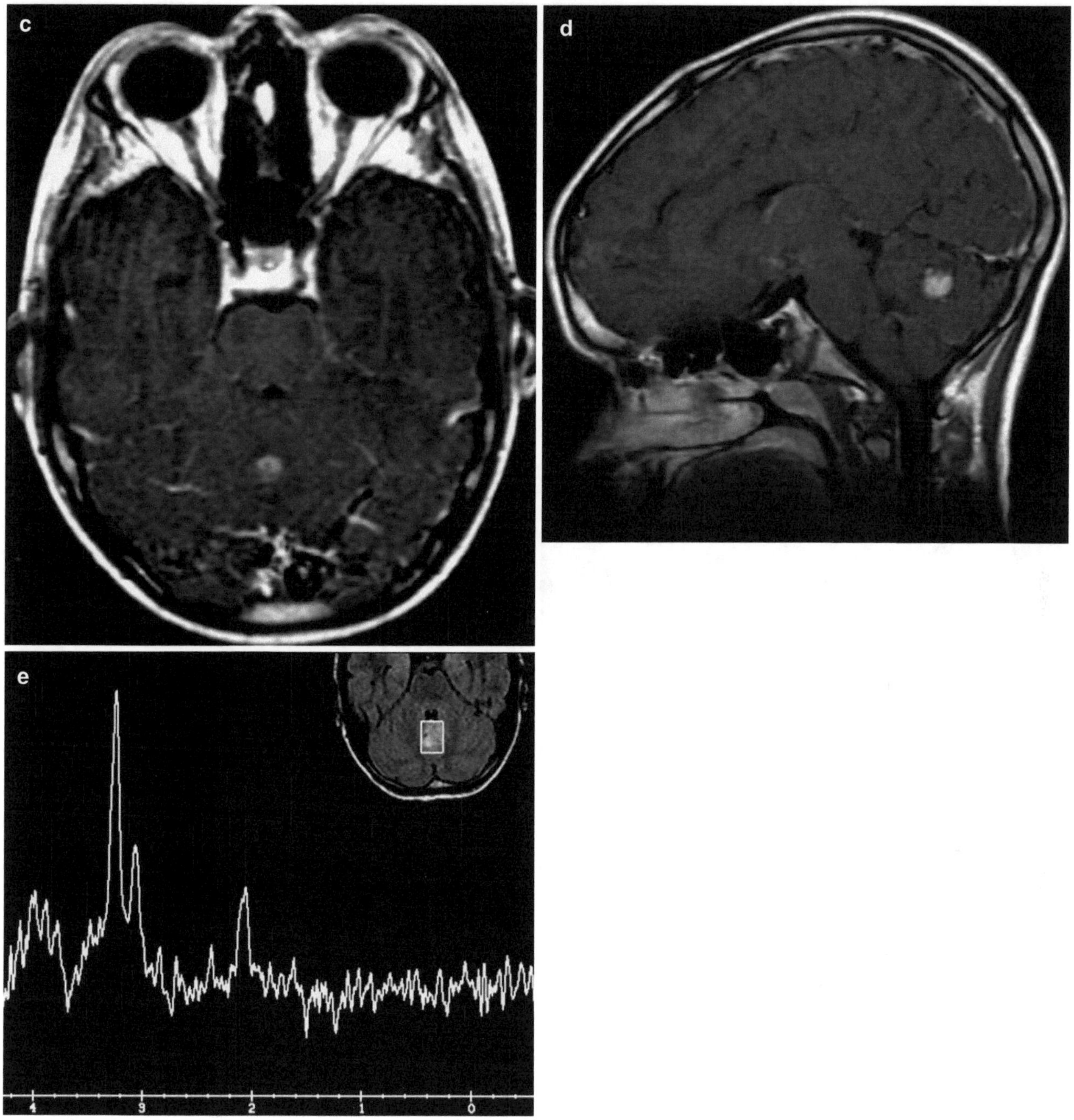

Fig. 2.17 (continued)

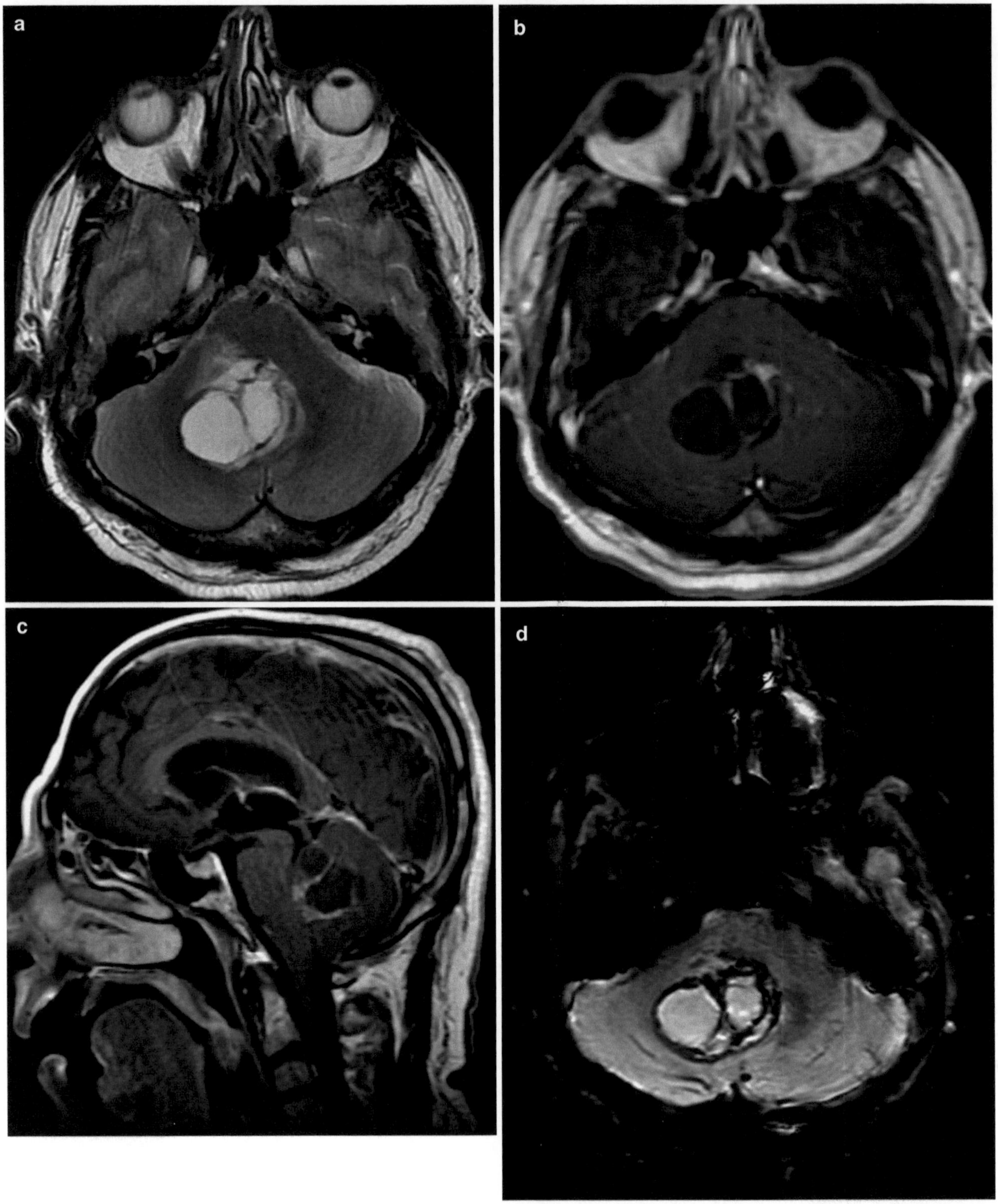

Fig. 2.18 Juvenile pilocytic astrocytoma. Axial T2 (**a**) and contrast axial (**b**) and sagittal (**c**) T1-weighted images in a 60-year-old male reveal a heterogeneously enhancing cystic tumor in the vermis that is slightly eccentric to the right. This tumor is more cystic than the previous case, with more focal anterior nodular enhancement, but also contains peripheral T2 hypointense calcifications as confirmed on axial susceptibility weighted image (**d**)

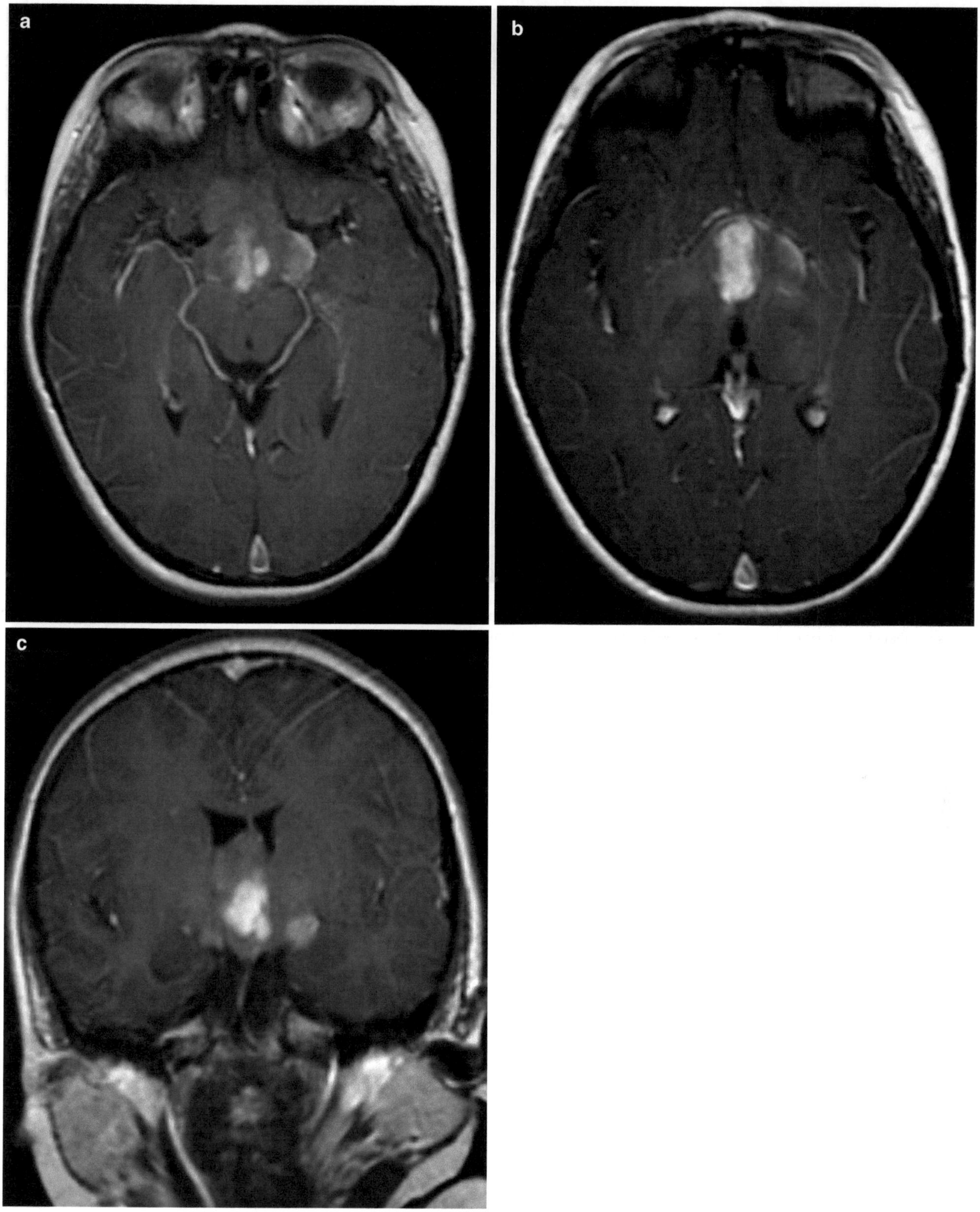

Fig. 2.19 Juvenile pilocytic astrocytoma. Contrast axial (**a** and **b**) and coronal (**c**) T1-weighted images in a 13-year-old female demonstrate a heterogeneously enhancing optic-hypothalamic tumor filling the suprasellar cistern and effacing the anterior third ventricle (More examples of optic pathway and optic-hypothalamic JPAs can be found in Chap. 3)

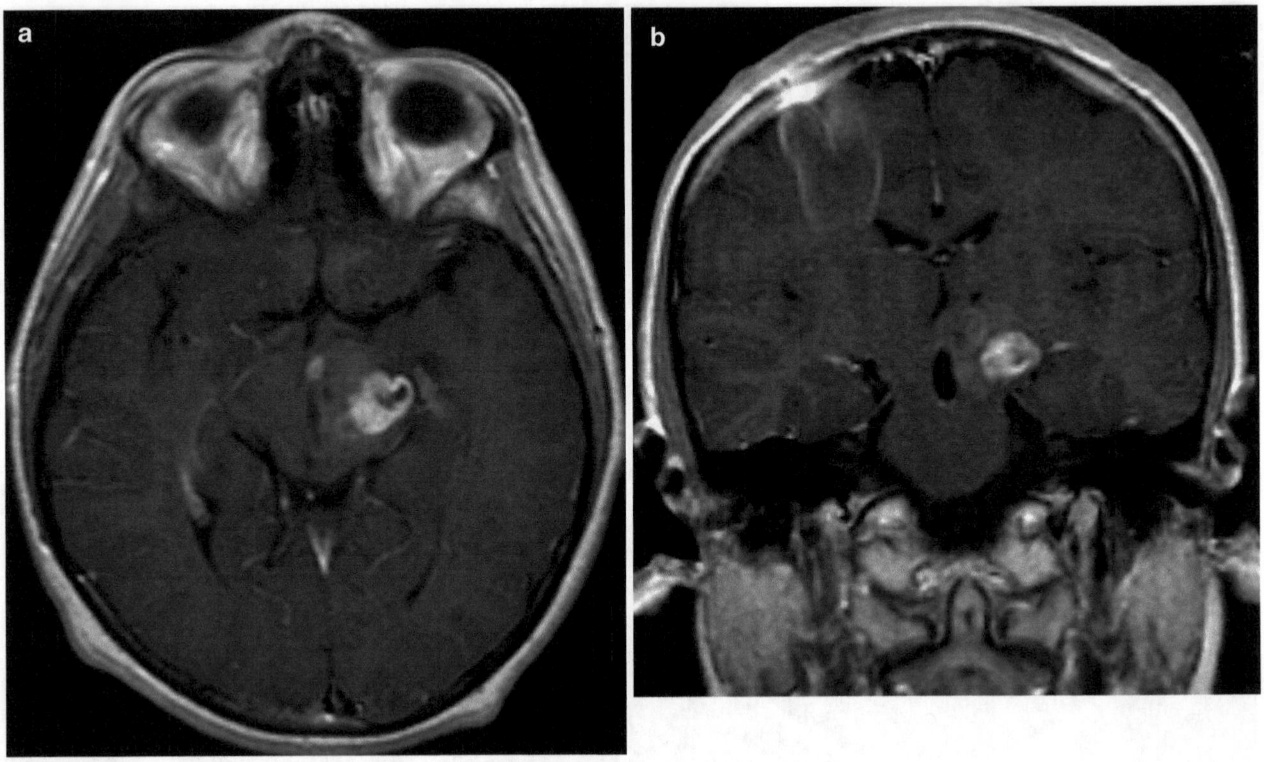

Fig. 2.20 Juvenile pilocytic astrocytoma. Contrast axial (**a**) and coronal (**b**) T1-weighted images in a 16-year-old male demonstrate a heterogeneously enhancing tumor in the left inferior medial basal ganglia and midbrain

Pineal Tumors

Pineoblastoma

A pineoblastoma is a grade IV malignant brain tumor that arises from primitive neuroectodermal cell lines [14]. Pineoblastomas and pineocytomas account for around 15 % of all pineal region malignancies [15]. Pineoblastomas have a mean age at diagnosis of 3 years old and occur at a 1:2 male to female ratio [16]. This tumor carries a poor prognosis with a median survival of around 16–25 months after diagnosis [14, 16].

Imaging features. Pineoblastomas are large pineal lesions with peripheral displacement of normal pineal gland calcification and poorly defined margins [15]. This heterogenous tumor commonly invades areas adjacent to the pineal gland and nearly all of them cause obstructive hydrocephalus [15, 16]. CSF dissemination with spinal metastasis is common. Contrast-enhanced magnetic resonance imaging (MRI) of the entire neuraxis is essential.

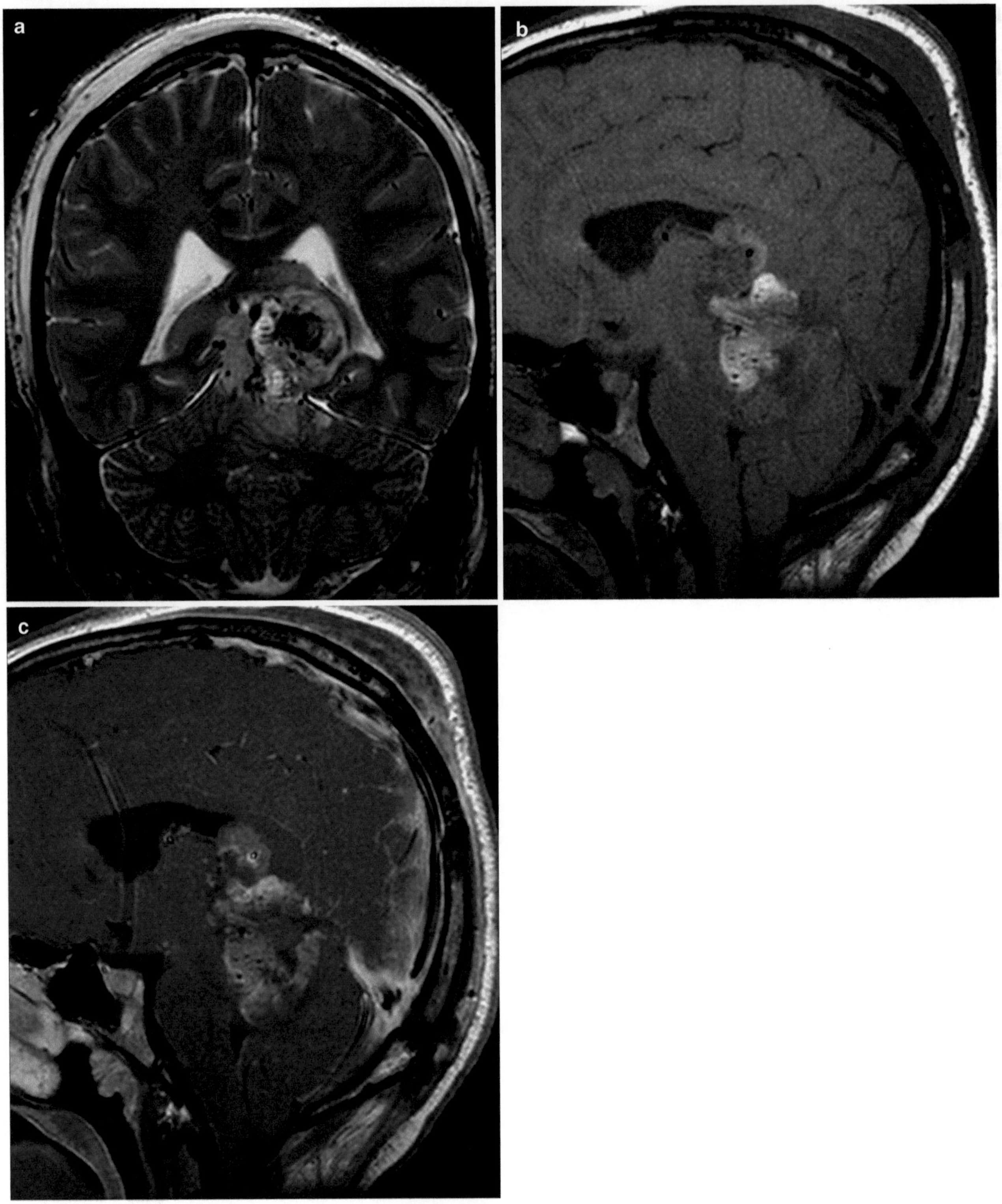

Fig. 2.21 Pineoblastoma. Coronal T2-weighted (**a**) and sagittal T1-weighted images without (**b**) and with (**c**) intravenous contrast in a 19-year-old female demonstrate a heterogeneously enhancing mass lesion centered in the pineal region with inferior extension in the superior cerebellar cistern and obstruction of cerebral aqueduct. The areas of T1 hyperintensity and T2 hyperintense are due to intratumoral hemorrhage, as well as calcifications

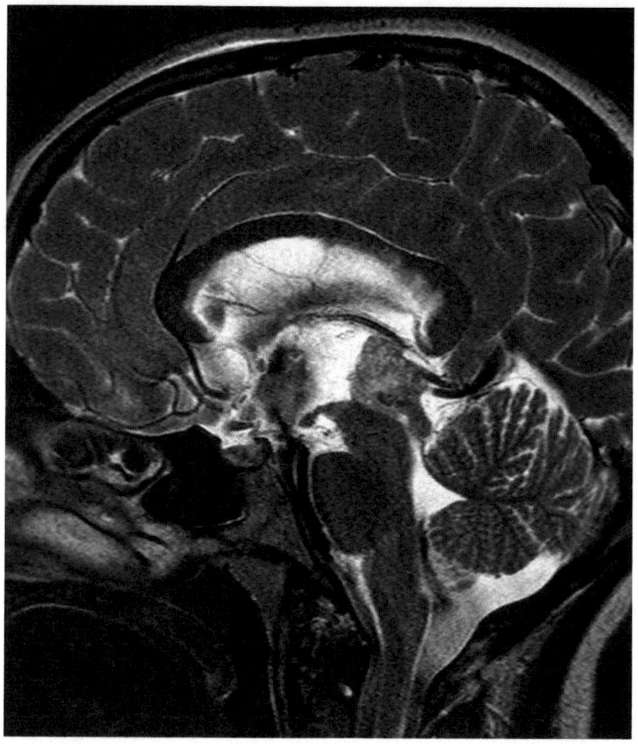

Fig. 2.22 Pineoblastoma. Sagittal T2-weighted image shows a heterogeneous pineal gland tumor. The patient is status post third ventriculostomy, with an exaggerated dark CSF flow void in the prepontine cistern through the patent ventriculostomy in the anterior inferior third ventricle

Germinoma

A germinoma is a grade III germ cell tumor of dysgerminomatous or seminomatous origin [17]. These tumors occur in various locations along the midline of the brain. Germinomas account for around 2–4 % of all pediatric intracranial tumors and are the most common tumor found in the pineal region [17]. This occurs most frequently in the young adult population with a peak incidence at 10–12 years [17]. Pure germinomas are extremely radiosensitive and have a excellent prognosis with a 5-year survival rate of around 90 % [18].

Imaging features. A majority of germinoma are well-demarcated tumors found along the midline near the third ventricle; 50–60 % occur in the pineal region; 25–35 % occur in the suprasellar region; and 5–10 % occur in the basal ganglia and thalami [17, 18]. The size of the tumor varies with location. Pineal region and suprasellar tumors are usually small on presentation whereas basal ganglia and thalamic lesions are large on presentation [18, 19]. This tumor has a strong uniform enhancement pattern and cystic, hemorrhagic, and necrotic components are not uncommon [19]. This tumor is diffusion restricted on diffusion-weighted imaging (DWI) due to its high cellularity [17, 19].

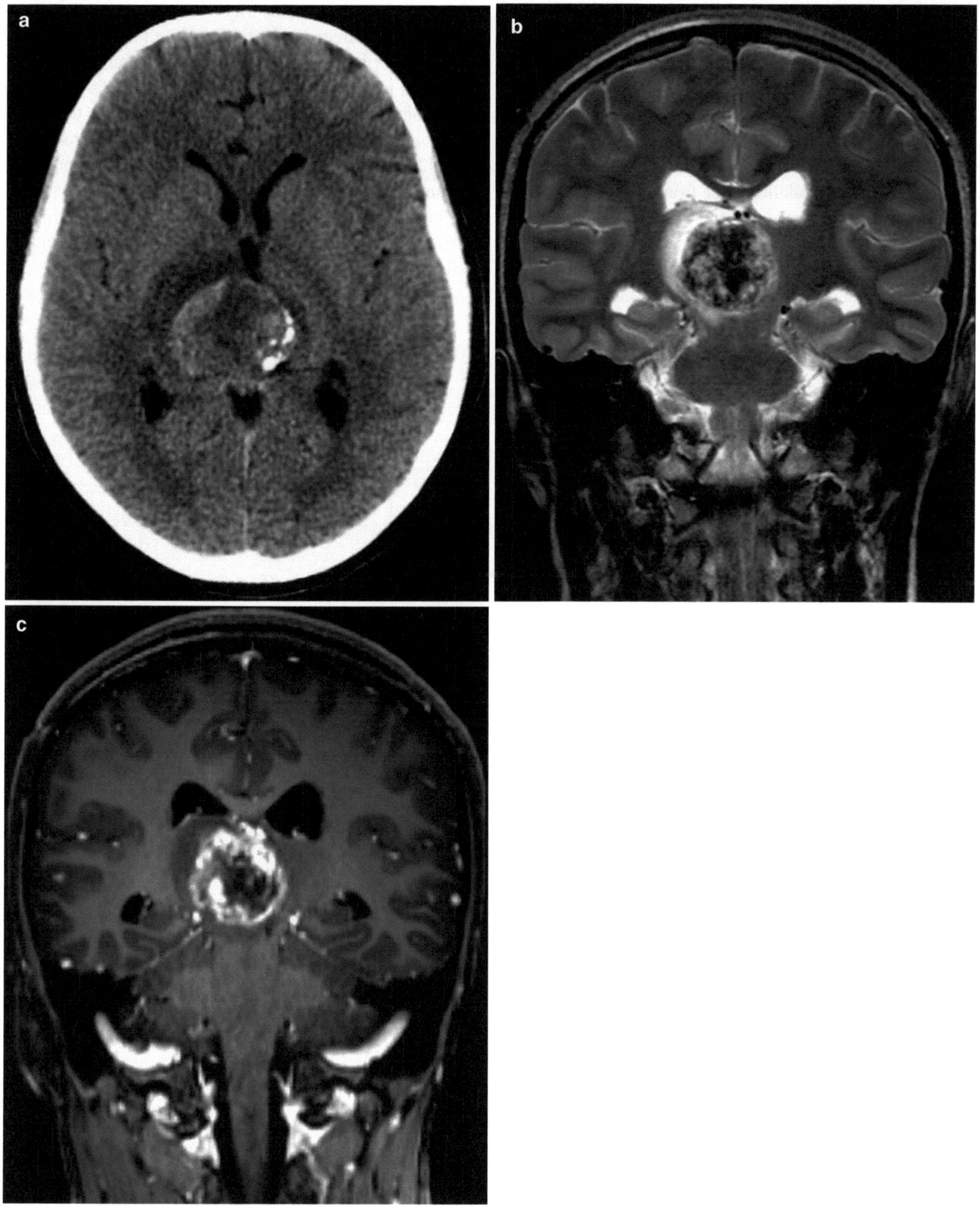

Fig. 2.23 Germinoma. Axial CT (**a**), coronal T2-weighted (**b**), and contrast T1-weighted (**c**) images in a 12-year-old male demonstrate an expansile tumor in the pineal region with left eccentric calcifications, central T2 hypointense blood products, and markedly heterogeneous enhancement

Pineocytoma

A pineocytoma is a rare grade II brain tumor that arises from the parenchyma of the pineal gland. [20, 21]. Although this tumor accounts for less than 1 % of all intracranial tumors, it is responsible for around 45 % of all pineal parenchymal brain tumors [20]. Pineocytoma most commonly occurs in young adults with a peak incidence from the second to third decade of life but can occur at any age [20]. This tumor is slow growing and has a good prognosis, with an overall 5-year survival rate of 86 % [20]. Surgical excision and stereotactic radiosurgery are usually the treatments of choice [20, 21].

Imaging features. A majority of these tumors can be visualized as well circumscribed, enhancing pineal lesions with what is described as "exploded" or peripheral displacement of normal pineal gland calcification [20, 21]. Pineocytomas are small tumors generally less than 3 cm in size that do not invade but may be seen compressing adjacent brain structures [20, 21]. Cystic change can be seen upon imaging of this tumor but rarely hemorrhage [21]. MR is the most sensitive imaging tool; post contrast sagittal and coronal images provide the best visualization of the pineal gland and associated lesions.

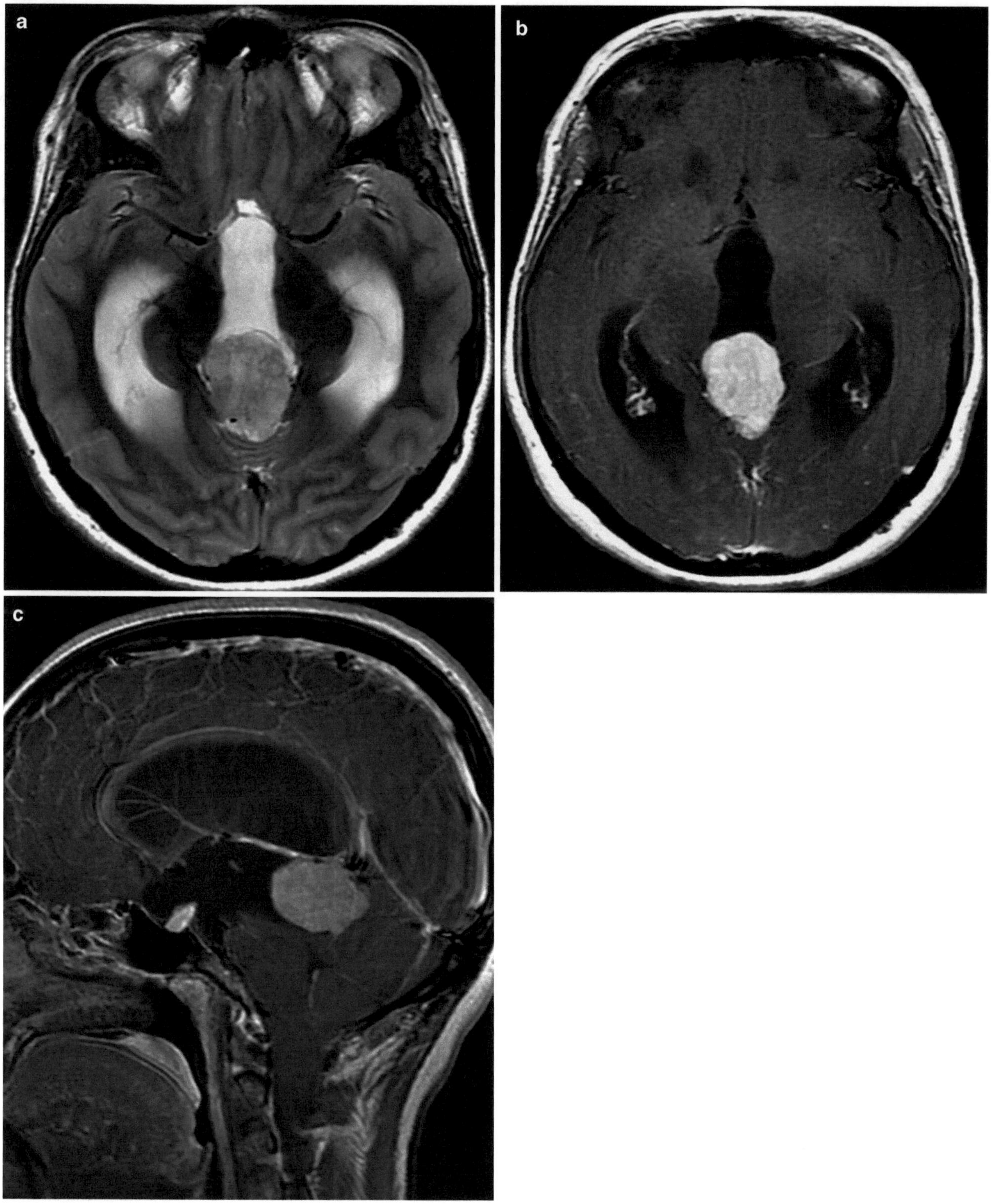

Fig. 2.24 Pineocytoma. Axial T2-weighted (**a**) and contrast axial (**b**) and sagittal (**c**) T1-weighted images reveal a T2 hyperintense, homogeneously enhancing pineal gland tumor. There is moderate obstructive hydrocephalus manifest by dilatation of the lateral ventricles including temporal horns and third ventricle

Intraventricular

Pediatric Ependymoma

This is a high-grade glial brain tumor made of ependymal cells. Pediatric ependymoma accounts for up to 5 % of all intracranial tumors in children and is the third most common posterior fossa tumor found in pediatric patients [23]. This tumor occurs most frequently between the ages 1 and 5 years and has a slight male predominance [23]. Pediatric ependymomas have a relatively poor prognosis [22, 23]. Gross total resection with chemotherapy and radiation therapy may improve patient prognosis [22].

Imaging features. Pediatric ependymomas are soft tumors that conform to the shape of the ventricle or cistern in which the tumors are located [24]. More than half of these lesions are located infratentorially and arise from the floor of the fourth ventricle [23]. Supratentorial parenchymal ependymomas tend to occur more commonly in the adult population. These irregularly shaped tumors may contain calcium, cysts, and/or hemorrhage and typically have a heterogenous enhancement pattern [24]. CSF dissemination may occur, therefore imaging of the spine is necessary to evaluate for drop metastasis [23, 24].

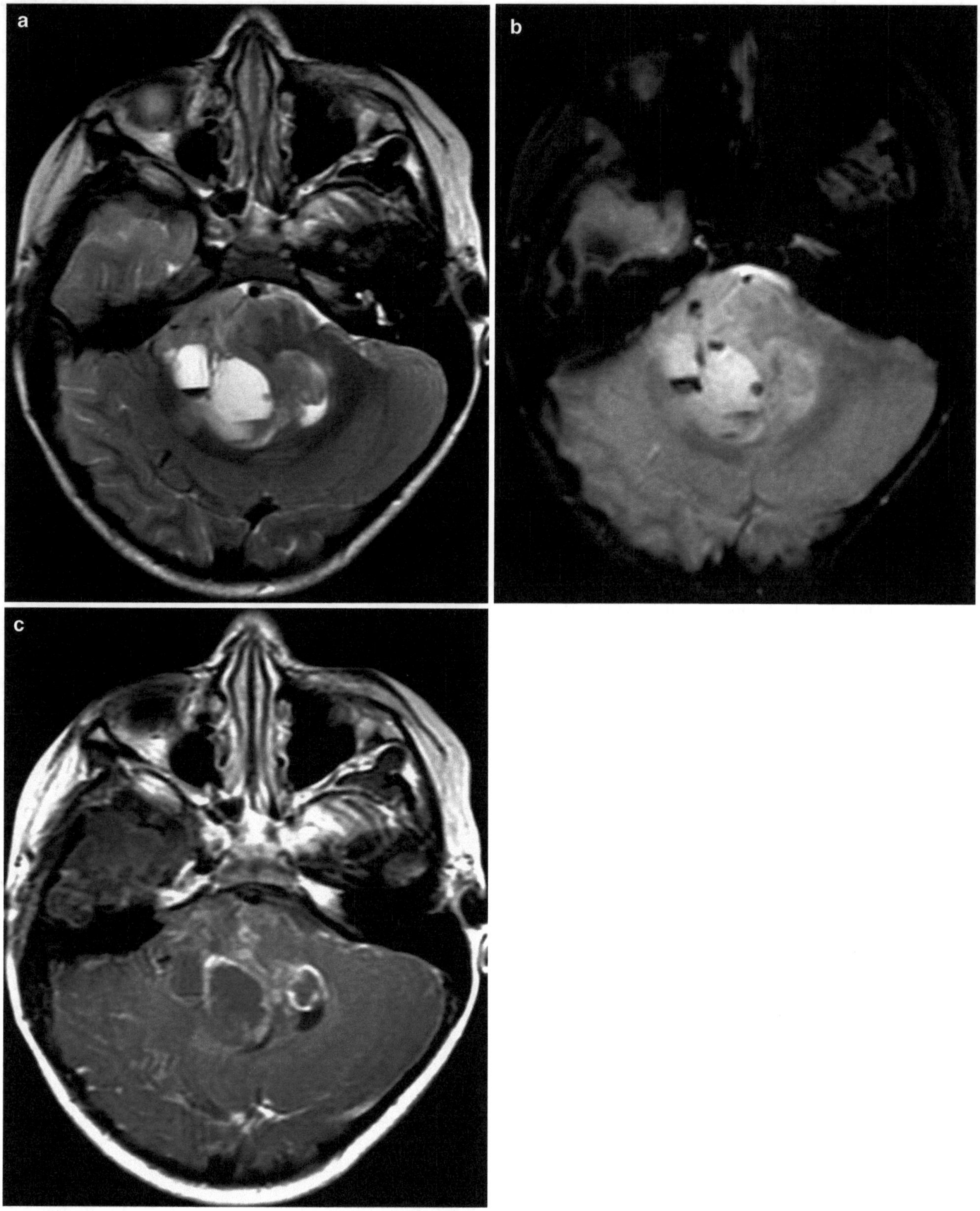

Fig. 2.25 Pediatric ependymoma. Axial T2-weighted (**a**), gradient-echo (**b**), and contrast axial (**c**) T1-weighted images in an 11-year-old female show a heterogeneously enhancing tumor in fourth ventricle with invasion in the brainstem, anterior lateral extension through the right foramen of Luschka. The layering T2- and gradient-echo hypointense material is consistent with hemorrhage and multiple small fluid-hemorrhage levels

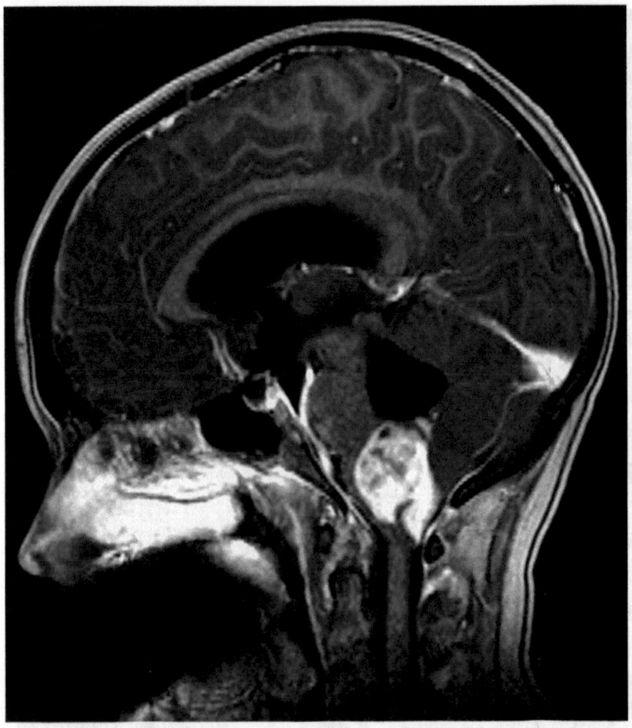

Fig. 2.26 Pediatric ependymoma. Sagittal contrast T1-weighted image in a 12-year-old male reveals a heterogeneously enhancing tumor in the fourth ventricle with caudal extension through the foramen of Magendie into the upper sinal canal

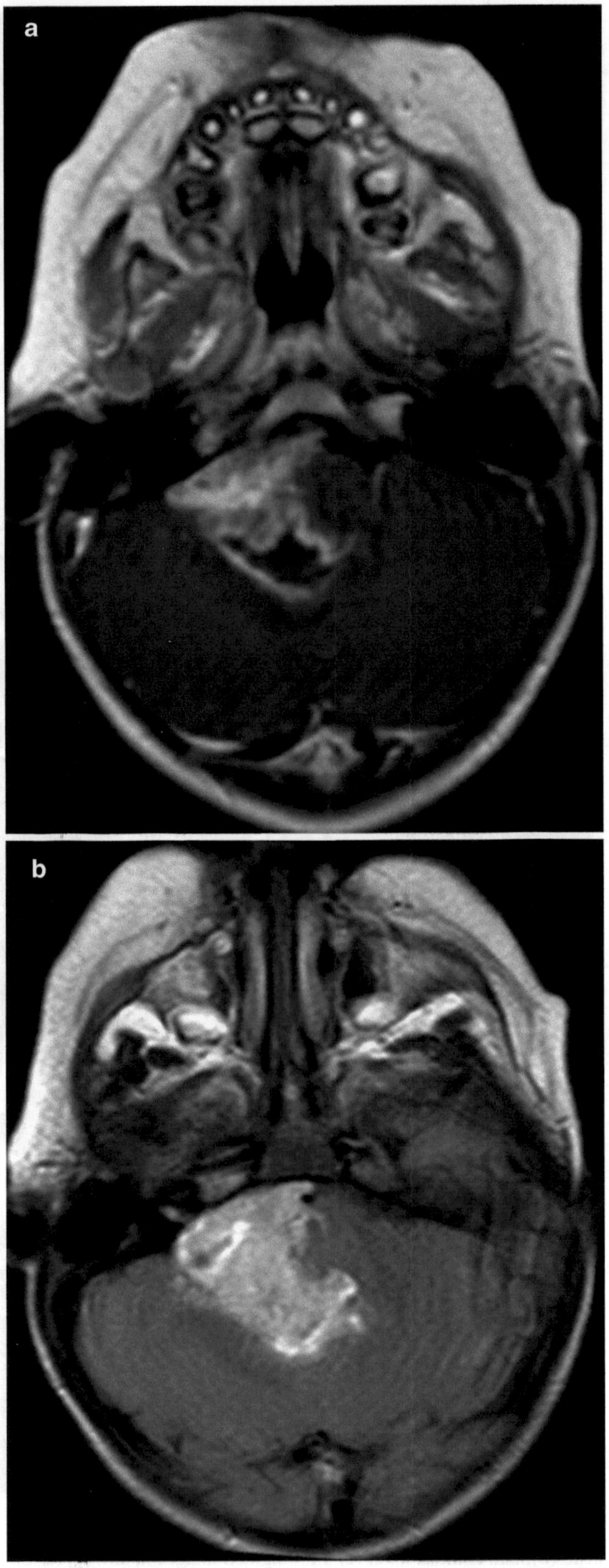

Fig. 2.27 Pediatric ependymoma. Axial contrast T1-weighted images (**a** and **b**) in an 8-year-old female demonstrate a recurrent heterogeneously enhancing mass in the fourth ventricle with anterior lateral extension through the right foramen of Luschka. As in the previous case, this plastic growth through foramina is typical for ependymomas

Medulloblastoma

Medulloblastoma is a grade IV primary neuroectodermal brain tumor [25]. This tumor is highly malignant and has a tendency to spread through the CSF and metastasize to different locations within the CNS [25]. This tumor accounts for around 15–20 % of all pediatric brain tumors and 30–40 % of all posterior fossa tumors in children [25]. Approximately 75 % of patients with medulloblastoma are diagnosed prior to the age of 10 [26]. Treatment consists of surgical resection and adjuvant chemotherapy, with radiation therapy reserved for high-risk patients with poor prognostic features [20, 25]. Patients with metastasis and/or gross residual tumor status post resection have a poor prognosis with a survival rate of 20 % [25, 26]

Imaging features. A majority of medulloblastoma are solid round tumors with homogeneous enhancement [26]. These tumors commonly arise from the roof of the fourth ventricle [27], in contrast to ependymomas that arise from the floor of the fourth ventricle [26]. This tumor is more commonly seen in the cerebellar hemispheres especially in older children and within the adult population [26]. Medulloblastoma may contain small intratumoral cysts and necrosis, whereas hemorrhage is rare [26, 27]. CSF dissemination and drop metastases are common in patients with medulloblastoma, therefore contrast-enhanced MR of brain and entire spine are essential.

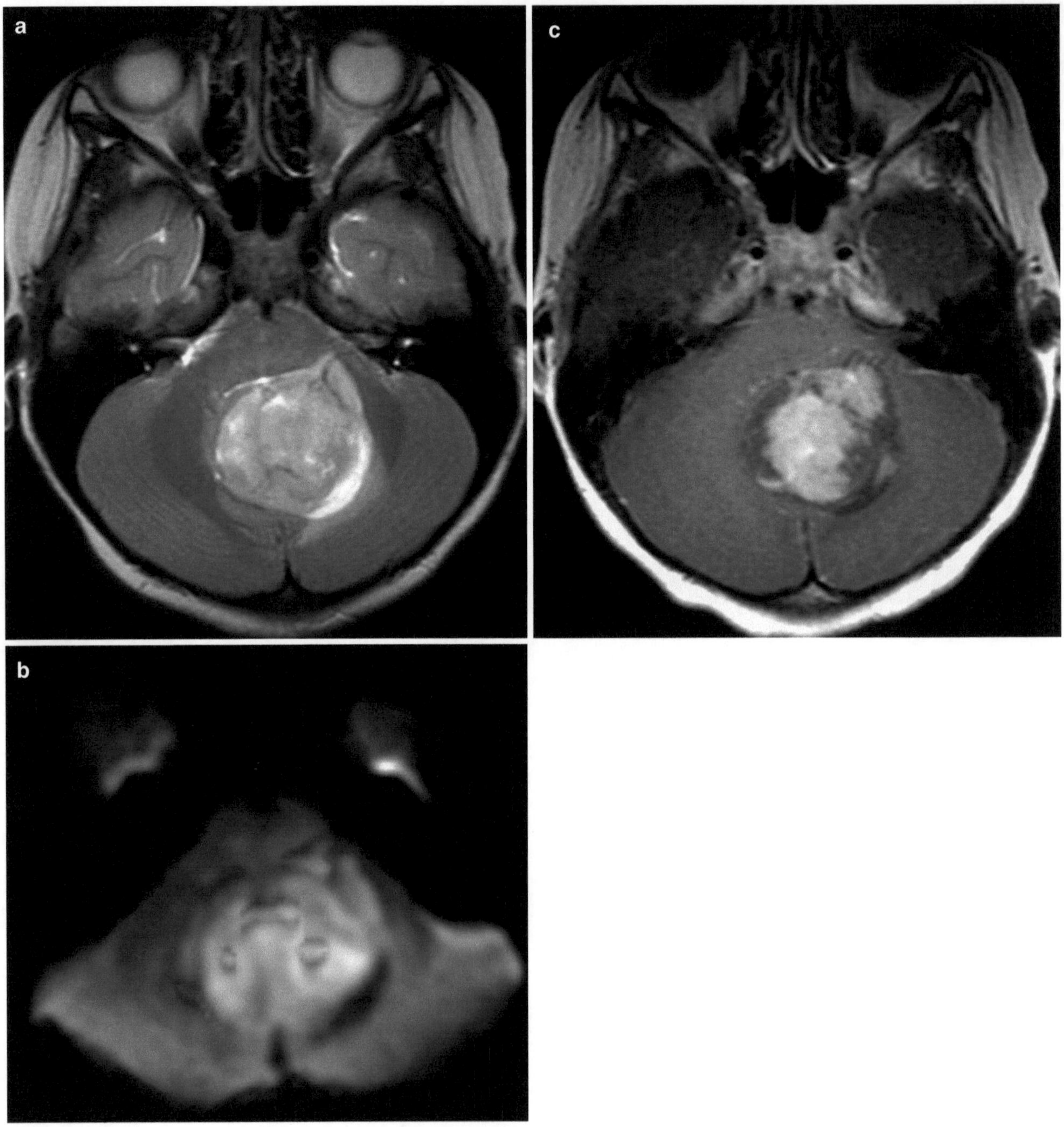

Fig. 2.28 Medulloblastoma. Axial T2-weighted (**a**), diffusion-weighted (**b**), and contrast T1-weighted (**c**) images in an 11-year-old female show a T2 hyperintense heterogeneously enhancing tumor in the midline posterior fossa. Diffusion restriction is characteristic for these small round blue cell tumors. Anterior displacement of the compressed fourth ventricle suggests an origin from the vermis or roof of the fourth ventricle (See the section on "Pediatric Ependymoma" above to compare tumors arising from the floor of and completely effacing the fourth ventricle)

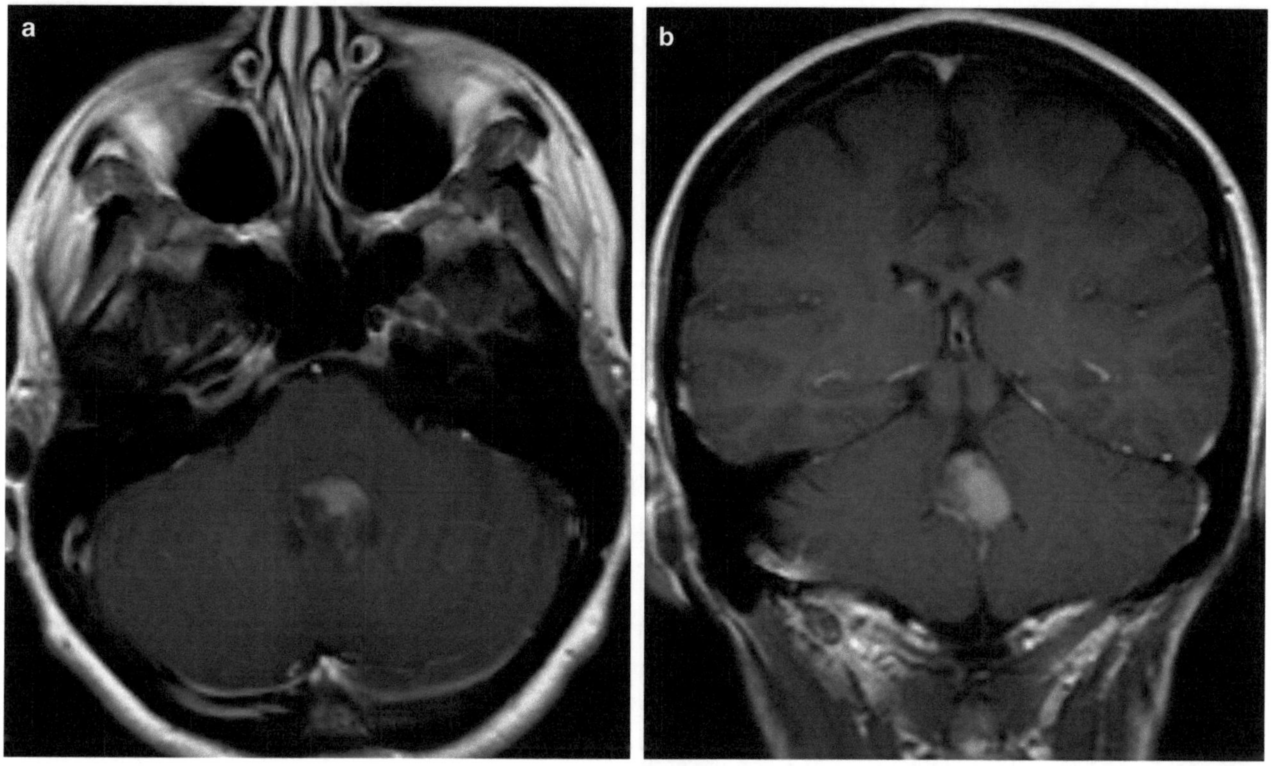

Fig. 2.29 Medulloblastoma. Contrast axial (**a**) and coronal (**b**) T1-weighted images in a 27-year-old female illustrate a small midline enhancing tumor in the fourth ventricle. Origin from the roof (favoring medulloblastoma) or the floor (favoring ependymoma) is difficult to discern in this case

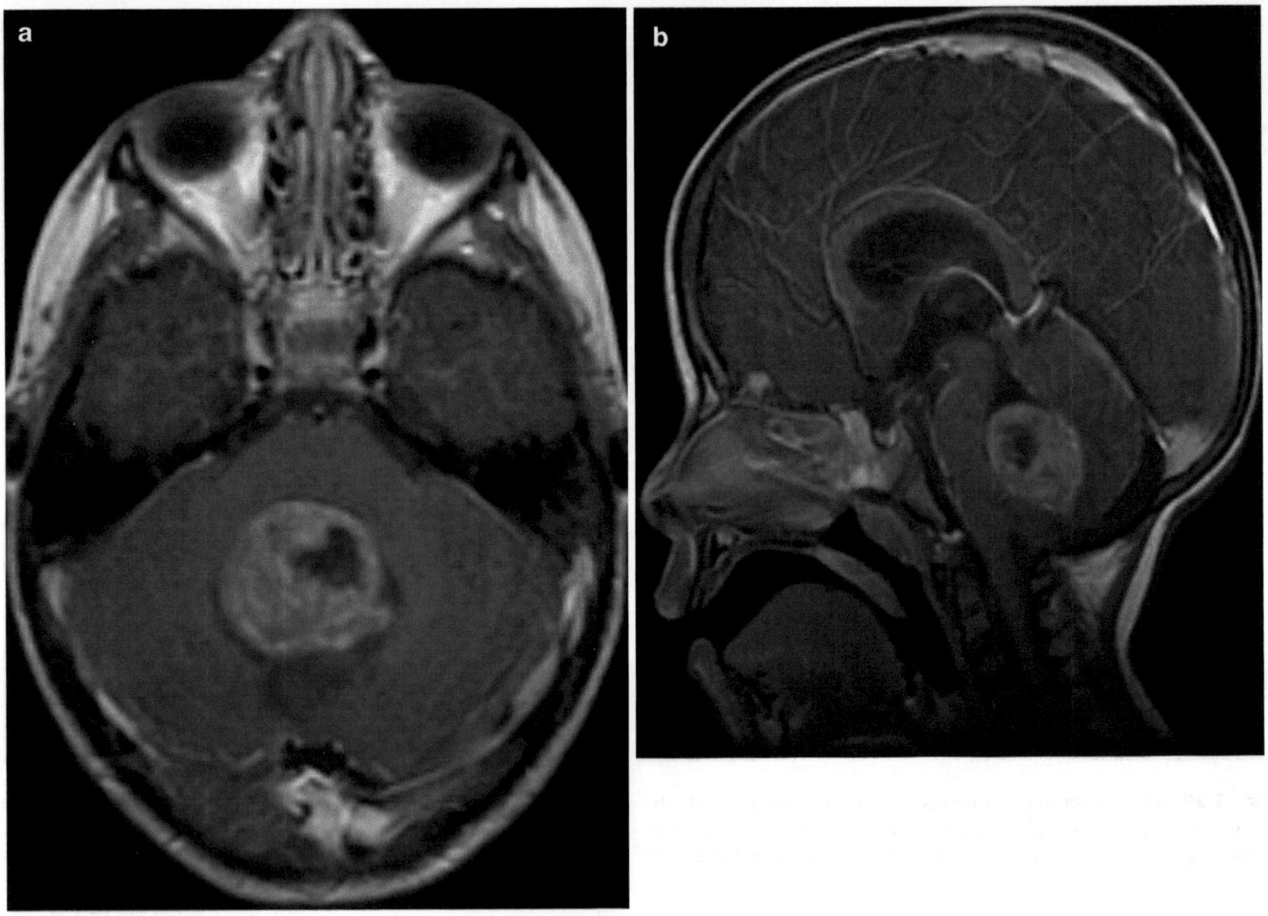

Fig. 2.30 Medulloblastoma. Contrast axial (**a**) and sagittal (**b**) T1-weighted images in a 7-year-old male show a heterogeneously enhancing midline tumor in the posterior fossa. Anterior displacement of the compressed fourth ventricle correctly suggests a medulloblastoma

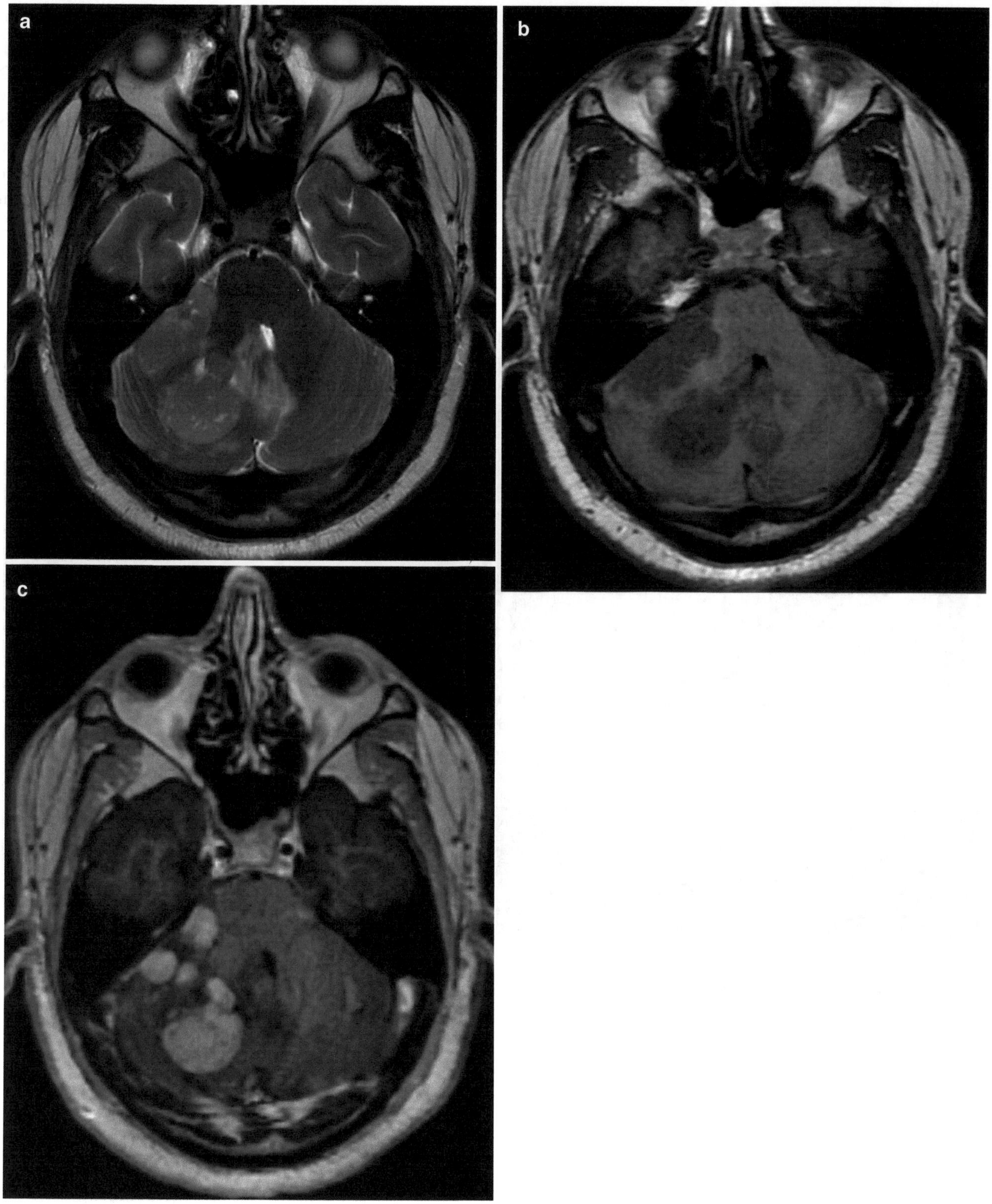

Fig. 2.31 Medulloblastoma. Axial T2-weighted (**a**) and T1-weighted flair images without (**b**) and with (**c**) intravenous contrast in 22-year-old female show multiple T2 hyperintense tumors in the vermis and right cerebellum. The multiple lesions confers high-risk stage for the patient, who subsequently underwent chemoradiation therapy after surgery

Subependymal Giant Cell Tumor

Subependymal giant cell tumor is grade I slow-growing neoplasm that is comprised of a variety of astroglial cell types. It is extremely rare to be diagnosed with this tumor type without tuberous sclerosis complex phenotype [28]. This is the most common CNS tumor in patients with tuberous sclerosis and accounts for 1.4 % of all pediatric brain tumors [28, 29]. Subependymal giant cell tumor typically occurs in patients younger than 20 years old [29]. Patients commonly present with symptoms of ventricular obstruction [28]. These tumors have a good prognosis and low recurrence rate after complete surgical resection [29].

Imaging features. Most subependymal giant cell tumors are well-circumscribed, enhancing lesions found abutting the ventricular wall in a patient with tuberous sclerosis [29]. It is almost always located adjacent to the foramen of Monro [29]. The tumor size may vary but often causes obstructive hydrocephalus when it approaches 3 cm [29]. Periventricular edema is a common finding secondary to ventricular obstruction [30]. Subependymal giant cell tumor may contain cysts, hemorrhage, and/or calcium [29].

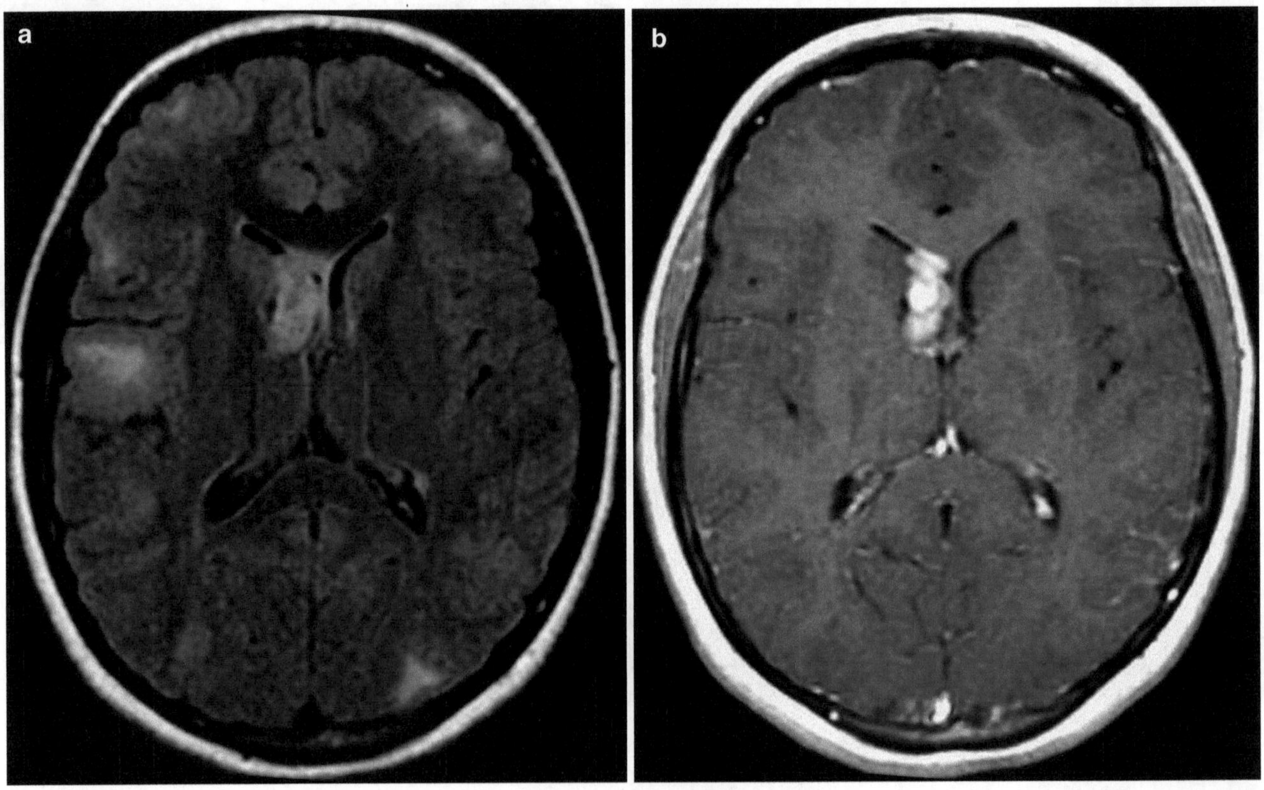

Fig. 2.32 Subependymal giant cell tumor. Axial FLAIR (**a**) and contrast T1-weighted (**b**) images demonstrate a nodular enhancing tumor in the right lateral ventricle adjacent to the foramen of Monro. The location of this tumor, and the presence of multiple bilateral cortical and subcortical FLAIR hyperintense tubers, is diagnostic for a subependymal giant cell tumor in a patient with tuberous sclerosis

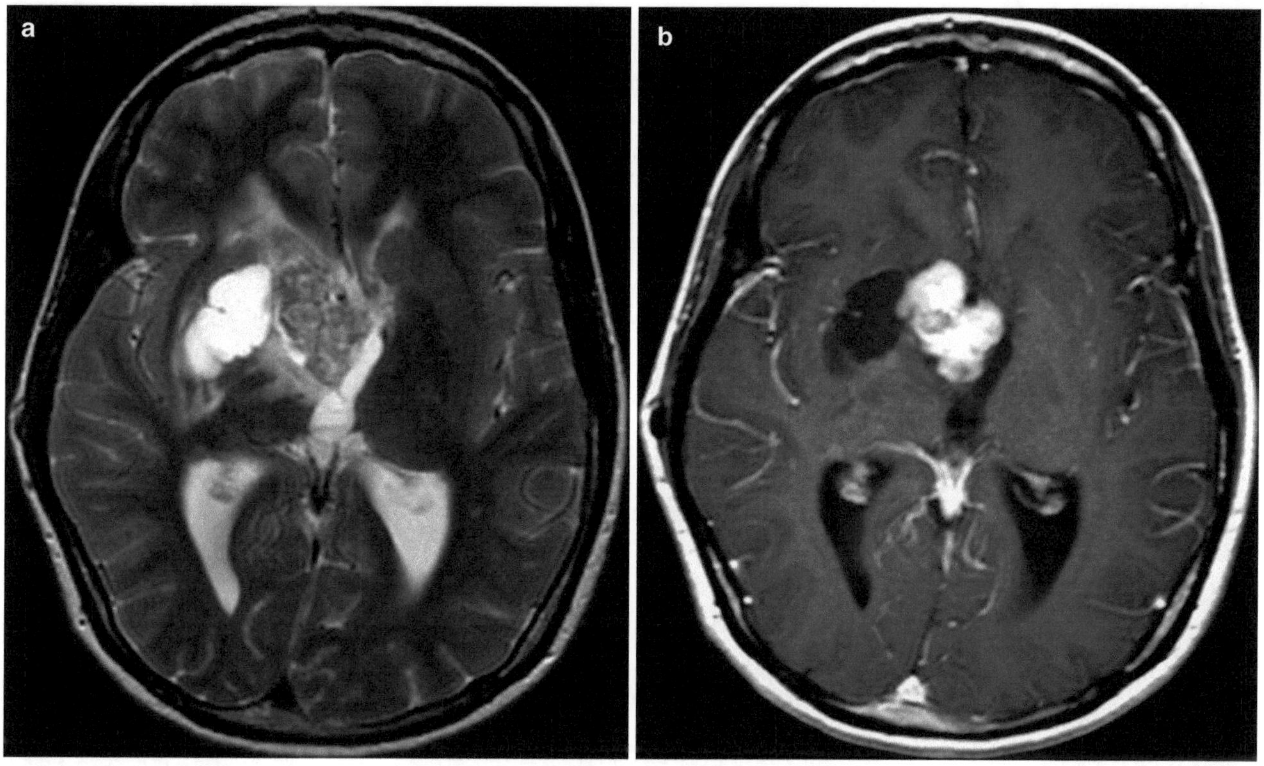

Fig. 2.33 Subependymal giant cell tumor. Axial T2-weighted (**a**) and contrast T1-weighted (**b**) images show a heterogeneously enhancing tumor in the right lateral ventricle and anterior third ventricle, again centered adjacent to the foramen of Monro

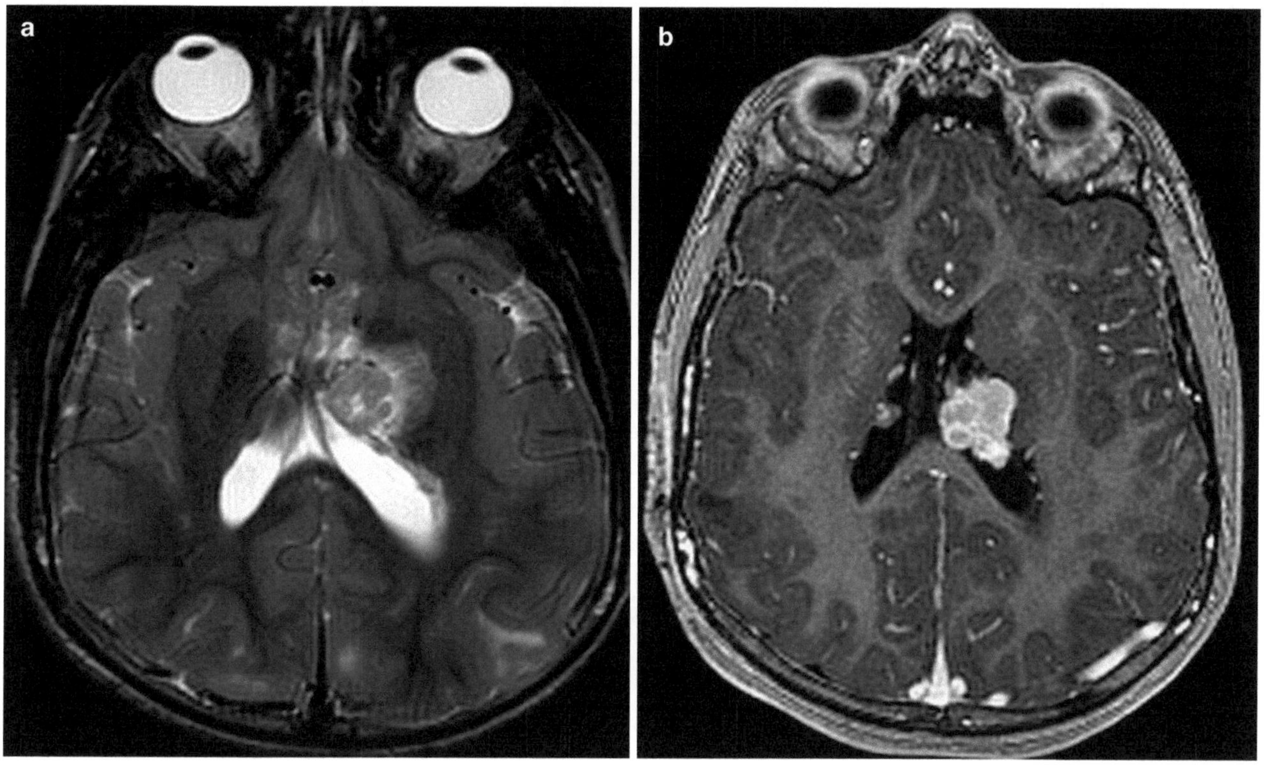

Fig. 2.34 Subependymal giant cell tumor. Axial T2-weighted (**a**) and contrast T1-weighted (**b**) images demonstrate a T2 hyperintense enhancing tumor in the left lateral ventricle posterior to the foramen of Monro with parenchymal invasion into the basal ganglia. (**a**) Hyperintense cortical/subcortical tubers are present

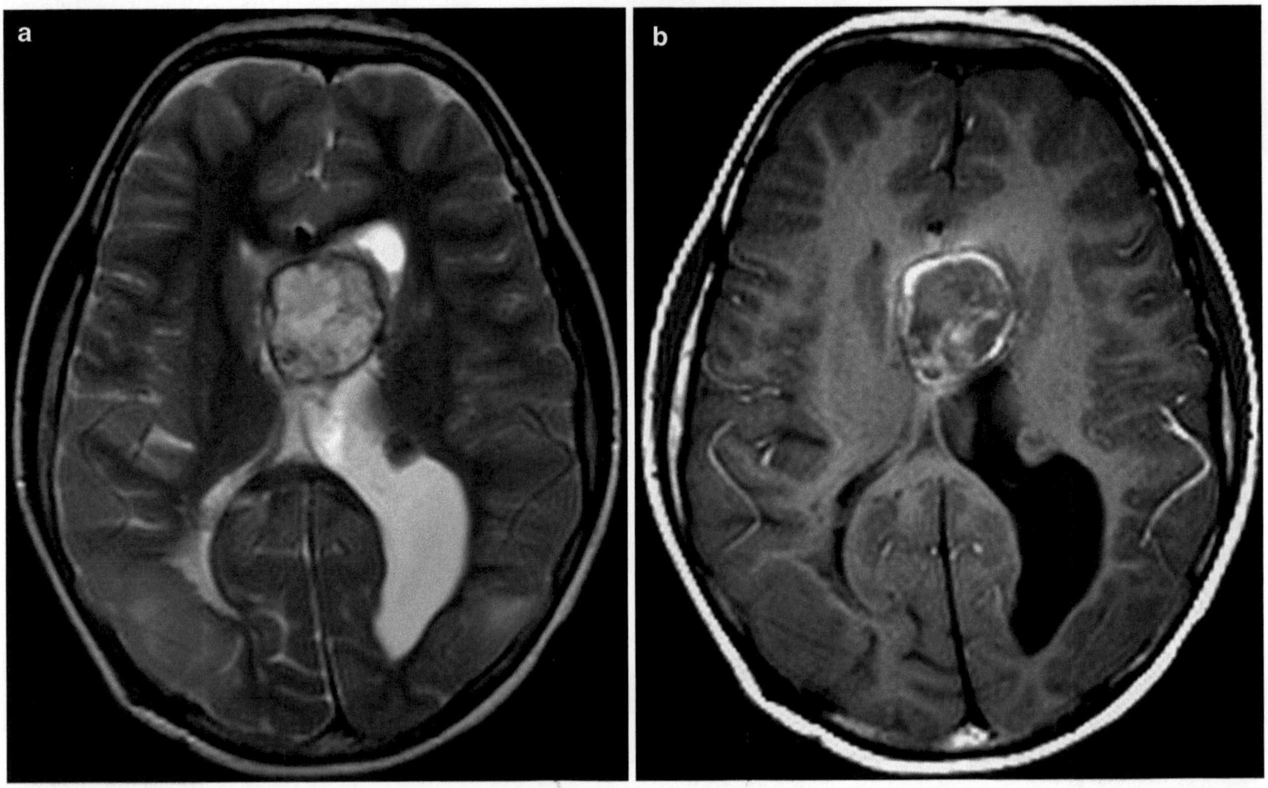

Fig. 2.35 Subependymal giant cell tumor. Axial T2-weighted (**a**) and contrast T1-weighted (**b**) images demonstrate an expansile T2 hyperintense tumor in the left lateral ventricle with peripheral T2 hypointense calcifications and/or blood products and heterogeneous enhancement. This may mimic a central neurocytoma, the subependymal nodules along the lateral wall of the body of the left lateral ventricle and the atrium of the right lateral ventricle, and the cortical/subcortical tubers in bilateral occipital lobes, indicate the patient has tuberous sclerosis

Choroid Plexus Papilloma

This is a grade I benign tumor comprised of epithelial cells within the choroid plexus [30]. Choroid plexus papilloma is the most common brain tumor in children under the age of one and accounts for up to 4 % of all pediatric brain tumors [30]. Age at diagnosis of choroid plexus papilloma depends upon location of tumor. Lateral ventricular location is more frequent in children, whereas the fourth ventricle location is more frequent in adults [30, 31]. This tumor is slow growing and has a good prognosis, with a 5-year survival rate of 100 % [30, 31].

Imaging features. Choroid plexus papillomas are commonly visualized as large lobulated lesions that enhance upon imaging [30]. Tumor location is a direct reflection of the locations and amounts of normal choroid plexus: these tumors do not occur anterior to the foramen of Monro and the anterior third ventricles as no choroid plexus is usually present there [30, 31]. This tumor is often large upon presentation and rarely invades brain parenchyma [31]. Hydrocephalus due to obstruction, overproduction of CSF, or impaired reabsorption is common [31]. This tumor may contain cysts, necrosis, calcium, or blood [30, 31]. Contrast-enhanced imaging of the entire CNS is recommended prior to surgical resection [30].

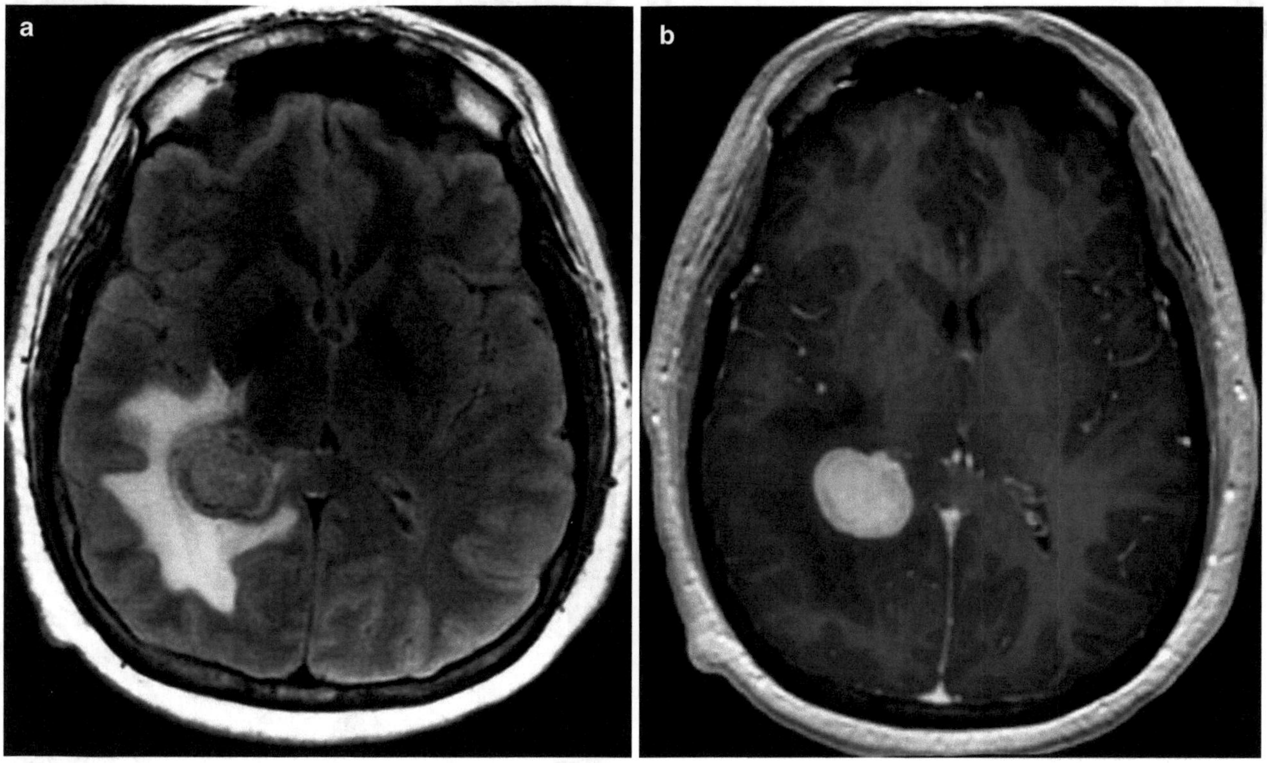

Fig. 2.36 Choroid plexus papilloma. Axial FLAIR (**a**) and contrast T1-weighted (**b**) images in a 24-year-old male show an enhancing tumor in the atrium of the right lateral ventricle and moderate surrounding brain edema. The location and enhancement may mimic an intraventricular meningioma in an adult

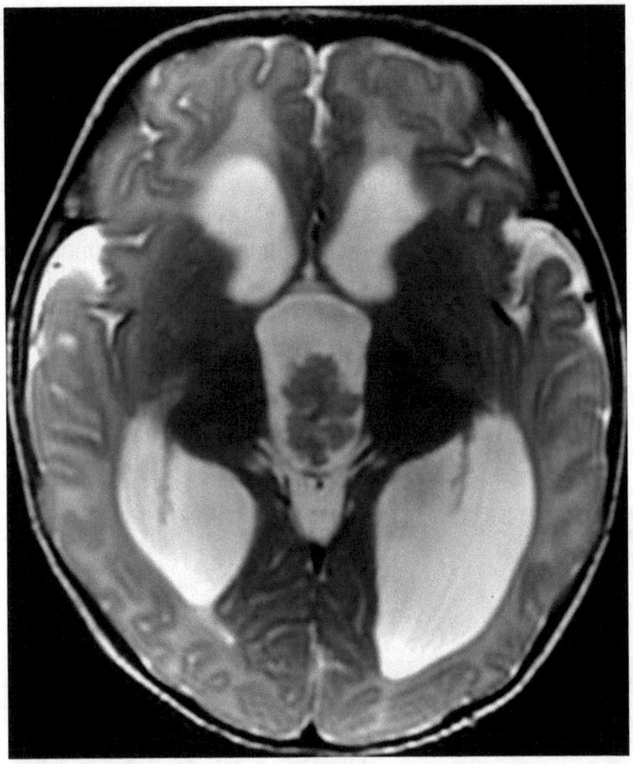

Fig. 2.37 Choroid plexus papilloma. Axial T2-weighted image in a 1-year-old male reveals a lobulated tumor in and obstructing the posterior third ventricle. Moderate hydrocephalus and interstitial edema are present

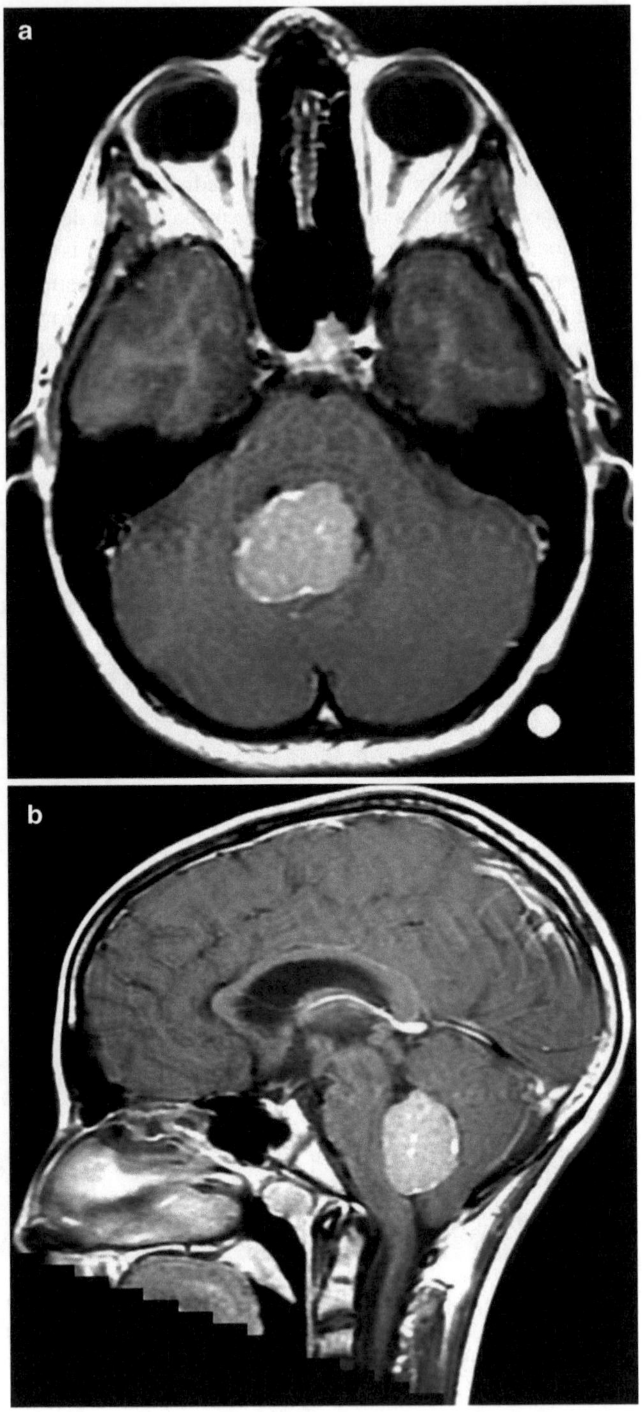

Fig. 2.38 Choroid plexus papilloma. Contrast axial (**a**) and sagittal (**b**) T1-weighted images in a 5-year-old female reveal a homogeneously enhancing midline posterior fossa tumor in the fourth ventricle (*See* "Medulloblastoma" and "Ependymoma" sections above for differential considerations)

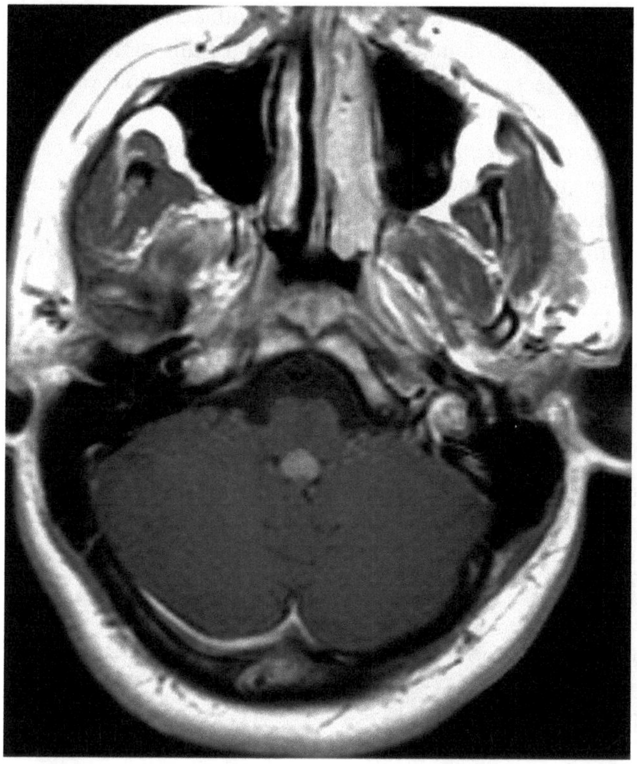

Fig. 2.39 Choroid plexus papilloma. Axial contrast T1-weighted image shows a small choroid plexus papilloma in the fourth ventricle of this 16-year-old male

Choroid Plexus Carcinoma

A choroid plexus carcinoma is a grade III malignant tumor that arises from epithelial cells of the choroid plexus [32]. This tumor type occurs most frequently in children younger than 5 years of age and occurs equally in both genders [32]. Clinical presentations of a patient with this tumor are typically symptoms of hydrocephalus, such as nausea, vomiting, and headache. Choroid plexus carcinoma is an aggressive tumor that carries a poor prognosis, with a 5-year survival of 40 % [32]. Recommended treatment for this tumor is gross total resection and chemotherapy with or without radiation therapy [30, 32].

Imaging features. MR images of choroid plexus carcinoma typically demonstrate large, enhancing intraventricular mass lesions [30]. These tumors may contain calcium and/or hemorrhage [30, 32]. Drop metastasis may occur, therefore imaging of the entire CNS is recommended.

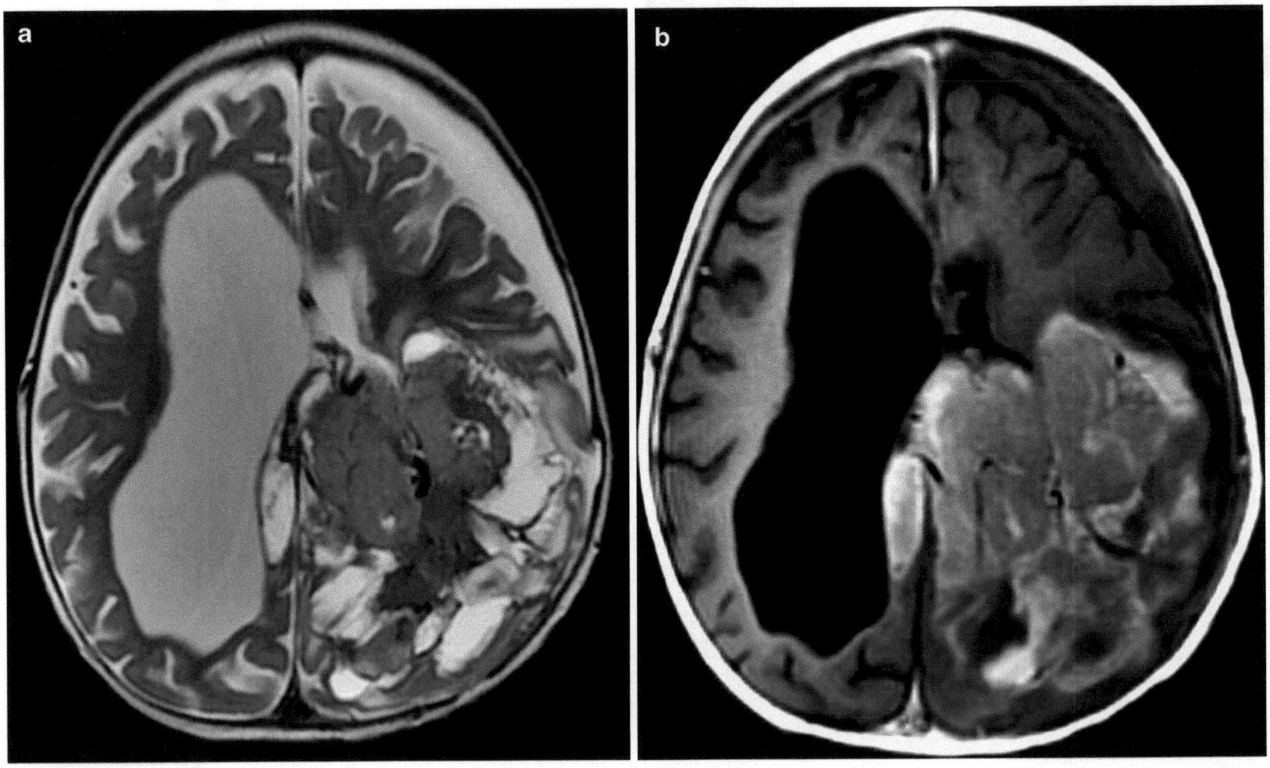

Fig. 2.40 Choroid plexus carcinoma. Axial T2-weighted (**a**) and contrast T1-weighted (**b**) images in a 1-year-old male show a large, heterogeneously enhancing tumor centered in the mid to posterior body of the left lateral ventricle with eccentric cystic/necrotic changes and probable invasion into the adjacent brain. Prominent flow voids (anterior margin and center of tumor in **a**) are characteristic for these highly vascularized tumors

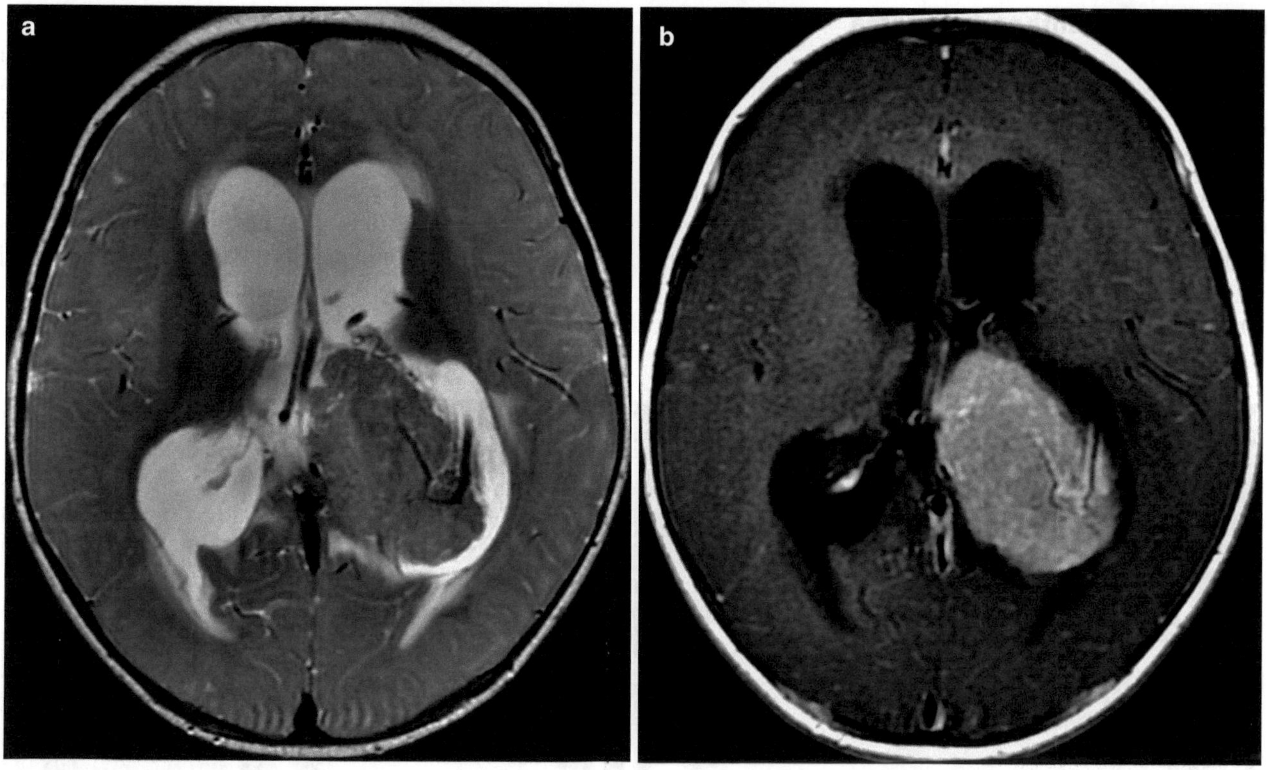

Fig. 2.41 Choroid plexus carcinoma. Axial T2-weighted (**a**) and contrast T1-weighted (**b**) images of a 7-month-old male reveal a heterogeneously enhancing tumor in the left lateral ventricle with a prominent feeding artery entering from the lateral margin

Pleomorphic Xanthoastrocytoma

This is a grade II benign astrocytoma that is made of pleomorphic cells that have xanthomatous change [33]. Pleomorphic xanthoastrocytoma (PX) accounts for less than 1 % of all astrocytomas [34]. A majority of these tumors are found in patients younger than 18 years of age [34]. This tumor occurs equally in both genders. Patients with PX have a fair prognosis with a 70 % survival rate at 10 years [33, 34].

Imaging features. Pleomorphic xanthoastrocytomas are peripherally located cortical/meningeal masses that have an enhancing dural tail [33, 34]. These tumors are frequently located supratentorially within the temporal lobe. More than half of PX are cystic masses with an enhancing mural nodule [33]. This tumor appears to be well circumscribed, however tumor often extends into surrounding brain parenchyma [33]. There is often minimal to no associated edema [33]. The presence of hemorrhage, calcium, and/or bone erosion is rare [34].

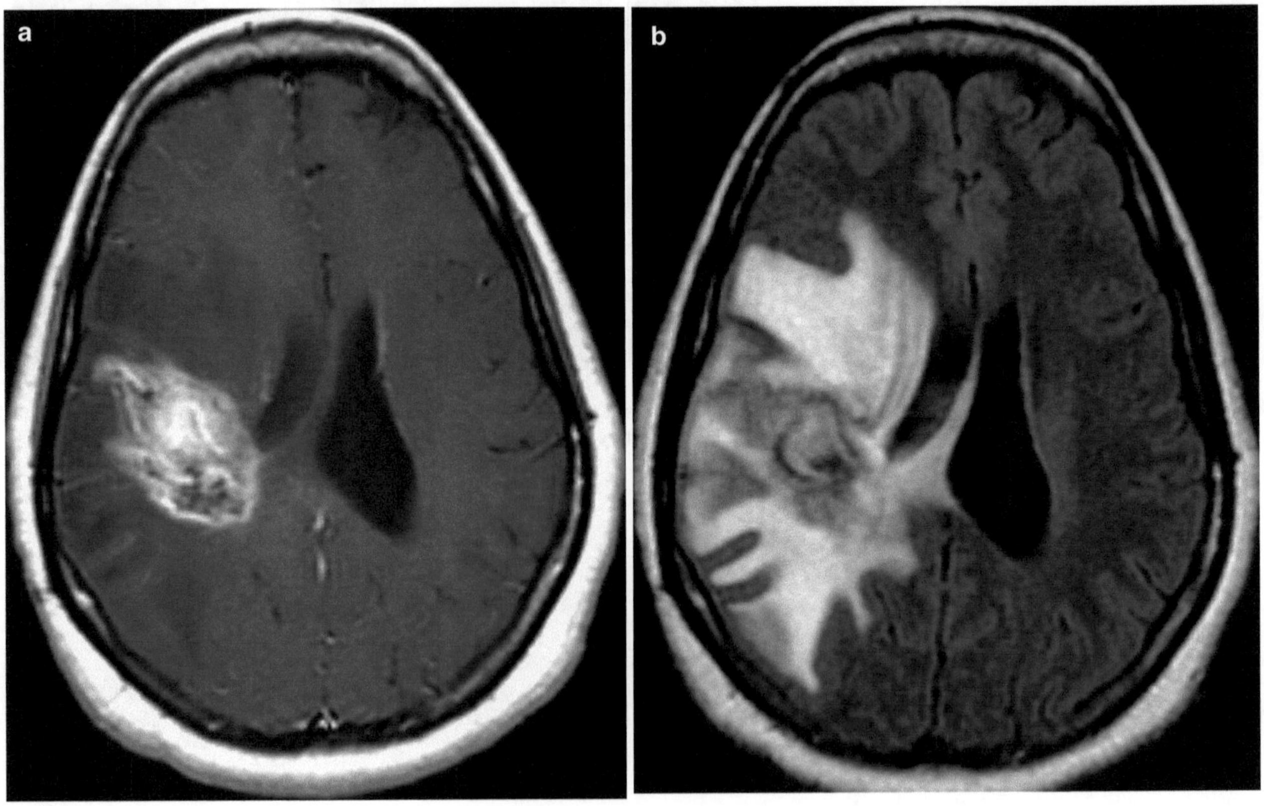

Fig. 2.42 Pleomorphic xanthoastrocytoma. Axial contrast T1-weighted (**a**) and FLAIR (**b**) images in a 25-year-old female show a heterogeneously enhancing tumor in the right frontal parietal operculum with marked surrounding FLAIR hyperintense edema-type changes

References

1. Osborne AG. Neoplasms and tumorlike lesions. In: Mascarenaz AD, Dearth CL, Kaerli M, editors. Diagnostic imaging: brain. Salt Lake City: Amirsys; 2005. p. 76–8.
2. Arbol D, Gandotra P, Maqbool M, et al. Dysembryoplastic neuroepithelial tumor: a rare brain tumor presenting with atypical radiological findings. JK Science. 2007;9:145–7.
3. Daumas-Duport C, Scheisytzthauer BW, Chodkiewicz JP, et al. Dysembryoplastic neuroepithelial tumor: a surgically curable tumor of young patients with intractable partial seizures. Report of thirty-nine cases. Neurosurgery. 1988;23:545–6.
4. Kwon JW, Kim IO, Cheon JE, et al. Cerebellopontine angle ganglioglioma: MR findings. AJNR Am J Neuroradiol. 2001;22:1377–9.
5. Osborne AG. Neoplasms and tumorlike lesions. In: Mascarenaz AD, Dearth CL, Kaerli M, editors. Diagnostic imaging: brain. Salt Lake City: Amirsys; 2005. p. 66–8.
6. Parwani AV, Stelow BS, Pambuccian SE, et al. Atypical teratoid/rhabdoid tumor of the brain cytopathologic characteristics and differential diagnosis. Cancer Cytopathol. 2005;105:65–70.
7. Osborne AG. Neoplasms and tumorlike lesions. In: Mascarenaz AD, Dearth CL, Kaerli M, editors. Diagnostic imaging: brain. Salt Lake City: Amirsys; 2005. p. 100–2.
8. Bruggers CS, Friedman HS, Fuller GN, et al. Comparison of serial PET and MRI scans in a pediatric patient with a brainstem glioma. Pediatr Blood Cancer. 1993;21:301–6.
9. Osborne AG. Neoplasms and tumorlike lesions. In: Mascarenaz AD, Dearth CL, Kaerli M, editors. Diagnostic imaging: brain. Salt Lake City: Amirsys; 2005. p. 12–4.
10. Kaplan AM, Albright AL, Zimmerman RA, et al. Brainstem gliomas in children. A Children's Cancer Group review of 119 cases. Pediatr Neurosurg. 1996;24:85–92.
11. Villarejo F, de Diego JMB, de la Riva AG. Prognosis of cerebellar astrocytomas in children. Childs Nerv Syst. 2008;24:203–10.
12. Osborne AG. Neoplasms and tumorlike lesions. In: Mascarenaz AD, Dearth CL, Kaerli M, editors. Diagnostic imaging: brain. Salt Lake City: Amirsys; 2005. p. 30–3.
13. Desai KI, Nadkarni TD, Muzumdar DP, et al. Prognostic factors for cerebellar astrocytomas in children: a study of 102 cases. Pediatr Neurosurg. 2001;35:311–7.
14. Gilheeney SW, Saad A, Chi S, et al. Outcome of pediatric pineoblastoma after surgery, radiation and chemotherapy. J Neurooncol. 2008;89:89–95.
15. Gaillard F, Jones J. Masses of the pineal region: clinical presentation and radiologic features. Postgrad Med J. 2010;86:597–607.
16. Osborne AG. Neoplasms and tumorlike lesions. In: Mascarenaz AD, Dearth CL, Kaerli M, editors. Diagnostic imaging: brain. Salt Lake City: Amirsys; 2005. p. 84–6.
17. Osborne AG. Neoplasms and tumorlike lesions. In: Mascarenaz AD, Dearth CL, Kaerli M, editors. Diagnostic imaging: brain. Salt Lake City: Amirsys; 2005. p. 132–4.
18. Packer RJ, Cohen K, Cooney K. Intracranial germ cell tumors. Oncologist. 2000;5:312–20.
19. Chang AH, Fuller GN, Debnam JM, et al. MR imaging of papillary tumor of the pineal region. AJNR Am J Neuroradiol. 2008;29:187–9.
20. Osborne AG. Neoplasms and tumorlike lesions. In: Mascarenaz AD, Dearth CL, Kaerli M, editors. Diagnostic imaging: brain. Salt Lake City: Amirsys; 2005. p. 88–90.
21. Fakhrana S, Escott EJ. Pineocytoma mimicking a pineal cyst on imaging: true diagnostic dilemma or a case of incomplete imaging? AJNR Am J Neuroradiol. 2008;29:159–63.
22. Bouffet E, Perilongo G, Canete A, Massimino M. Intracranial ependymomas in children: a critical review of prognostic factors and a plea for cooperation. Med Pediatr Oncol. 1998;30:319–29; discussion 329–31.
23. Osborne AG. Neoplasms and tumorlike lesions. In: Mascarenaz AD, Dearth CL, Kaerli M, editors. Diagnostic imaging: brain. Salt Lake City: Amirsys; 2005. p. 52–4.
24. Yuh EL, Barkovich AJ, Gupta N. Imaging of ependymomas: MRI and CT. Childs Nerv Syst. 2009;25:1203–13.
25. Menon G, Nair S, Muthurethinam T, et al. Medulloblastoma in children: prognostic factors and predictors of outcome. J Pediatr Neurosci. 2006;1:16–20.
26. Osborne AG. Neoplasms and tumorlike lesions. In: Mascarenaz AD, Dearth CL, Kaerli M, editors. Diagnostic imaging: brain. Salt Lake City: Amirsys; 2005. p. 92–4.
27. Meyers SP, Kemp SS, Tarr RW. MR imaging features of medulloblastoma. AJR Am J Roentgenol. 1992;158:859–65.
28. Berhouma M. Management of subependymal giant cell tumors in tuberous sclerosis complex: the neurosurgeon's perspective. World J Pediatr. 2010;6:103–10.
29. Osborne AG. Neoplasms and tumorlike lesions. In: Mascarenaz AD, Dearth CL, Kaerli M, editors. Diagnostic imaging: brain. Salt Lake City: Amirsys; 2005. p. 38–40.
30. Koeller KK, Sandberg GD, Armed Forces Institute of Pathology. From the archives of AFIP: cerebral intraventricular neoplasms:radiologic-pathologic correlation. Radiographics. 2002;22:1473–505.
31. Osborne AG. Neoplasms and tumorlike lesions. In: Mascarenaz AD, Dearth CL, Kaerli M, editors. Diagnostic imaging: brain. Salt Lake City: Amirsys; 2005. p. 60–2.
32. Osborne AG. Neoplasms and tumorlike lesions. In: Mascarenaz AD, Dearth CL, Kaerli M, editors. Diagnostic imaging: brain. Salt Lake City: Amirsys; 2005. p. 64–5.
33. Koeller KK, Henry JM, Armed Forces Institute of Pathology. From the archives of AFIP: superficial gliomas: radiologic-pathologic correlation. Radiographics. 2001;21:1533–56.
34. Osborne AG. Neoplasms and tumorlike lesions. In: Mascarenaz AD, Dearth CL, Kaerli M, editors. Diagnostic imaging: brain. Salt Lake City: Amirsys; 2005. p. 34–6.

Sellar and Parasellar Masses

3

Gitanjali V. Patel, Sasan Karimi, and Robert J. Young

Lesions located within the sella and parasellar region of the brain may present with similar clinical symptoms and imaging findings. Anatomic location and key imaging characteristics can aid in the differentiation of these tumors. Major anatomic references within the sella and parasellar region include the pituitary gland, pituitary stalk, optic chiasm, hypothalamus, cavernous sinus, sphenoid sinus, and the meninges. Although the most common tumors located within this region are pituitary adenoma, it is important to consider other less common entities that will also be discussed in this chapter [1]. Normal pituitary may vary in size with gender and age. Premenopausal women tend to have a larger pituitary gland than men and postmenopausal women [1, 2]. Magnetic resonance imaging (MRI) is generally the modality of choice for identification of lesions within this region. There are a few imaging pitfalls and it is important to be aware that nearly 15–20 % of lesions found within the pituitary are asymptomatic incidental findings [2].

Pituitary Adenoma

Pituitary adenomas are benign tumors of the anterior pituitary that account for 10–15 % of all intracranial tumors [2]. These are the most common suprasellar masses found in adults. The majority occur in middle-aged females, with hyperfunctioning or secreting adenomas more likely to present earlier at a smaller size than nonfunctioning adenomas [3].

Pituitary Microadenoma

A microadenoma is ≤10 mm in diameter. Prolactin-secreting microadenomas are more common in patients 20–35 years old whereas microadenomas that secrete growth hormone are more common in patients 30–50 years old [4].

Microadenomas are commonly visualized as well-defined lesions that enhance less than the normal pituitary gland [4]. Dynamic contrast-enhanced MR may be useful as normal pituitary tissue normally enhances faster than microadenoma. Even when small, microadenomas may cause a mass effect that results in increased convexity of the superior margin of the pituitary gland or contralateral displacement of the infundibulum [4, 5].

G.V. Patel
Department of Radiology, Memorial Sloan-Kettering Cancer Center, 1275 York Avenue, MRI-1156, New York, NY 10065, USA
e-mail: gita.patel@gmail.com

S. Karimi (✉) • R.J. Young
Department of Radiology,
New York Presbyterian Hospital/Weill Cornell Medical College, New York, NY, USA

Neuroradiology Service, Department of Radiology,
Memorial Sloan-Kettering Cancer Center,
1275 York Avenue, MRI-1156, New York, NY 10065, USA
e-mail: karimis@mskcc.org; youngr@mskcc.org

S. Karimi (ed.), *Atlas of Brain and Spine Oncology Imaging*, Atlas of Oncology Imaging,
DOI 10.1007/978-1-4614-5653-7_3, © Springer Science+Business Media New York 2013

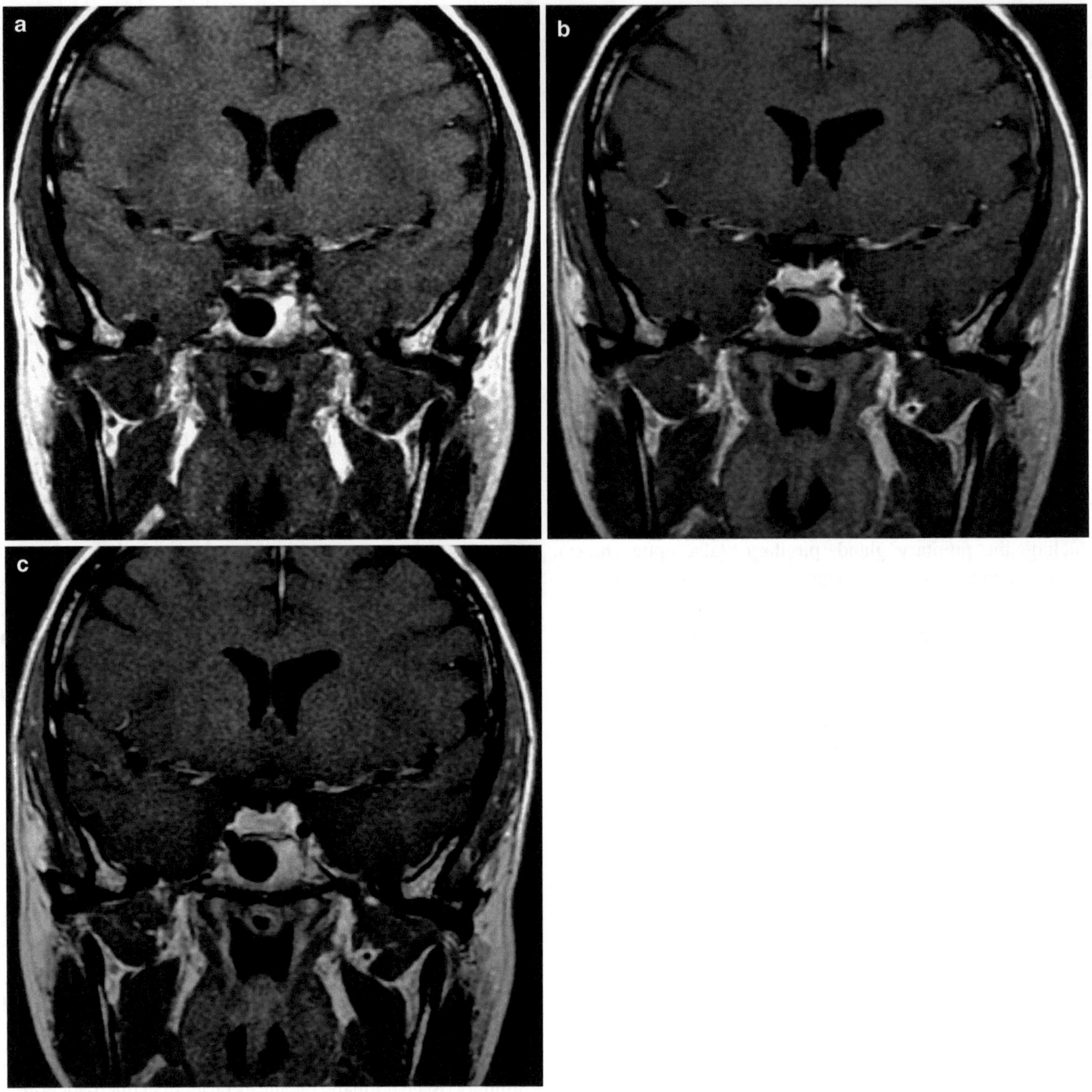

Fig. 3.1 Pituitary microadenoma. Pre-contrast (**a**), early dynamic contrast (**b**), and late dynamic contrast (**c**) coronal T1-weighted images show progressive enhancement of a microadenoma in the inferior left pituitary gland. The lesion is best seen on the early dynamic image; many microadenomas may be difficult to detect on routine non-dynamic contrast images when the differential enhancement has equalized with normal pituitary tissue

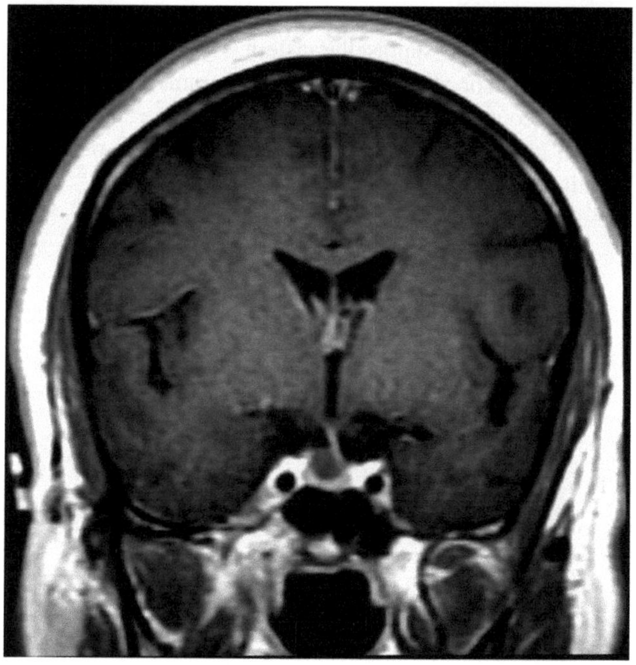

Fig. 3.2 Pituitary cyst. Coronal contrast T1-weighted image shows increased superior convexity of the right pituitary gland and contralateral displacement of the infundibulum by the nonenhancing right pituitary cyst that mimics a cystic microadenoma. Pathology only revealed acellular mucoid material

Pituitary Macroadenoma

A macroadenoma is larger than 10 mm in diameter [6, 14]. Macroadenomas may cause endocrine symptoms, or visual disturbances due to mass effect upon the optic chiasm or pre-chiasmatic optic nerves. Management of macroadenoma can vary from medical management to surgical resection, often through a trans-sphenoidal approach [7].

Macroadenomas are expansile masses that often grow superiorly into the suprasellar cistern. When large, they may impinge upon or compress the optic apparatus. Hemorrhagic, proteinaceous, and cystic changes may variably occur. Lateral growth in the cavernous sinus may limit otherwise curative surgical resection of these tumors [5, 6].

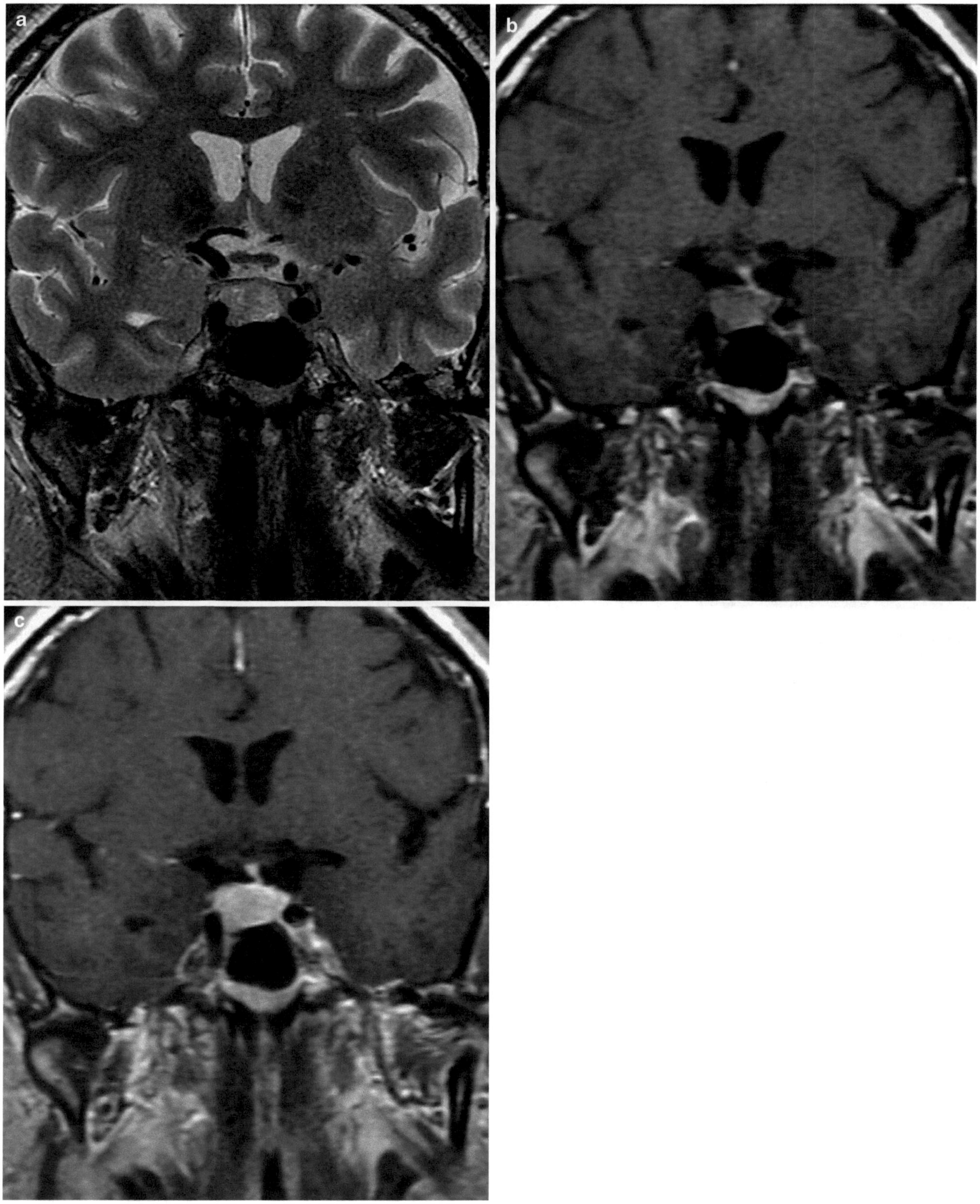

Fig. 3.3 Pituitary macroadenoma. Coronal T2-weighted (**a**) and early (**b**) and delayed (**c**) dynamic contrast T1-weighted images show a T2 hyperintense macroadenoma extending into the right cavernous sinus and displacing the infundibulum to the left. The macroadenoma is difficult to distinguish from normal pituitary tissue by the delayed image (**c**)

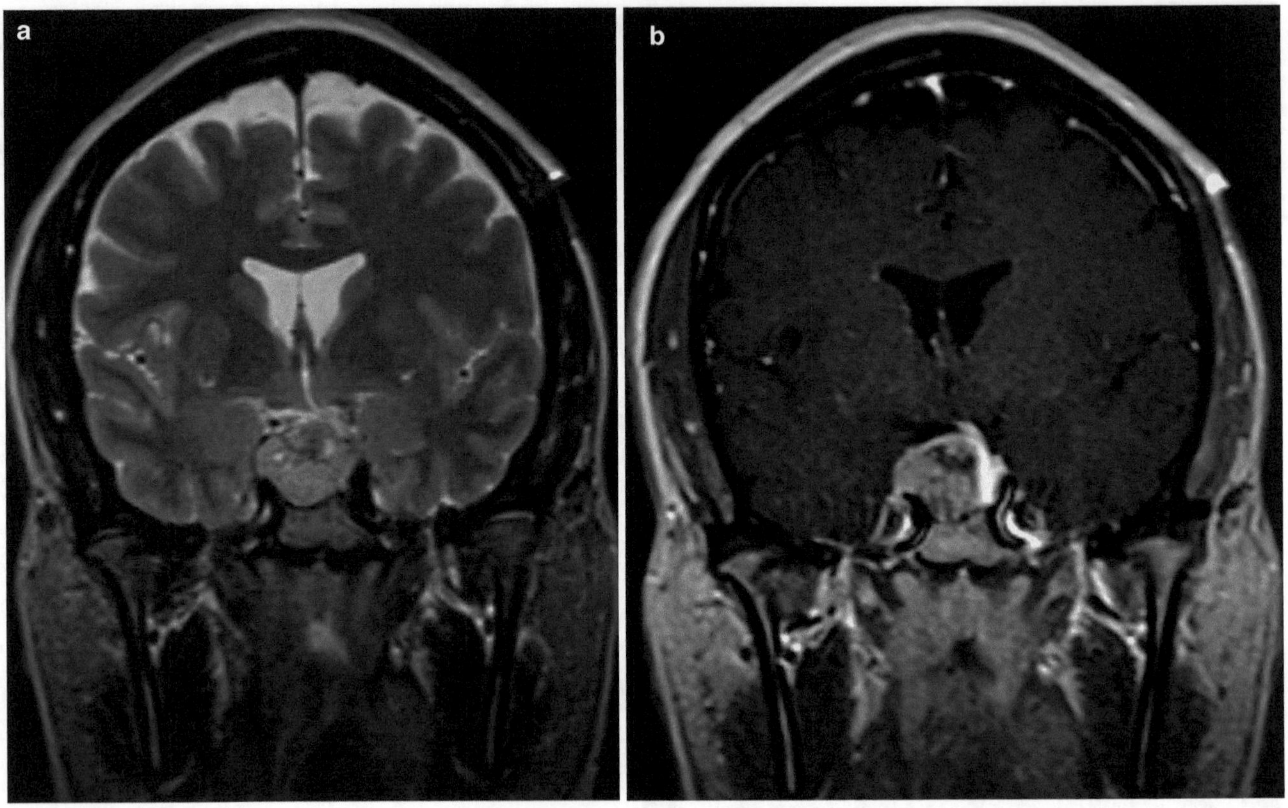

Fig. 3.4 Pituitary macroadenoma. Coronal T2-weighted (**a**) and contrast T1-weighted (**b**) images show a heterogeneously enhancing right pituitary macroadenoma invading into the right cavernous sinus, with suprasellar extension and contralateral displacement of the infundibulum. The macroadenoma is easier to distinguish from the normal, avidly enhancing pituitary gland in the left sella in (**b**)

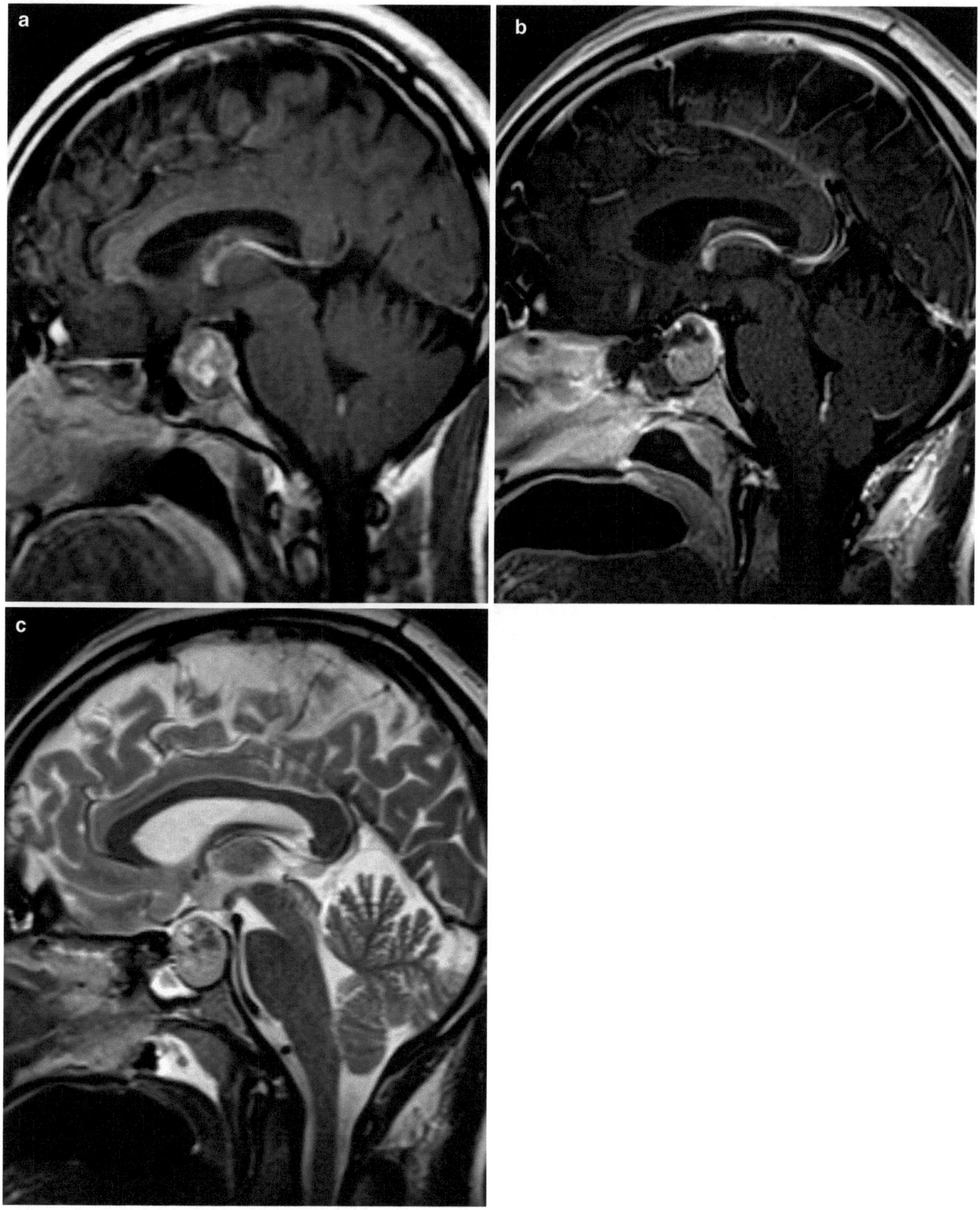

Fig. 3.5 Pituitary macroadenoma. Sagittal preoperative (**a**) and intraoperative (**b**) contrast T1-weighted images and intraoperative T2-weighted image (**c**) show subtotal resection of the macroadenoma extending into the suprasellar cistern. Curvilinear hyperintensity in (**a**) probably represents hemorrhagic and/or proteinaceous material within the macroadenoma

Invasive Pituitary Adenoma

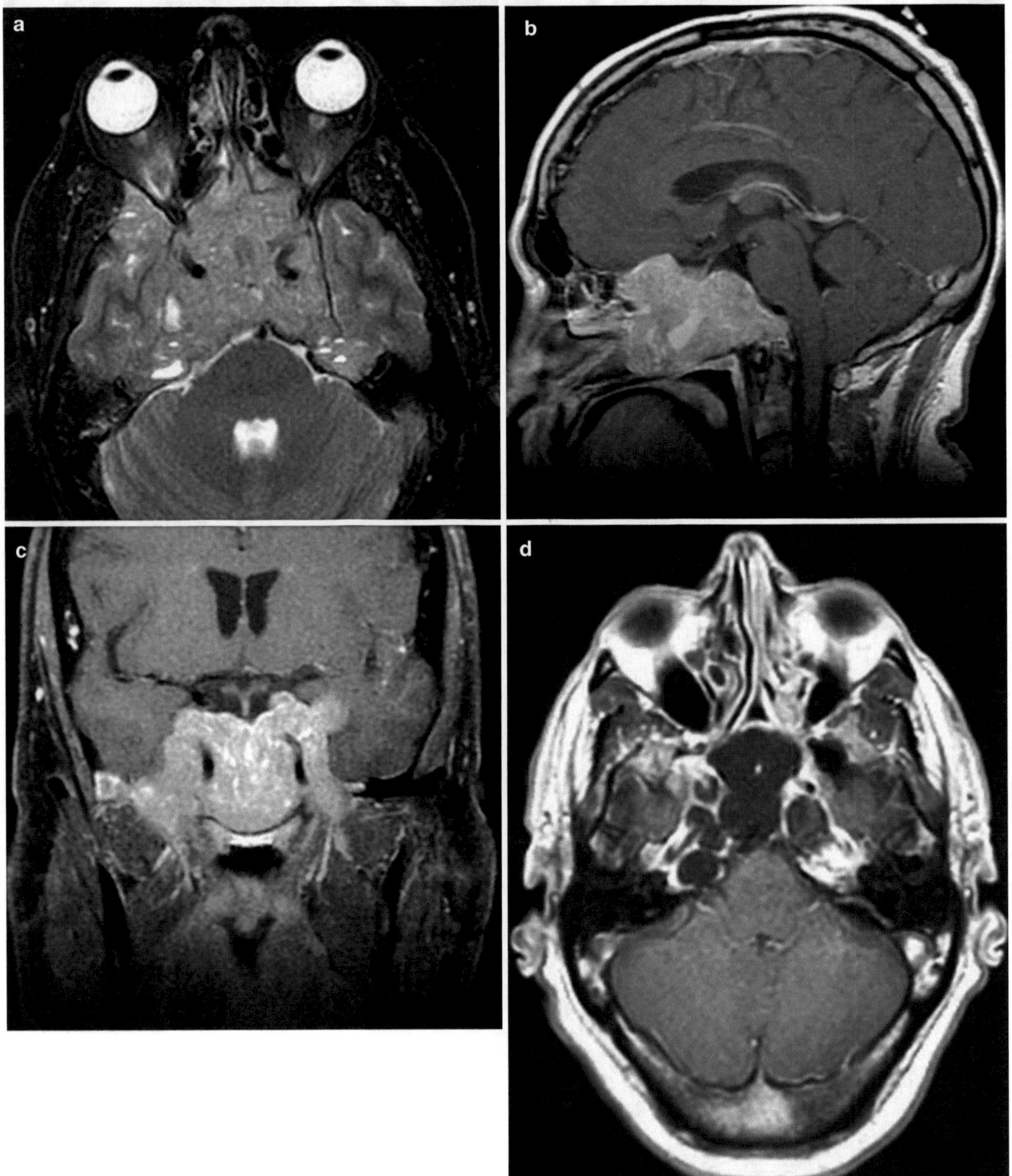

Fig. 3.6 Pretreatment axial T2 (**a**), sagittal T1 (**b**), and coronal T1 (**c**) post-contrast images of a patient with a large invasive pituitary adenoma infiltrating the central skull base. Small cystic changes are evident within the tumor on the axial T2-weighted image (**a**). Follow-up imaging 3 years after medical treatment demonstrates excellent treatment response as the mass has resolved leaving cystic and CSF-filled cavities with the skull base at sites of prior tumoral involvement. Axial (**d**) and sagittal T1 (**e**) post-contrast and coronal T2-weighted (**f**) images

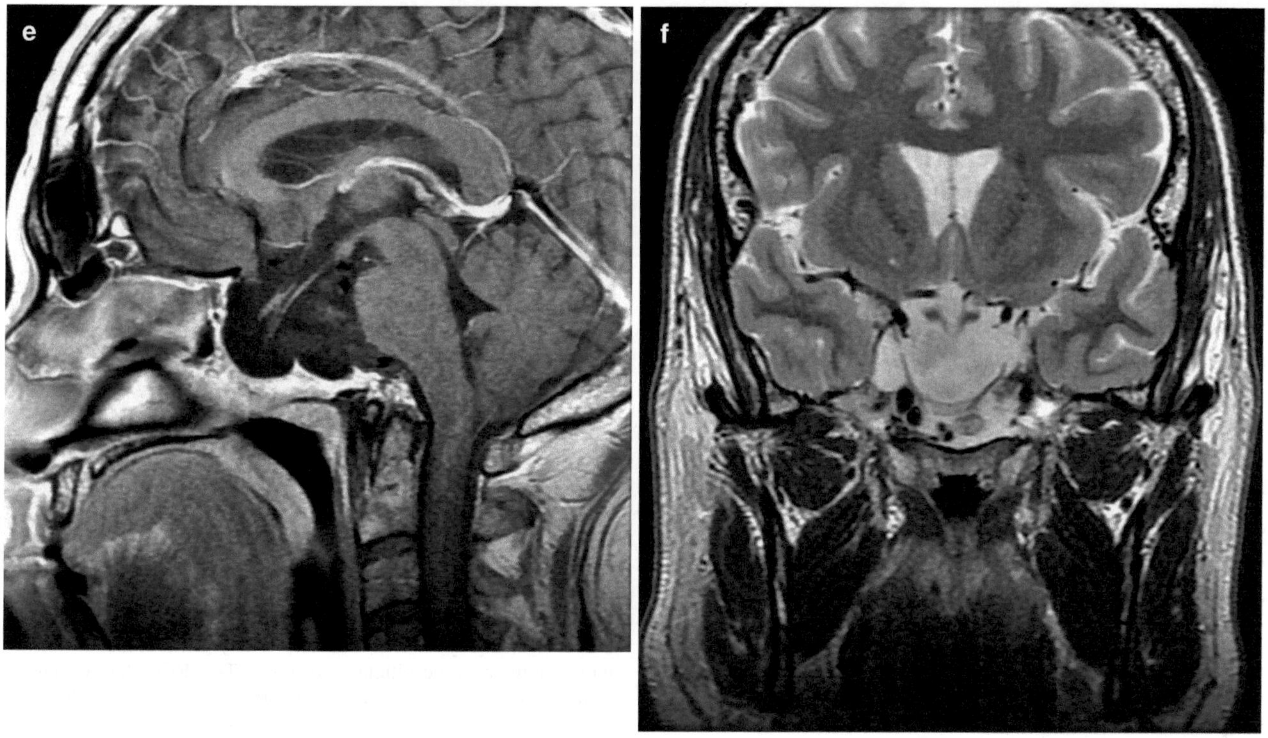

Fig. 3.6 (continued)

Rathke's Cleft Cyst

Rathke's cleft cyst (RCC) is a benign cyst that arises from the embryonic Rathke cleft. The cyst may contain a clear or mucoid material. RCCs are usually asymptomatic and are commonly found incidentally upon imaging or autopsy [8]. RCCs are most commonly diagnosed in the fifth decade of life and have a slight female predominance [9]. These cysts typically remain benign and management is usually conservative. If the patient is symptomatic aspiration or partial excision may be necessary.

Most RCCs are visualized as lobulated, well-defined, intrasellar, or suprasellar cysts that contain a small intracystic nodule [8]. More than 50 % of RCCs have a hypointense intracystic nodule upon T2-weighted imaging. RCCs typically do not enhance and rarely contain calcium. Around 40 % of these cysts are located completely within the sella and 60 % have suprasellar extension [9, 12].

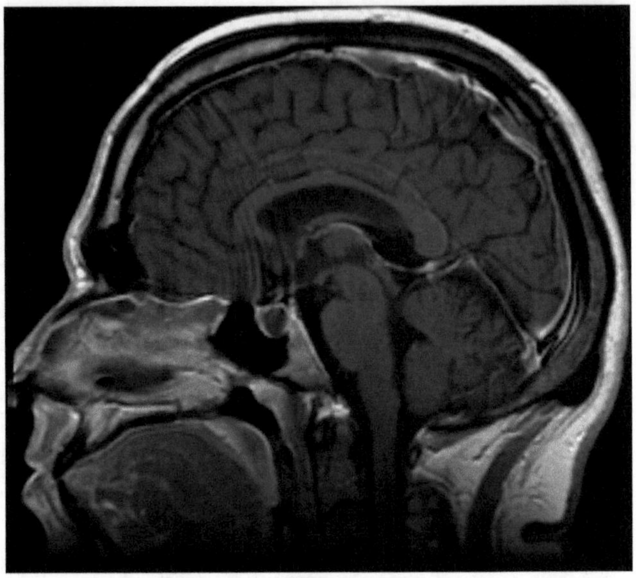

Fig. 3.7 Rathke cleft cyst. Sagittal contrast T1-weighted image shows a nonenhancing cystic lesion in the pituitary gland that could mimic a more common cystic pituitary adenoma. This RCC did not have the characteristic T1 hypointense, T2 hypointense intracystic nodule. Most craniopharyngiomas have cystic and solid-enhancing components (*see* "Craniopharyngioma")

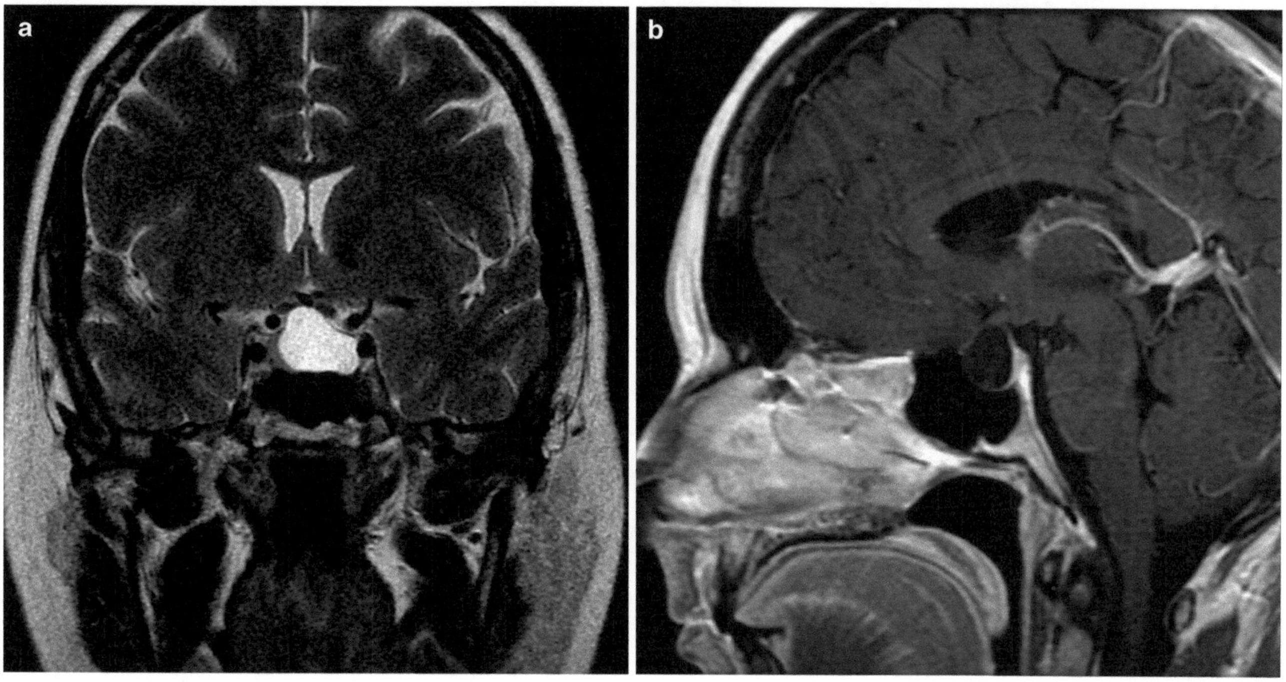

Fig. 3.8 Rathke cleft cyst. Coronal T2-weighted (**a**) and sagittal contrast T1-weighted (**b**) images demonstrate an expansile T2 hyperintense and T1 hypointense nonenhancing sellar and suprasellar lesion that impinges upon the prechiasmatic optic nerves. RCC fluid may show variable signal intensity; in this case, the fluid is slightly greater than normal cerebrospinal fluid on the T2-weighted image and equal on the T1-weighted image

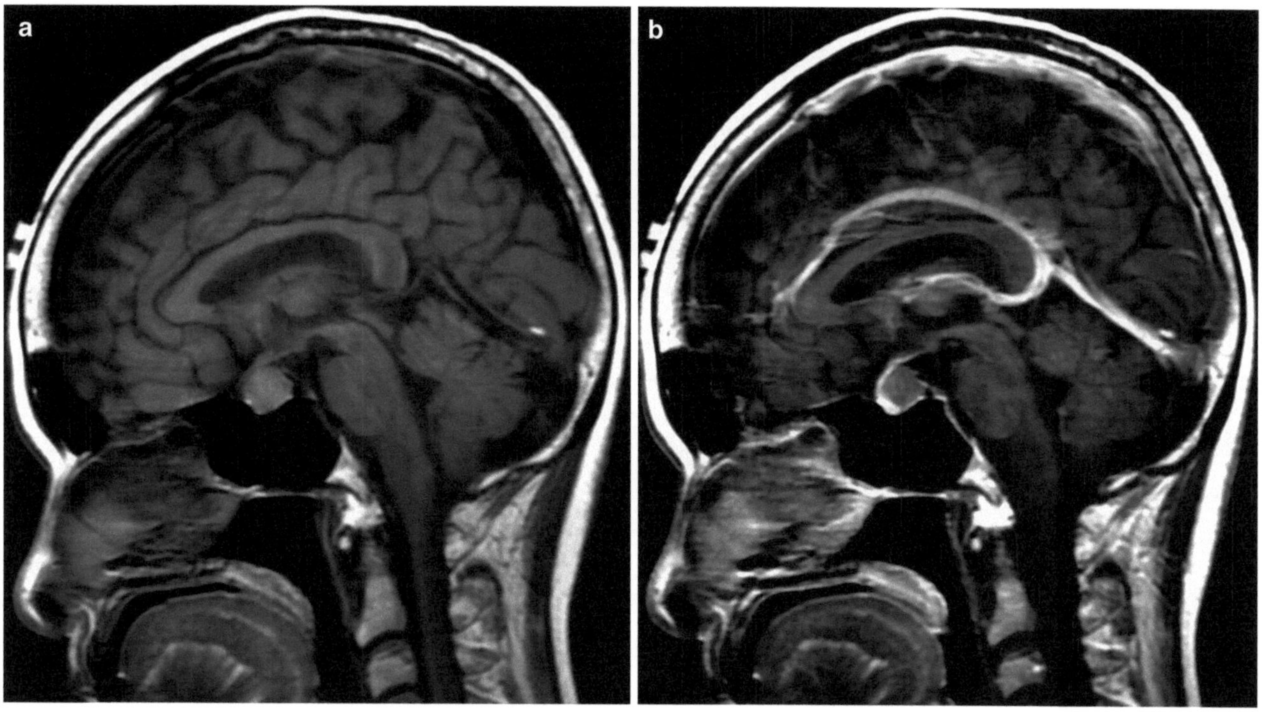

Fig. 3.9 Rathke cleft cyst. Sagittal T1-weighted images before (**a**) and after (**b**) contrast show a hyperintense, nonenhancing RCC

Craniopharyngioma

Craniopharyngioma are benign tumors that originate from embryonal cells originating from the Rathke cleft and/or craniopharyngeal duct epithelium [10]. This is the most common intracranial tumor in the pediatric population that is not of glial origin [11]. Craniopharyngiomas account for around half of all sellar tumors that occur in childhood [10]. This tumor type has no gender predominance and occurs in patients age 5–15 years old and patients older than age 50 [11]. Patients may present with visual and/or endocrine disturbances. Prognosis varies with tumor size; tumors with a diameter greater than 5 cm have a worse prognosis than tumors with diameters less than 5 cm [10].

Craniopharyngiomas are typically mixed solid and cystic lesions that contain calcium. Findings on pre-contrast T1-weighted MRI usually show a suprasellar lesion with high signal intensity [12]. These tumors may span to include the anterior, middle, and/or posterior cranial fossa. For surgical purposes, the location of the craniopharyngioma may be described as being sellar, prechiasmatic, or retrochiasmatic. Nonenhanced computed tomography (CT) may be useful to detect the presence of calcium if MR diagnosis is inconclusive [12].

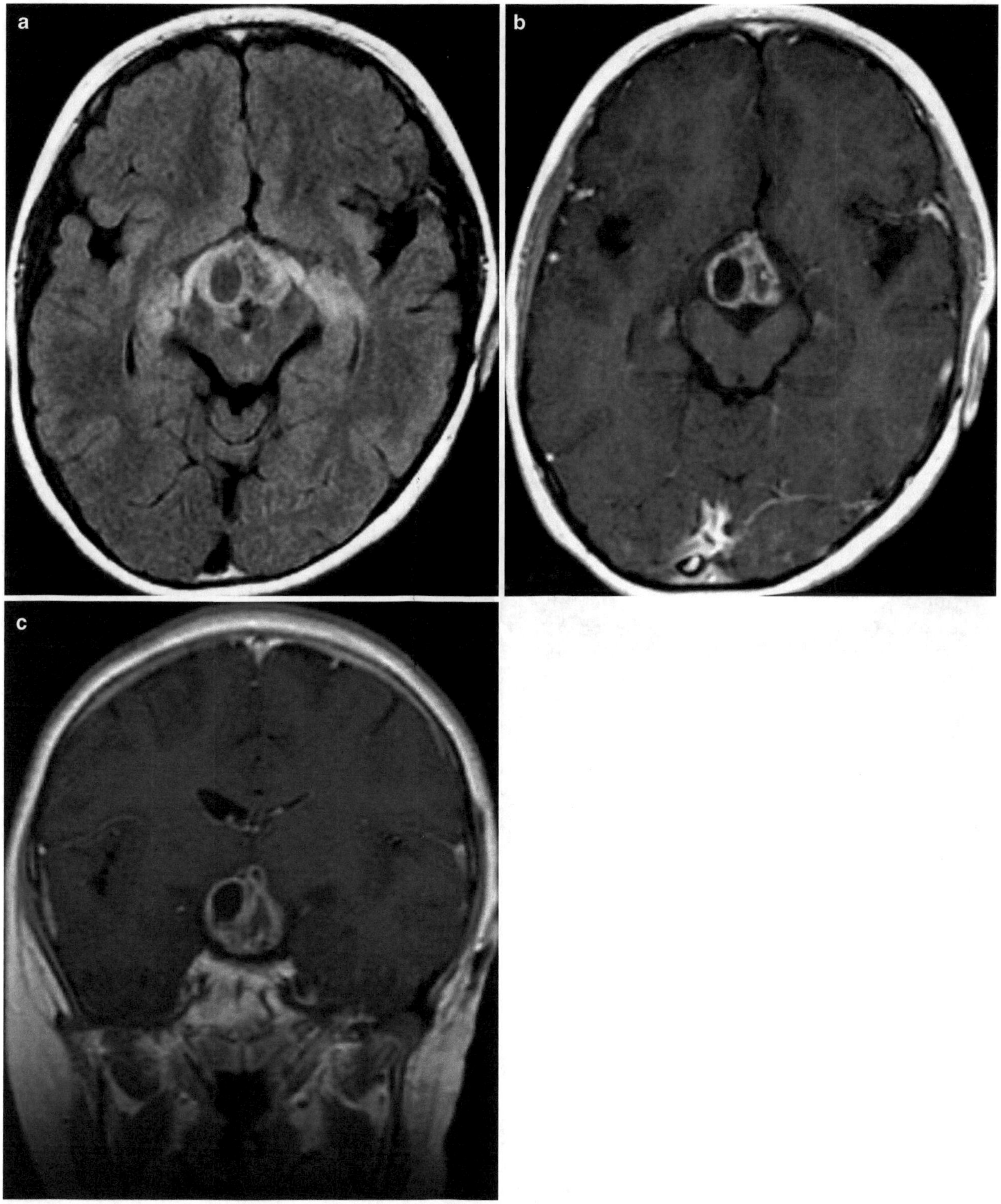

Fig. 3.10 Craniopharyngioma. Axial fluid attenuated inversion recovery (FLAIR) image (**a**) and axial (**b**) and coronal (**c**) contrast T1-weighted images show a solid and cystic suprasellar craniopharyngioma in a 7-year-old patient. Adjacent FLAIR hyperintense changes extend into the optic tracts and mesial temporal lobes (**a**)

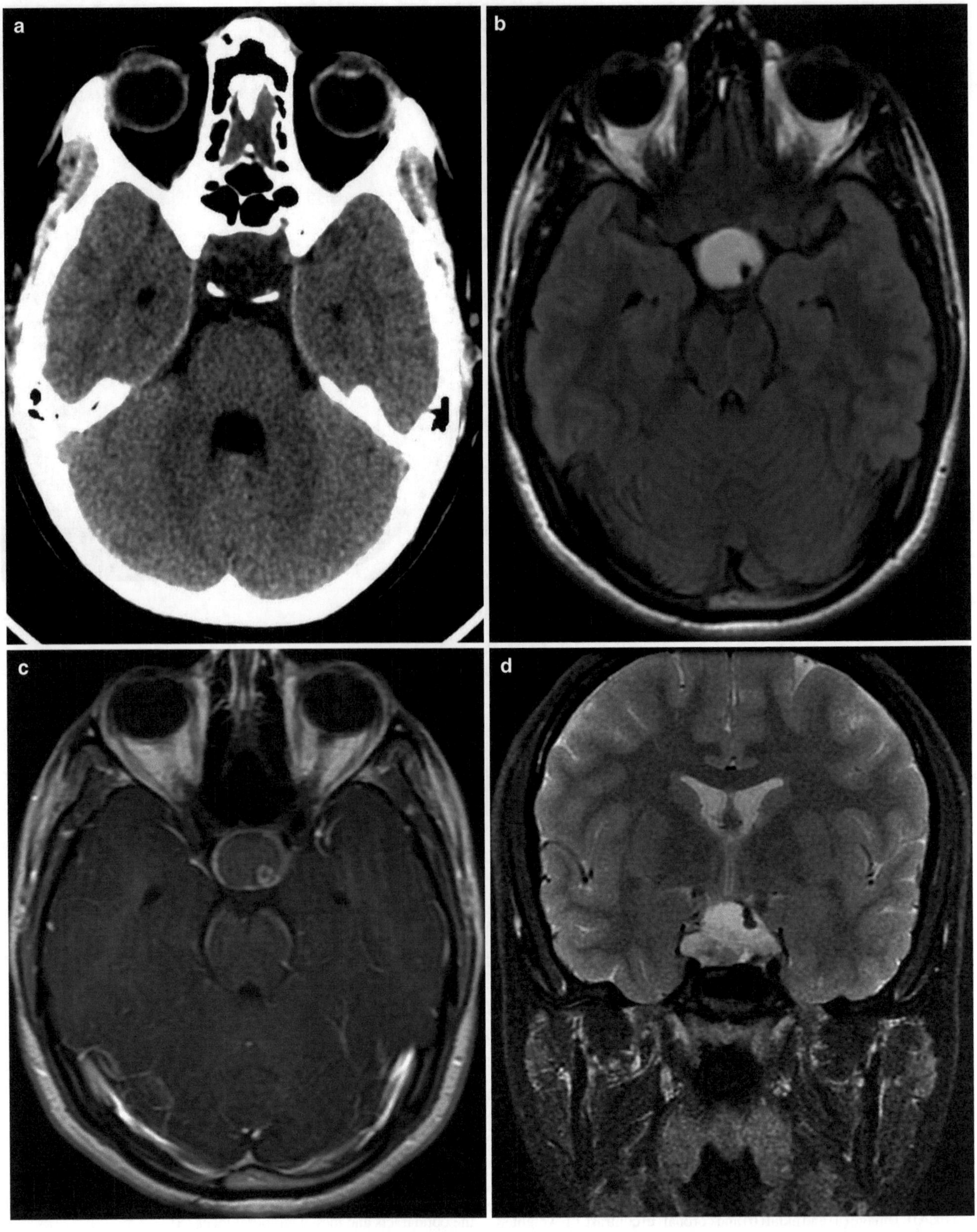

Fig. 3.11 Craniopharyngioma. Axial CT (**a**), axial FLAIR (**b**), and contrast T1-weighted (**c**) images and coronal T2-weighted image (**d**) reveal a T2/FLAIR hyperintense sellar and suprasellar adamantinomatous craniopharyngioma in a 16-year-old patient. There is lateral extension into the cavernous sinuses. The eccentric T2/FLAIR hypointense calcification and eccentric nodular enhancement are characteristic for adamantinomatous craniopharyngiomas compared to heterogeneously enhancing cystic pituitary macroadenomas (*see* "Pituitary Macroadenoma"). Adamantinomatous craniopharyngiomas peak in children at 5–14 years old

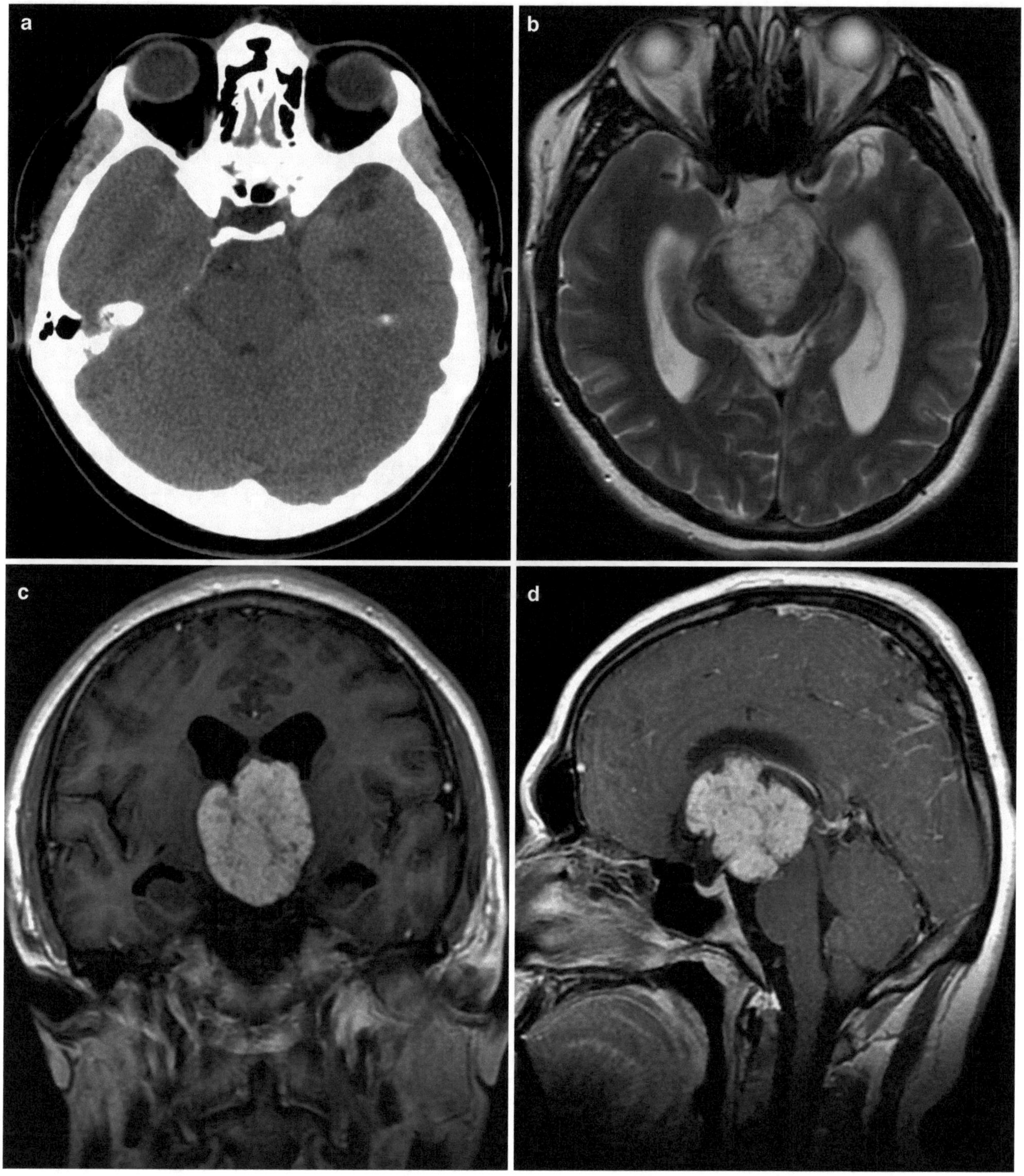

Fig. 3.12 Craniopharyngioma. Axial CT (**a**) and axial T2-weighted (**b**) images and coronal (**c**) and sagittal (**d**) contrast T1-weighted images show an expansile heterogeneously enhancing papillary craniopharyngioma in a 20-year-old patient. The tumor is centered in the suprasellar cistern and third ventricle, with splaying of the cerebral peduncles (**b**) and obstructive hydrocephalus manifest with dilatation of the lateral ventricles including the temporal horns. Squamous-papillary craniopharyngiomas are more common in adults at the smaller of the bimodal age peaks at 65–74 years old, and are more likely to be solid-enhancing compared to the solid and cystic adamantinomatous craniopharyngiomas in children

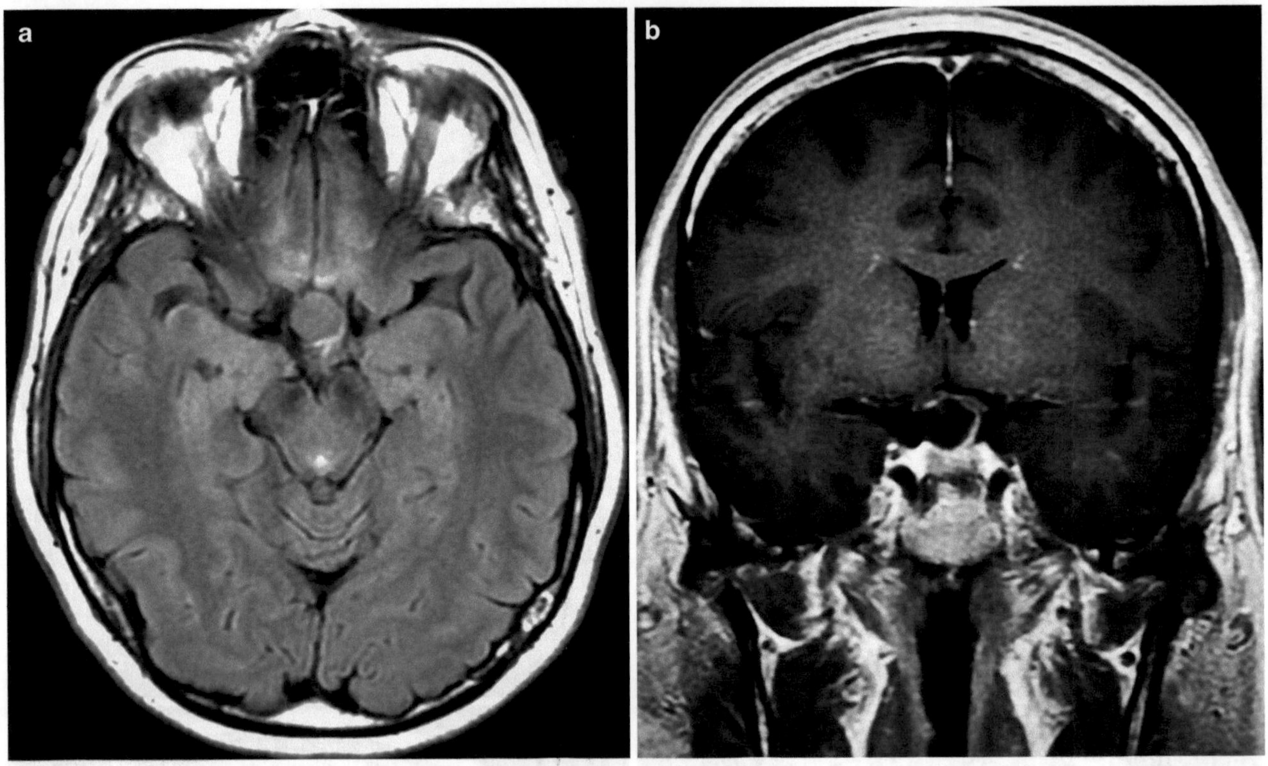

Fig. 3.13 Craniopharyngioma. Axial FLAIR (**a**) and coronal contrast T1-weighted (**b**) images show a cystic FLAIR hyperintense suprasellar adamantinomatous craniopharyngioma in a 49-year-old patient. These tumors are usually cystic and solid – the mild nodular peripheral enhancement along the superior margin adjacent to the right prechiasmatic optic nerve helps exclude a nonenhancing RCC (*see* "Rathke's Cleft Cyst"). The adamantinomatous subtype is more common in children

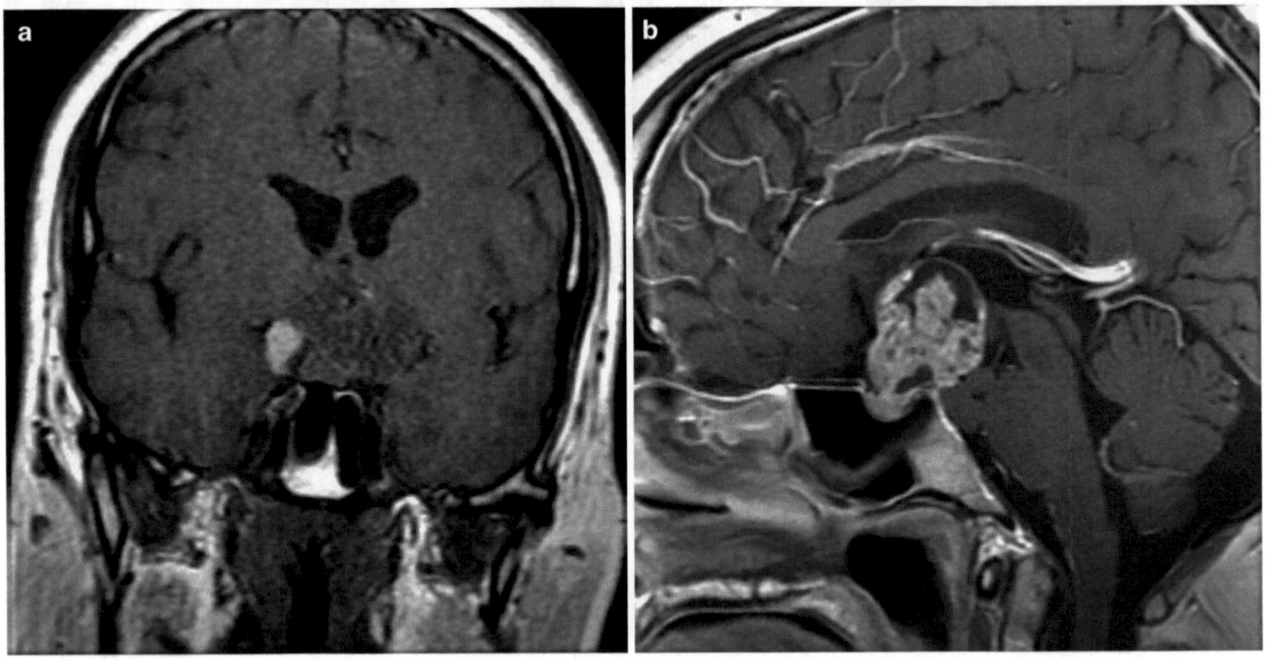

Fig. 3.14 Craniopharyngioma. Coronal (**a**) and contrast sagittal (**b**) T1-weighted images show a heterogeneously enhancing tumor centered in the suprasellar cistern with right eccentric pre-contrast T1 hyperintense blood products

Optic Pathway Glioma

Optic pathway gliomas are responsible for 5 % of all brain tumors. They comprise up to 15 % of supratentorial lesions within the pediatric population [13]. These are usually benign low-grade astrocytomas, although they are difficult to treat because of their location. In 10–20 % or more of patients with optic pathway gliomas, stigmata of neurofibromatosis type 1 are also found [13]. Compared to neurofibromatosis type 1–related tumors, sporadic optic pathway gliomas are more likely to have worse outcomes, impair vision, involve the optic chiasm, extend beyond the optic pathway, have larger size, and cystic nonenhancing components.

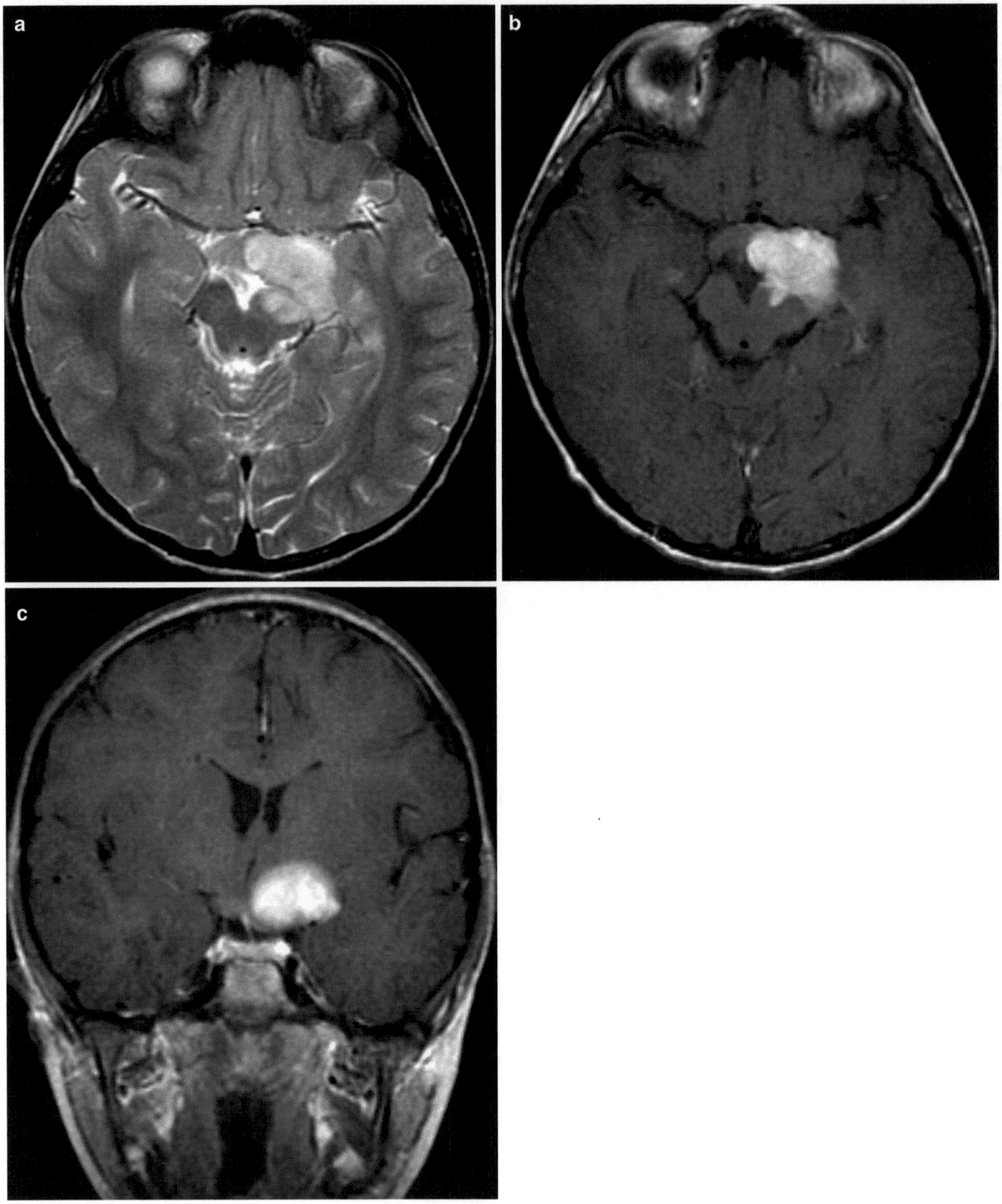

Fig. 3.15 Optic pathway glioma. Axial T2-weighted (**a**) and contrast axial (**b**) and coronal (**c**) T1-weighted images in a 4-year-old patient with a left optic chiasmatic-hypothalamic glioma. The expansile enhancing tumor extends posteriorly from the left optic chiasm along the optic tract and hypothalamus, inferiorly into the cerebral peduncle, and laterally into the mesial temporal lobe (*not shown*). Chiasmatic-hypothalamic gliomas in children younger than 5 years and older than 20 years old may demonstrate aggressive growth, despite the usually low-grade pathology. Posterior location may also indicate a poor outcome. This child received chemotherapy due to his age, tumor location, and slow growth over a year; radiation therapy is often deferred when possible in small children

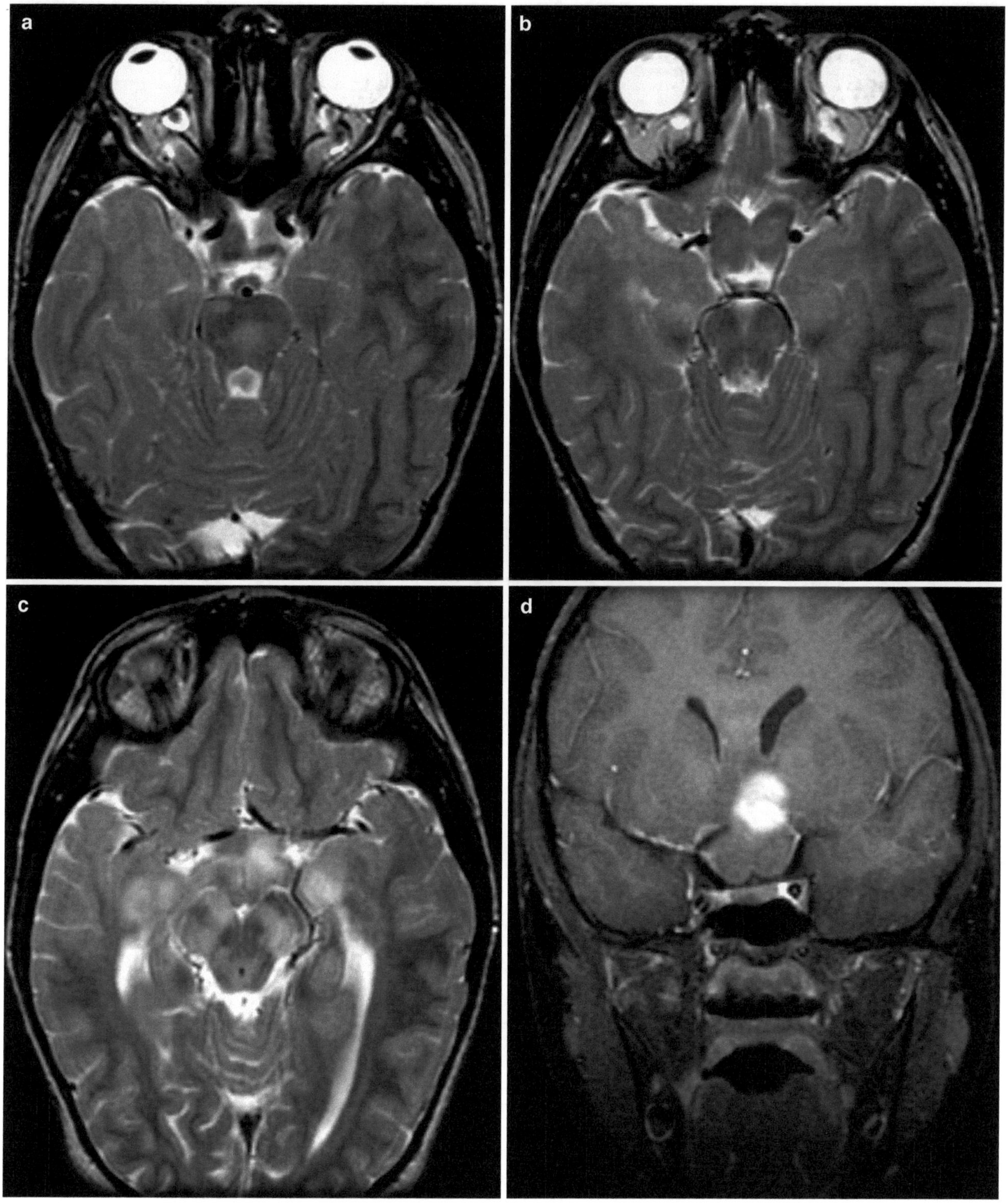

Fig. 3.16 Optic pathway glioma. Axial T2-weighted images (**a–c**) reveal expansile T2 hyperintense tumors in the prechiasmatic optic nerves (from anterior to posterior), chiasm, tracts, and pathways in a 7-year-old patient with bilateral chiasmatic-hypothalamic and optic pathway tumors. Additional areas of T2 hyperintensity in the brainstem and in the cerebral and cerebellar white matter (*not shown*) are consistent with vacuolar changes from underlying neurofibromatosis type 1. Coronal contrast fat-saturated T1-weighted image (**d**) 3 months later showed progression manifest by new enhancement in the optic chiasm and hypothalamus that prompted initiation of chemotherapy

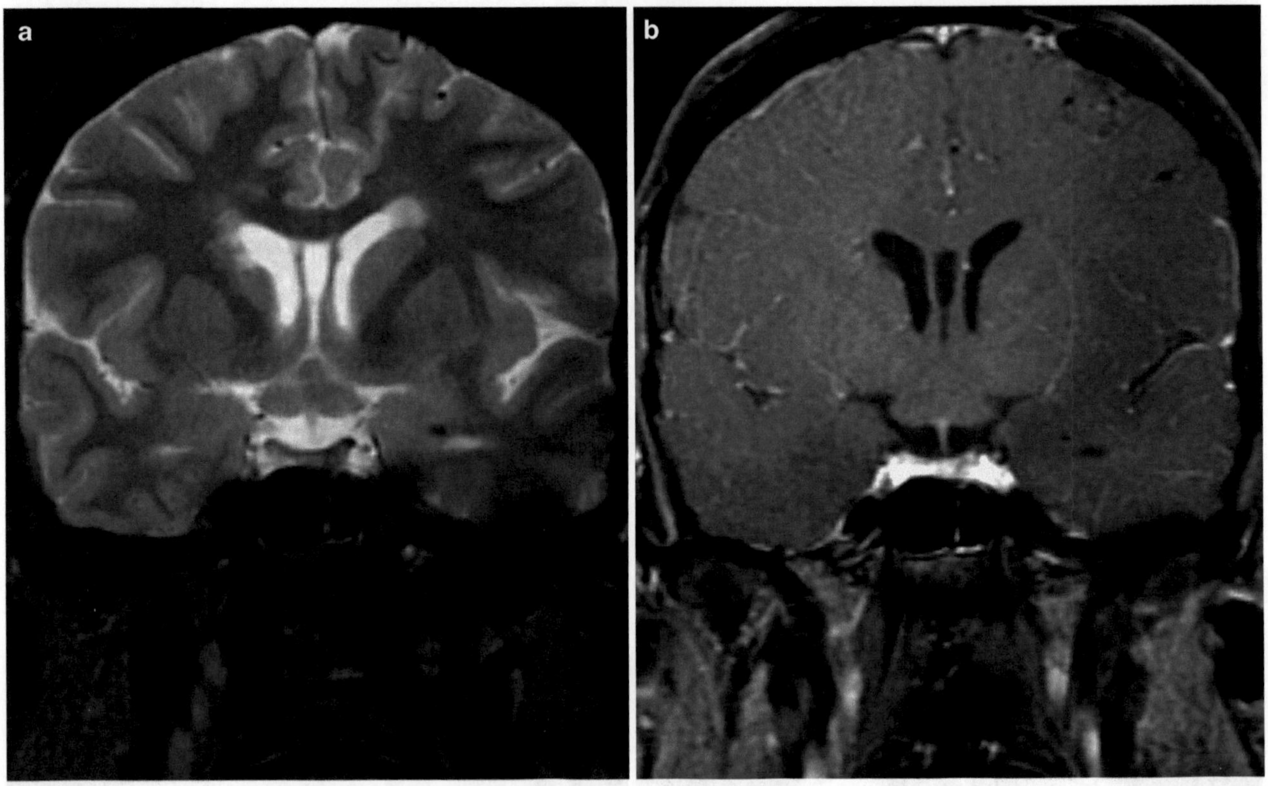

Fig. 3.17 Optic pathway glioma. Coronal fat-saturated T2-weighted (**a**) and contrast T1-weighted (**b**) images reveal an expansile nonenhancing glioma in the optic chiasm of a 19-year-old with neurofibromatosis type 1. Note the absence of normal internal carotid artery and proximal circle of Willis flow voids consistent with Moyamoya syndrome, one of many vascular lesions that may occur in neurofibromatosis type 1 (*see* Fig. 2.17a for normal arterial flow voids on a coronal T2-weighted image)

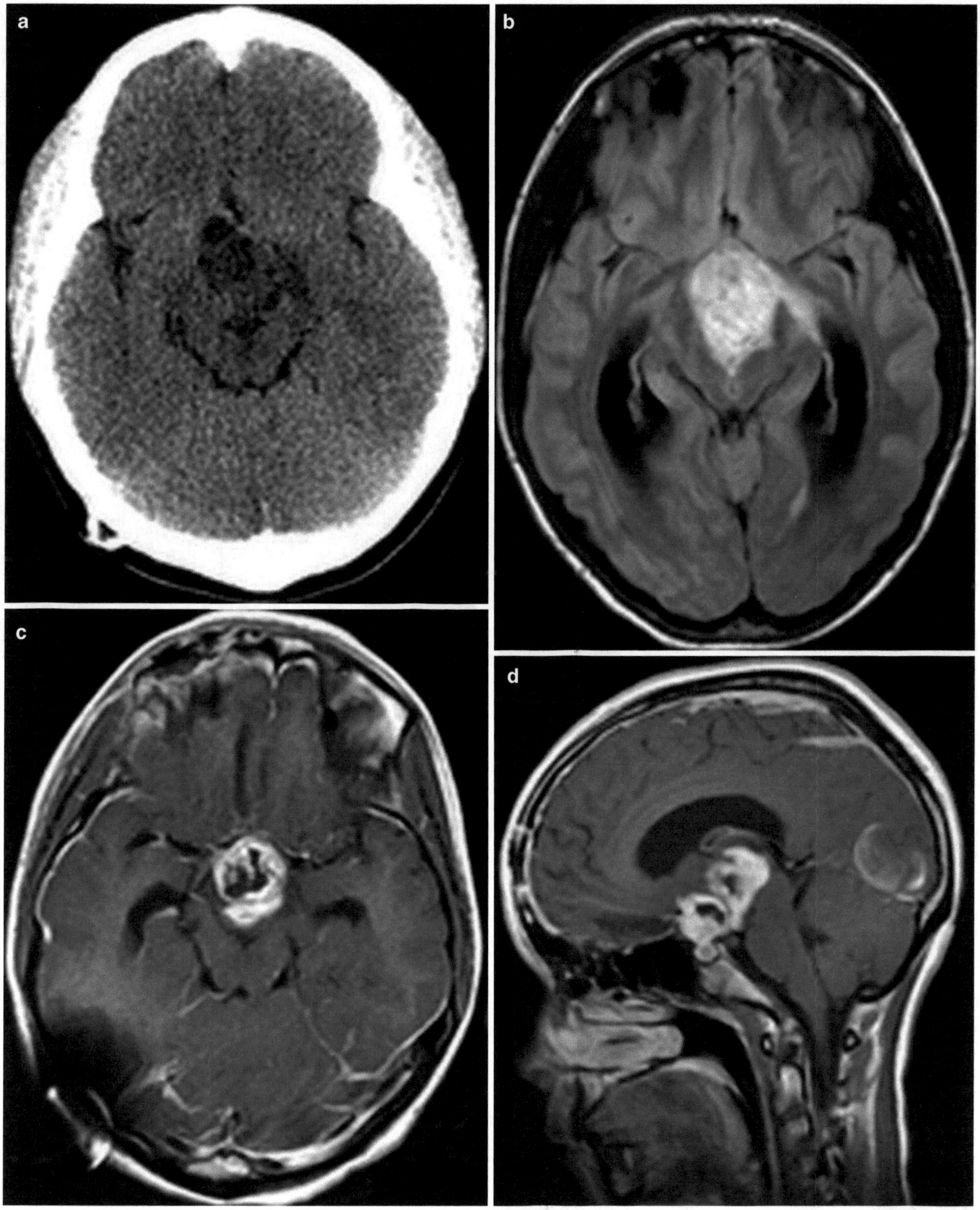

Fig. 3.18 Optic pathway glioma. Axial noncontrast CT (**a**), FLAIR (**b**), contrast axial (**c**), and sagittal (**d**) T1-weighted images and coronal T2-weighted image (**e**) reveal an expansile complex cystic and solid, heterogeneously enhancing mass lesion in the region of the optic chiasm, hypothalamus, and optic tracts. Mass effect from the tumor compresses the third ventricle, causing obstructive hydrocephalus with dilatation of the lateral ventricles including the temporal horns

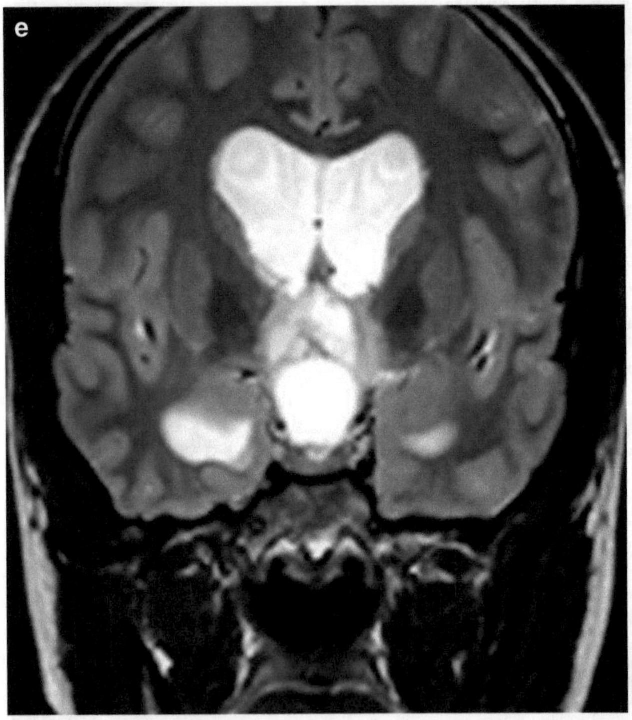

Fig. 3.18 (continued)

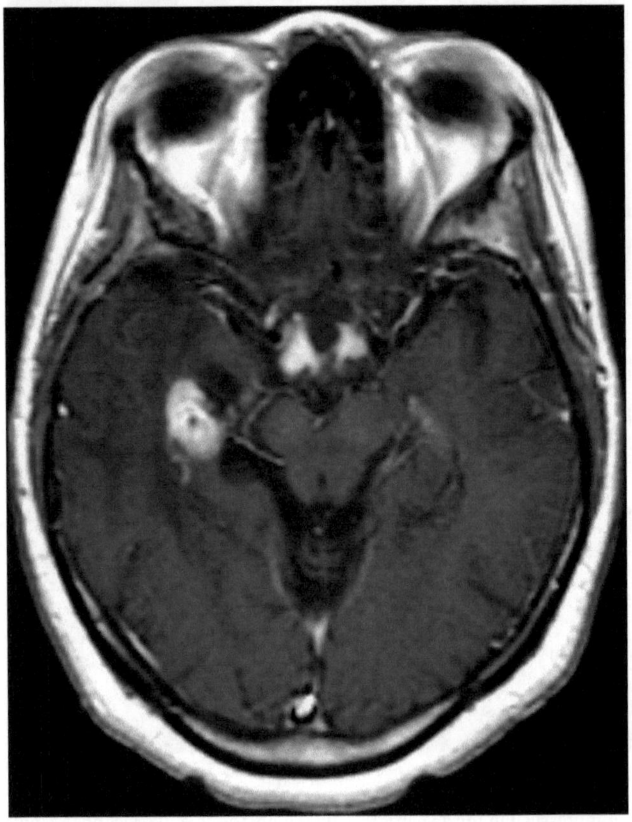

Fig. 3.19 Optic pathway glioma. Axial contrast T1-weighted image shows enhancing tumors in the bilateral optic tracts and in the right mesial temporal lobe near the lateral geniculate nucleus. Contiguous lesions were also present in the optic chiasm and hypothalamus (*not shown*)

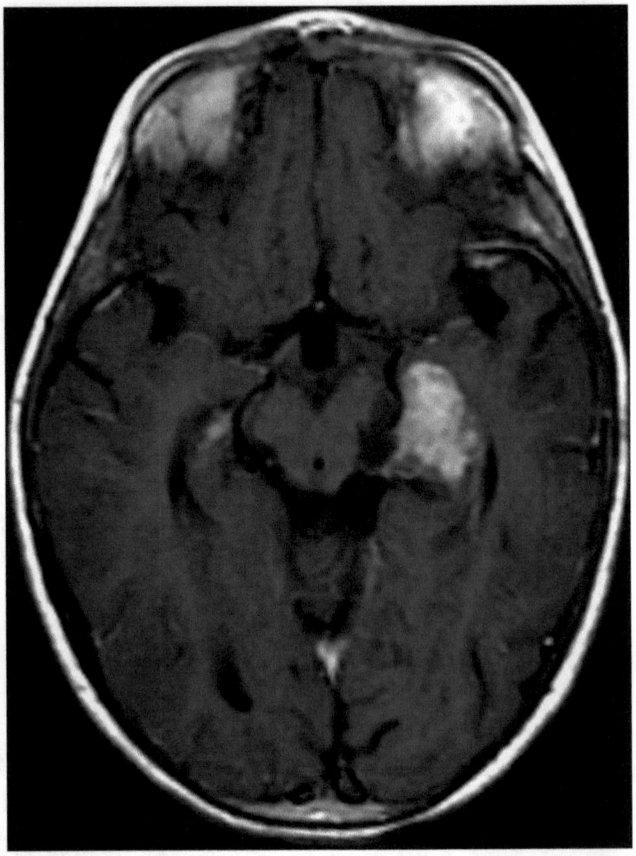

Fig. 3.20 Optic pathway glioma. Axial contrast T1-weighted image shows an enhancing tumor in the left mesial temporal lobe near the lateral geniculate nucleus with sparing of the remaining optic pathway

Pituitary Hypophysitis

Pituitary hypophysitis or autoimmune hypophysitis is visualized as radiographically similar to nonsecreting adenomas of the pituitary gland [14]. There are two histological subtypes of hypophysitis: lymphocytic and granulomatous [14]. Lymphocytic is the most commonly encountered subtype. Lymphocytic hypophysitis occurs most commonly in the female population with a 1:9 male:female ratio [15]. These lesions are often mistaken for adenomas, and are often diagnosed after subtotal resection and histologic correlation [14]. Pituitary hypophysitis is most commonly seen on MR as a thick, uniformly enhancing infundibulum with or without a pituitary mass lesion [14].

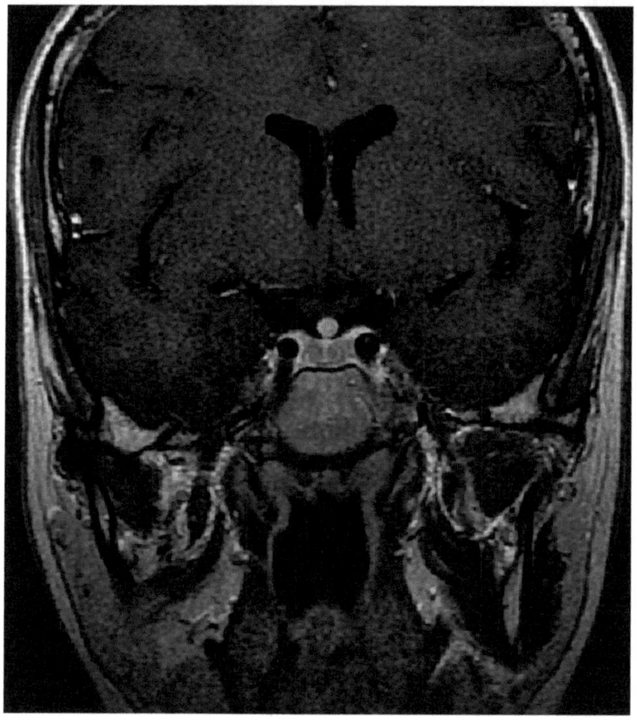

Fig. 3.21 Lymphocytic hypophysitis. Coronal contrast T1-weighted image shows thickening of the midline infundibulum to 0.5 cm with normal pituitary gland. In this postpartum 31-year-old woman who had developed diabetes insipidus with polydipsia and polyuria during her third trimester, the thickened infundibulum although nonspecific is consistent with pregnancy-related autoimmune lymphocytic hypophysitis. The infundibulum returned to a normal size (<3 mm) several months later

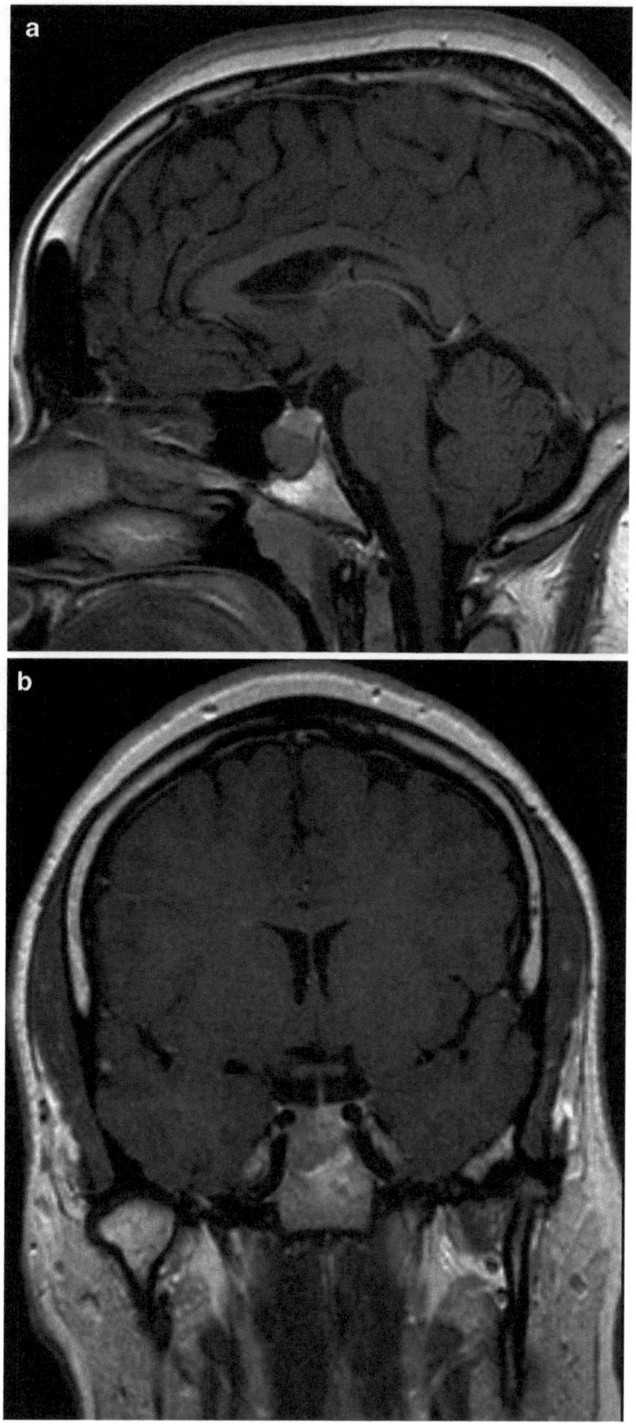

Fig. 3.22 Lymphocytic hypophysitis. Sagittal (**a**) and coronal (**b**) contrast T1-weighted images in a 25-year-old woman demonstrate an enhancing tumor in the sella that grows down into the sphenoid sinus. Pathology revealed a prolactin-expressing pituitary macroadenoma with coexisting lymphocytic hypophysitis

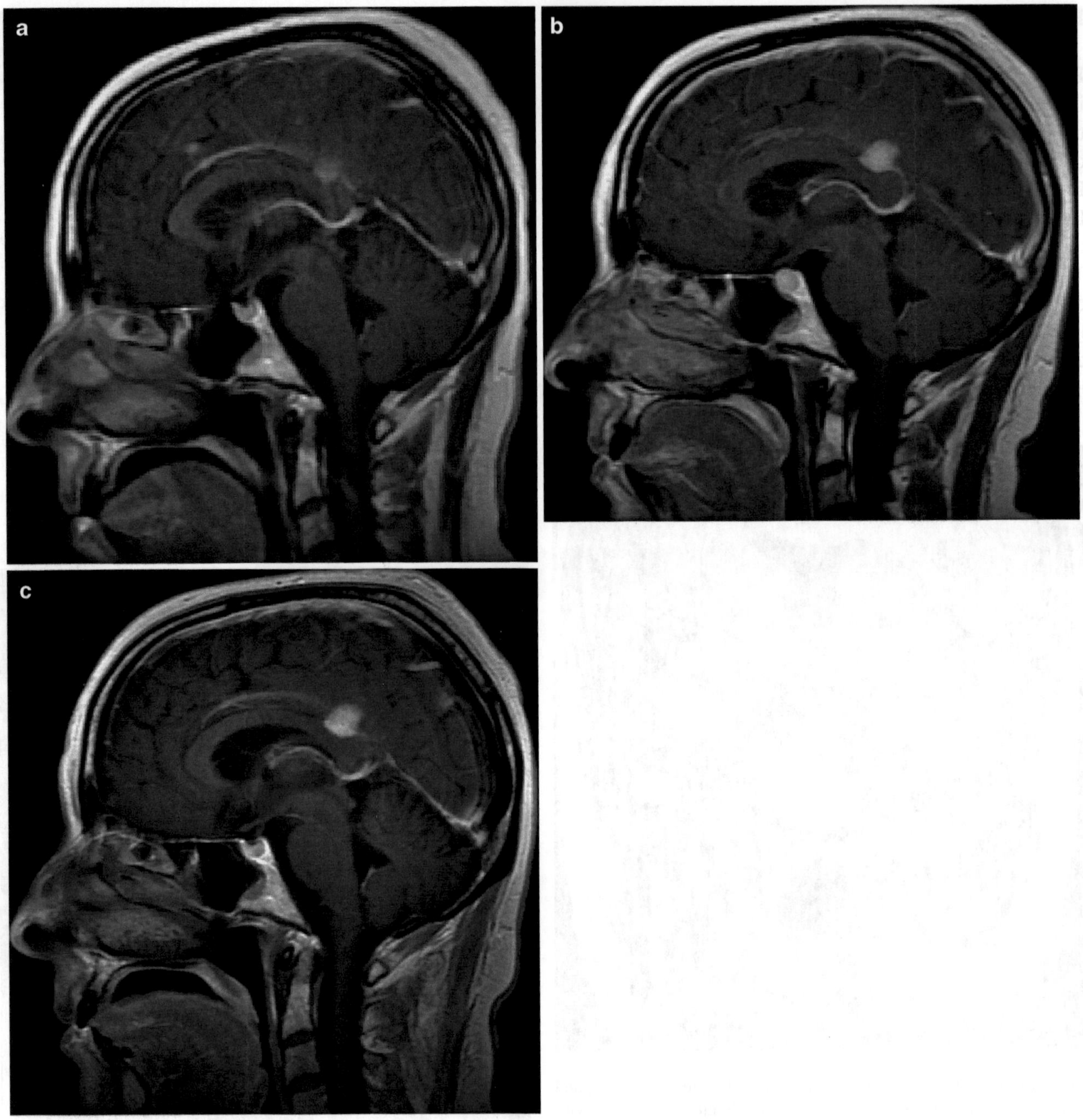

Fig. 3.23 Ipilimumab hypophysitis. Sagittal contrast T1-weighted images obtained before (**a**), during (**b**), and after (**c**) ipilimumab administration in a patient with melanoma. Diffuse homogeneous enlargement of the pituitary gland in (**b**) normalizes in (**c**) after discontinuation of the inciting drug. An enhancing metastasis in the posterior cingulate gyrus in (**a**) increases in (**b**) and then stabilizes in (**c**)

Tuber Cinereum Hamartoma

Tuber cinereum hamartoma is a congenital malformation that can be described as a collection of neurons and glial cells that are located in the tuber cinereum region of the hypothalamus [16]. Tuber cinereum hamartomas are responsible for a third of patients diagnosed with precocious puberty due to excess release of luteinizing hormone-releasing hormone [16, 17]. Although a majority of patients present with symptoms of precocious puberty, seizures are also a common initial presentation. Tuber cinereum hamartoma usually present between the ages of 1 and 3 years old and have no gender predominance [18]. Patients are usually treated medically with hormone suppressants, and surgery is only indicated if medical management fails [16, 18]. Tuber cinereum hamartoma are usually visualized as small, round, nonenhancing lesions on MR and rarely contain cysts or calcium [16].

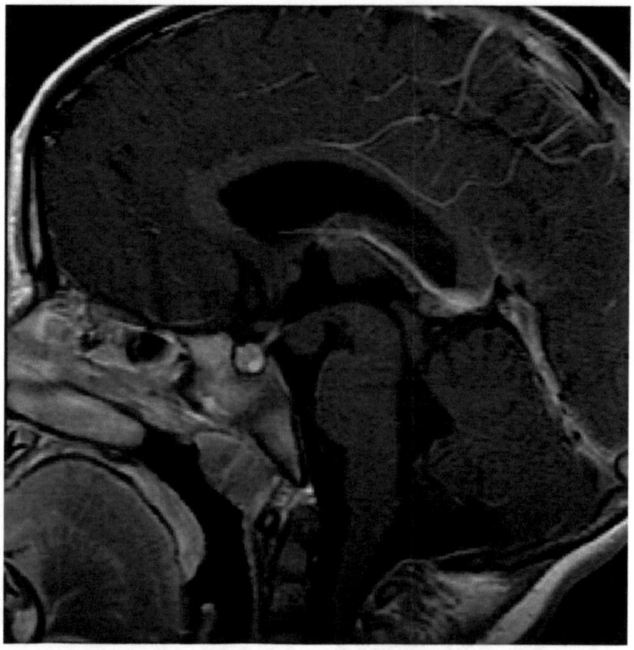

Fig. 3.24 Tuber cinereum hamartoma. Sagittal contrast T1-weighted image shows a nodular lesion located posterior to the infundibulum and anterior to the mammillary bodies along the floor of the anterior third ventricle. The location, lack of enhancement, and isointensity to normal gray matter are diagnostic for a parahypothalamic hamartoma of the tuber cinereum. These are usually found at 10–20 years, more commonly in boys than in girls. Parahypothalamic hamartomas often appear pedunculated and are more likely associated with precocious puberty, whereas intrahypothalamic hamartomas appear sessile, may cause distortion of the floor of the third ventricle, and are more likely associated with gelastic seizures

Langerhans Cell Histiocytosis

Langerhans cell histiocytosis (LCH) is a disease spectrum that evolves as a result of the overproduction of a particular line of dendritic cells that have similar characteristics to Langerhans cells [19]. It is a rapidly progressing disease that can affect virtually any organ within the body and rarely affects the central nervous system (CNS) [19]. The most common CNS manifestation of this disease on MR is a well-circumscribed granuloma located within the sella. Clinical manifestations of this disorder commonly include hormone deficiencies due to invasion of the anterior pituitary [19].

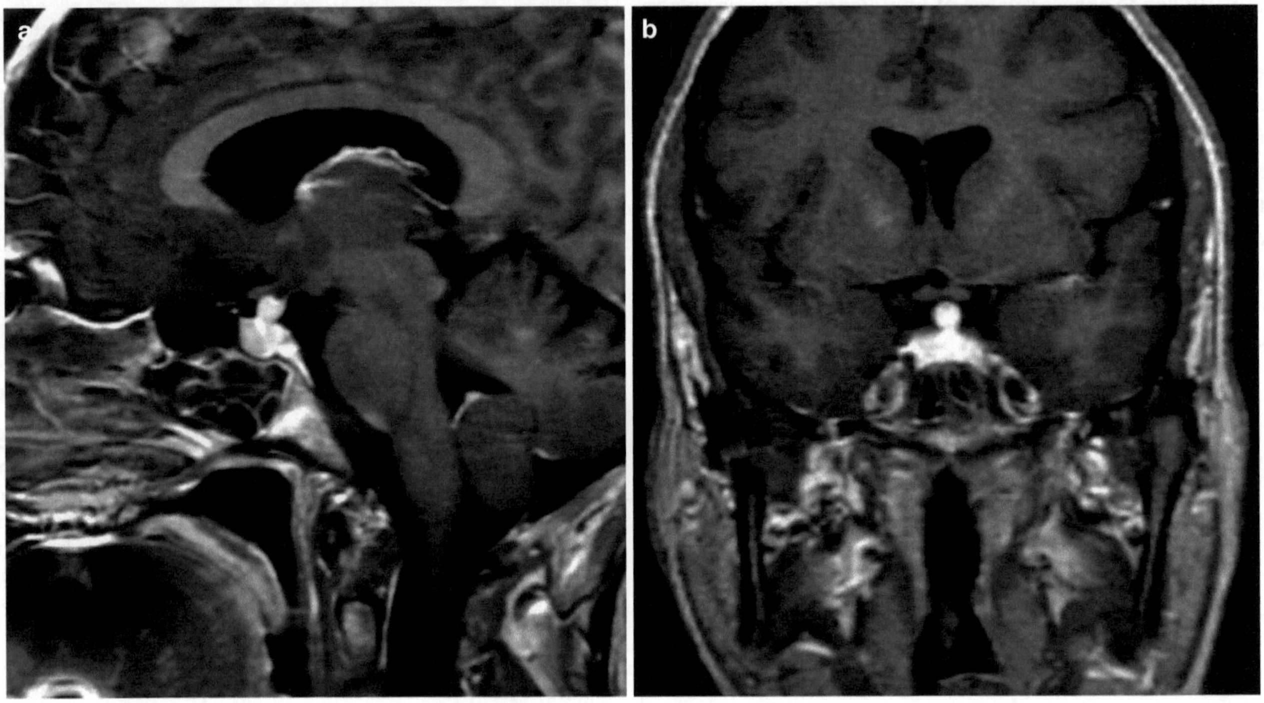

Fig. 3.25 Langerhans cell histiocytosis. Contrast sagittal (**a**) and coronal (**b**) T1-weighted images show thickening of the infundibulum, which is normally less than 3 mm. Loss of the posterior pituitary bright spot (due to vasopressin-containing granules) on pre-contrast images (*not shown*) is consistent with disruption of the normal hypothalamic hypophyseal pathway. One quarter of LCH patients may present with diabetes insipidus. This patient had lytic calvarial lesions consistent with disseminated LCH (*not shown*)

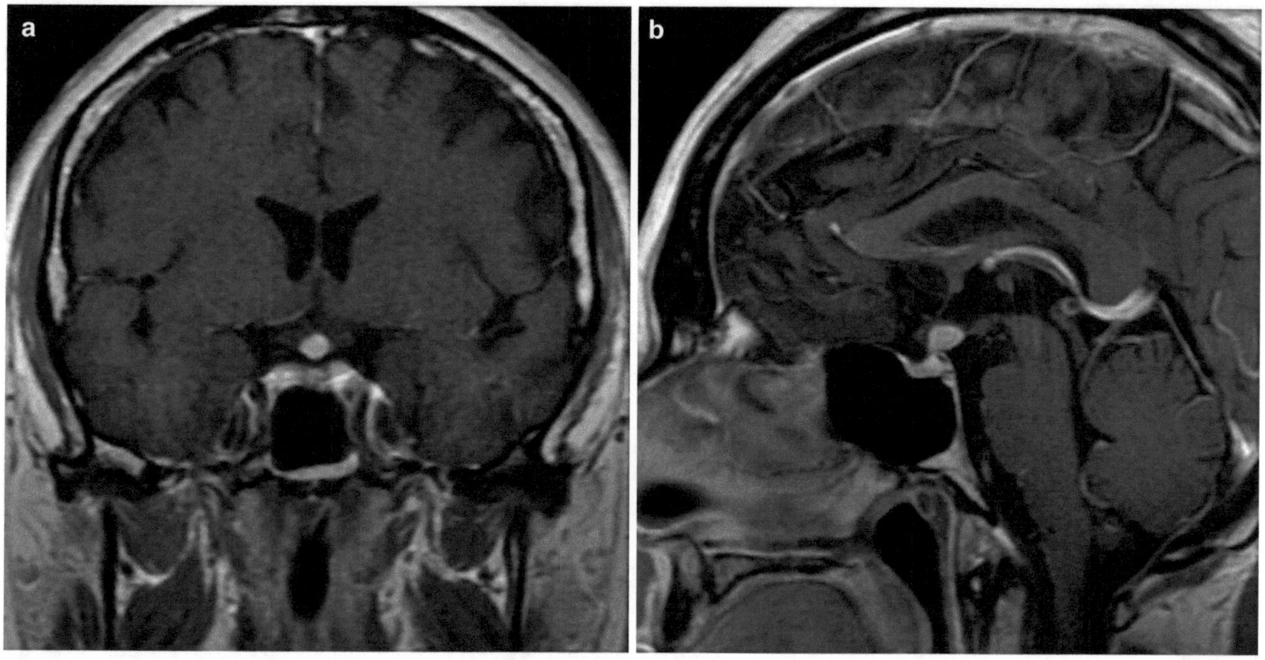

Fig. 3.26 Langerhans cell histiocytosis. Contrast coronal (**a**) and sagittal (**b**) T1-weighted images demonstrate thickening of the infundibulum in a 51-year-old patient (*see* Fig. 3.26). Other possibilities include metastasis, germ cell tumor (in a child), tuberculosis, and sarcoidosis

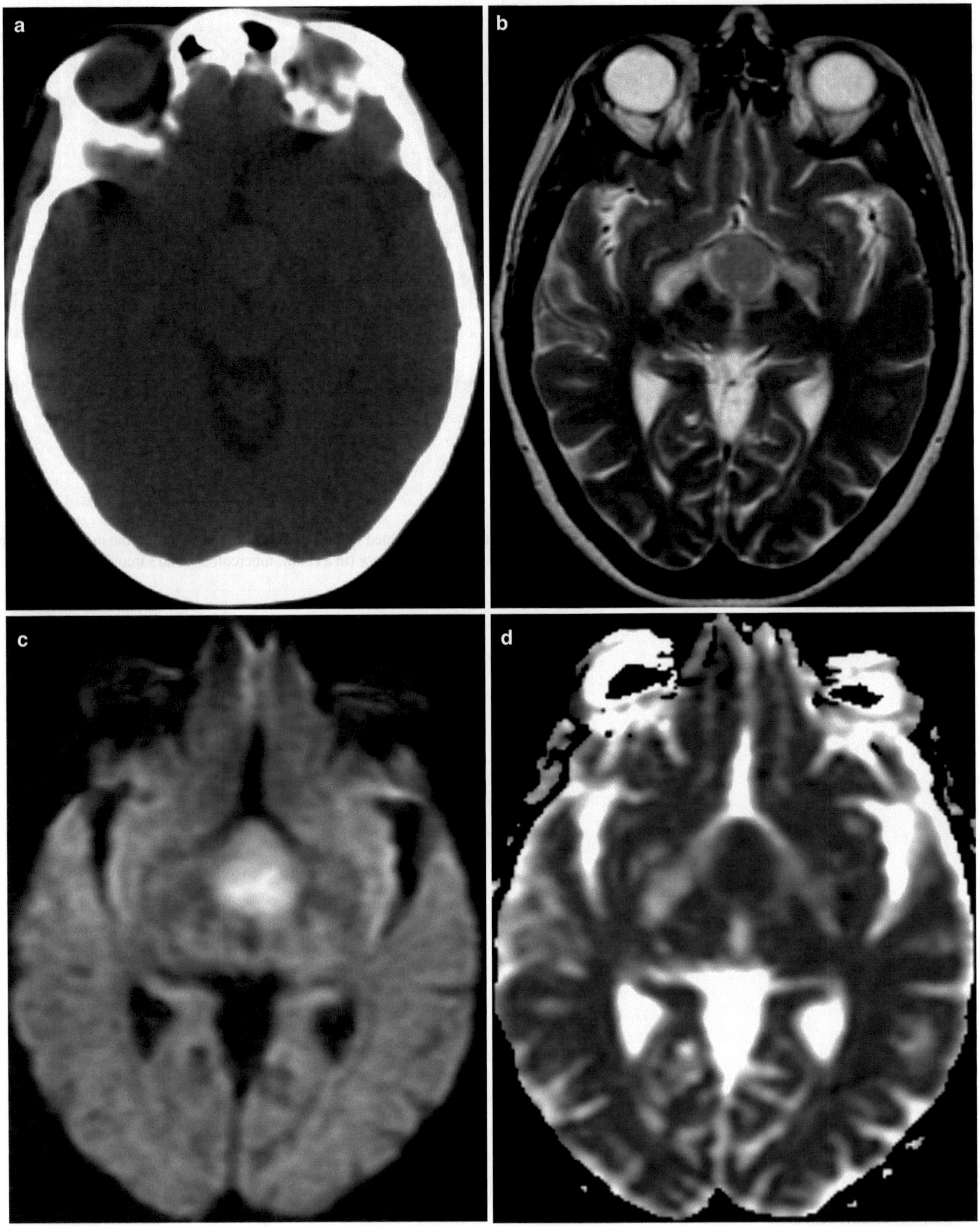

Fig. 3.27 Lymphoma of infundibulum. Axial noncontrast CT (**a**) shows a slightly hyperdense mass of the infundibulum, which is slightly hyperintense on a T2-weighted image (**b**) and diffusion restricted on a diffusion-weighted image (**c**) and apparent diffusion coefficient map (**d**). Contrast axial (**e**) and coronal (**f**) T1-weighted images demonstrate homogeneous enhancement in this lymphoma, where the diffusion restriction is typical for tightly packed cells and high nucleus:cytoplasm ratio, similar to other small, round, blue-cell tumors

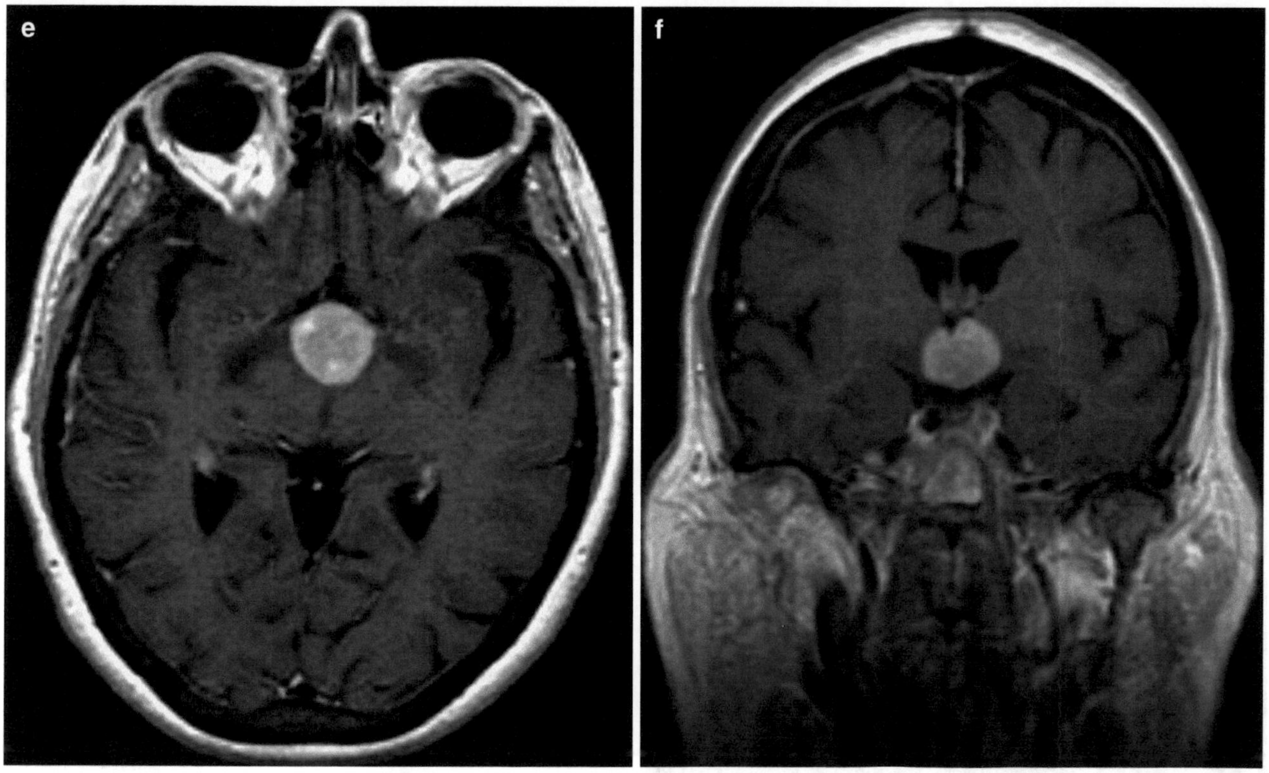

Fig. 3.27 (continued)

Meningioma

A meningioma is a benign slow-growing lesion that arises from the meninges. Meningioma that occurs in the sella/parasellar region of the brain often occur within the midline in the planum sphenoidale or tuberculum sella region [20]. Patients with these lesions usually present with unilateral loss of visual acuity due to compression of optic structures [20]. Surgical resection is only necessary if clinical symptoms are present. Asymptomatic meningioma should be followed by serial imaging. This lesion is most commonly visualized as a dural-based enhancing lesion with the presence of cortical hyperostosis [20, 21].

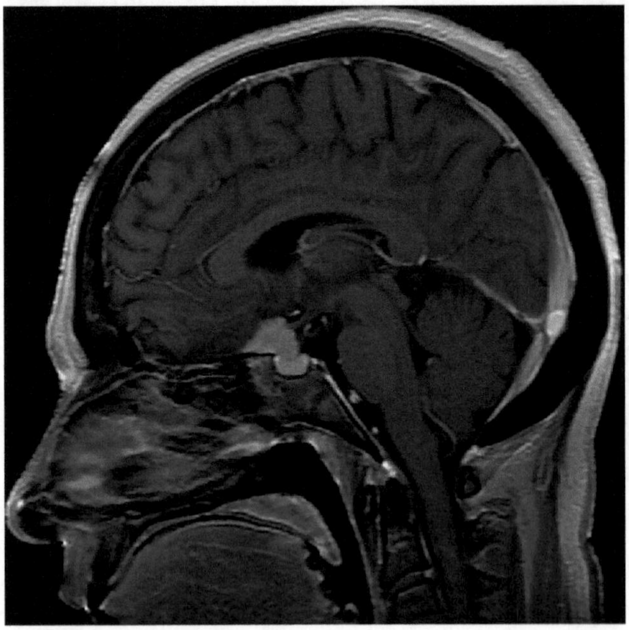

Fig. 3.28 Planum sphenoidale and tuberculum sella meningioma. Contrast sagittal T1-weighted image shows an enhancing extra-axial tumor in the suprasellar cistern with anterior extension and a broad dural base against the planum sphenoidale, and posterior inferior extension over the tuberculum sella toward the sella. Subtle hyperostosis or "blistering" of the dark cortical bone of the planum sphenoidale is diagnostic for a meningioma

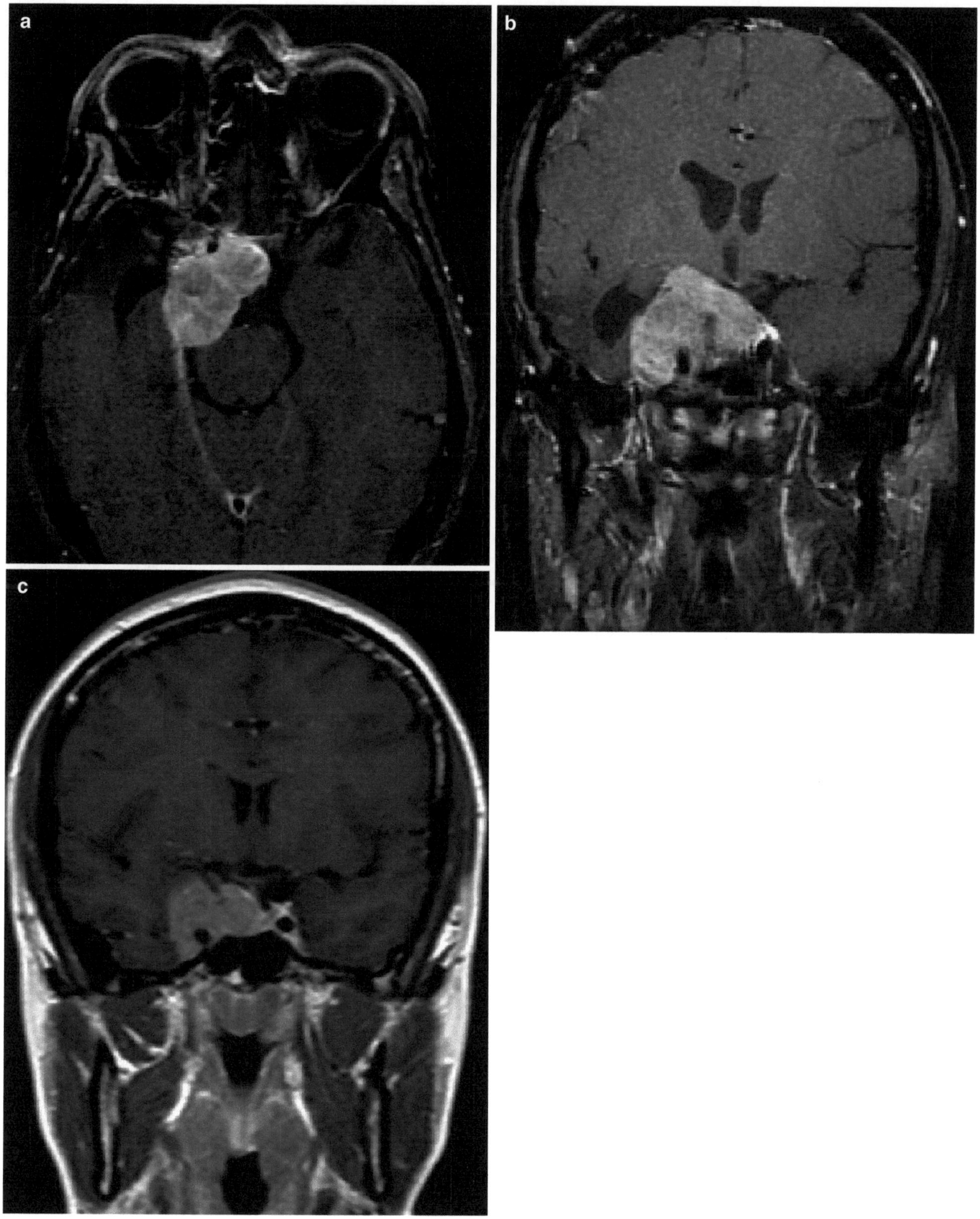

Fig. 3.29 Paracavernous sinus meningioma. Contrast axial (**a**) and coronal T1-weighted images with (**b**) and without (**c**) fat saturation demonstrate an expansile extra-axial enhancing tumor centered in the right cavernous sinus and paracavernous sinus region. There is medial extension into the sella and suprasellar cistern, with mass effect upon the infundibulum, lateral extension into the middle cranial fossa, and posterior extension along the petroclival ligament into the basal and prepontine cisterns

References

1. Johnsen DE, Woodruff WW, Allen IS, et al. MR imaging of the sellar and juxtasellar regions. Radiographics. 1991;11:727–58.
2. Osborne AG. Sella and pituitary. In: Mascarenaz AD, Dearth CL, Kaerli M, editors. Diagnostic imaging: brain. Salt Lake City: Amirsys; 2005. p. 4–7.
3. Bronstein MD, Paraiba DB, Jallad RS. Management of pituitary tumors in pregnancy. Nat Rev Endocrinol. 2011;7:301–10.
4. Osborne AG. Sella and pituitary. In: Mascarenaz AD, Dearth CL, Kaerli M, editors. Diagnostic imaging: brain. Salt Lake City: Amirsys; 2005. p. 20–2.
5. Cottier JP, Destriex C, Brunereau L, et al. Cavernous sinus invasion by pituitary adenoma: MR imaging. Radiology. 2000;215:463–9.
6. Osborne AG. Sella and pituitary. In: Mascarenaz AD, Dearth CL, Kaerli M, editors. Diagnostic imaging: brain. Salt Lake City: Amirsys; 2005. p. 24–6.
7. Berkmann S, Fandino J, Zosso S, et al. Intraoperative magnetic resonance imaging and early prognosis for vision after transsphenoidal surgery for sellar lesions. J Neurosurg. 2011;115:518–27.
8. Byun WB, Kim OL, Kim DS. MR imaging findings of Rathke's cleft cysts: significance of intracystic nodules. AJNR Am J Neuroradiol. 2000;21:485–8.
9. Osborne AG. Sella and pituitary. In: Mascarenaz AD, Dearth CL, Kaerli M, editors. Diagnostic imaging: brain. Salt Lake City: Amirsys; 2005. p. 16–8.
10. Gupta DK, Ojha BK, Sarkar C, et al. Recurrence in craniopharyngiomas: analysis of clinical and histological features. J Clin Neurosci. 2006;13:438–42.
11. Osborne AG. Sella and pituitary. In: Mascarenaz AD, Dearth CL, Kaerli M, editors. Diagnostic imaging: brain. Salt Lake City: Amirsys; 2005. p. 32–4.
12. Shin JL, Asa SL, Woodhouse LJ, et al. Cystic lesions of the pituitary: clinicopathological features distinguishing craniopharyngioma, Rathke's cleft cyst, and arachnoid cyst. J Clin Endocrinol Metabol. 1999;84:3972–82.
13. Kornreich L, Blaser S, Schwarz M, et al. Optic pathway glioma: correlation of imaging findings with the presence of neurofibromatosis. AJNR Am J Neuroradiol. 2001;22: 1963–9.
14. Gutenberg A, Larsen J, Lupi I, et al. A radiologic score to distinguish autoimmune hypophysitis from nonsecreting pituitary adenoma preoperatively. AJNR Am J Neuroradiol. 2009;30:1766–72.
15. Osborne AG. Sella and pituitary. In: Mascarenaz AD, Dearth CL, Kaerli M, editors. Diagnostic imaging: brain. Salt Lake City: Amirsys; 2005. p. 40–1.
16. Saleem SN, Said A-HM, Lee DH. Lesions of the hypothalamus: MR imaging diagnostic features. Radiographics. 2007;27: 1087–108.
17. Arita K, Ikawa F, Kurisu K, et al. The relationship between magnetic resonance imaging findings and clinical manifestations of hypothalamic hamartoma. J Neurosurg. 1999;91: 212–22.
18. Osborne AG. Sella and pituitary. In: Mascarenaz AD, Dearth CL, Kaerli M, editors. Diagnostic imaging: brain. Salt Lake City: Amirsys; 2005. p. 12–4.
19. Grois N, Prayer D, Prosch H, et al. Neuropathology of CNS disease in Langerhans cell histiocytosis. Brain. 2005;128:829–38.
20. Massachusetts General Hospital. Tuberculum sellae meningioma. Accessible at: http://neurosurgery.mgh.harvard.edu/cranialbase-center/c94.htm. Accessed 1 Dec 2011.
21. Osborne AG. Skull, scalp, and meninges. In: Mascarenaz AD, Dearth CL, Kaerli M, editors. Diagnostic imaging: brain. Salt Lake City: Amirsys; 2005. p. 56–8.

Neoplastic Disease of the Spine

4

Alan Victor Krauthamer, Sasan Partovi, and John Lyo

The spinal axis may be divided into three compartments: extradural, intradural extramedullary, or intramedullary. When evaluating spinal pathology, it is essential to first determine the compartment affected by the lesion in order to arrive at an appropriate diagnosis. Different neoplasms affect different compartments by virtue of their corresponding anatomic contents. For example, primary bone neoplasms such as osteoblastoma occur in the extradural compartment where the bony vertebral elements reside. As a result, one may use location as a reliable discriminatory factor in the quest for accurate diagnosis. That said, the same exact pathology may often times affect different compartments in isolation or simultaneously. For example, metastatic disease may involve any of the compartments including the intramedullary space. Some tumors may affect more than one compartment simultaneously. The classic example of this is a peripheral nerve sheath tumor such as a schwannoma. These neoplasms often involve the intradural extramedullary space, but also extend beyond the confines of the spinal canal into the extradural space via the adjacent neural foramina or vice versa.

As a general rule, to accurately determine a lesion's location, one should pay close attention to its margins, as well as to its effect on the subjacent cerebrospinal fluid (CSF) space. Extradural neoplasms tend to have a clear CSF interface between them and the spinal cord and often times narrow the intervening CSF space. In contrast, intradural extramedullary lesions tend to widen the ipsilateral CSF space by displacing and often compressing the spinal cord or cauda equina nerve roots in the contralateral direction. Finally, intramedullary neoplasms typically result in space-occupying expansion of the spinal cord, resulting in circumferential narrowing of the CSF space and often remodeling of the subjacent vertebra leading to spinal canal widening.

The goal of this chapter is to provide the reader with a comprehensive understanding of the various neoplasms occurring within each spinal compartment so that in association with other factors such as clinical presentation, age, and gender, they may generate an appropriate differential diagnosis and ultimately arrive at the correct diagnosis. Complications affecting the spinal axis in association with high-dose radiotherapy will be addressed as a separate topic at the conclusion of the chapter.

A.V. Krauthamer (✉)
Department of Radiology,
New York Presbyterian Hospital/Weill Cornell Medical College,
New York, NY, USA

Department of Radiology, Division of Neuroradiology,
Memorial Sloan-Kettering Cancer Center,
1275 York Avenue, MRI-1156, New York, NY 10065, USA
e-mail: avkmd1@gmail.com

S. Partovi
Department of Radiology, Memorial Sloan-Kettering Cancer Center,
1275 York Avenue, MRI-1156, New York, NY 10065, USA
e-mail: sasanp@gmx.de

J. Lyo
Department of Radiology,
New York Presbyterian Hospital/Weill Cornell Medical College,
New York, NY, USA

Department of Radiology, Neuroradiology Service,
Memorial Sloan-Kettering Cancer Center,
1275 York Avenue, MRI-1156, New York, NY 10065, USA
e-mail: lyoj@mskcc.org

S. Karimi (ed.), *Atlas of Brain and Spine Oncology Imaging*, Atlas of Oncology Imaging,
DOI 10.1007/978-1-4614-5653-7_4, © Springer Science+Business Media New York 2013

Extradural Neoplasms

Enostosis/Bone Island

Enostoses are most commonly referred to as bone islands. They are incidentally discovered, asymptomatic, benign developmental lesions consisting of lamellated compact bone with a haversian system embedded within the medullary cavity typically just beneath the cortex [1]. They tend to occur within the axial skeleton, particularly within the spine, pelvis, and ribs. They vary in size but are usually less than 1 cm. Lesions greater than 2 cm are often referred to as giant bone islands. The margins of these lesions are usually irregular or spiculated; however, the adjacent trabecular bone is strikingly normal, helping to distinguish them from osteoblastic metastasis that may have a similar appearance. Other helpful distinguishing characteristics include size, stability, and absence of radiotracer uptake on bone scintigraphy. Yet, this is not an absolute rule, as bone islands may sometimes enlarge over time and some larger bone islands have been shown to accumulate radiotracer activity on bone scintigraphy due to increased osteoblastic activity [1].

On magnetic resonance imaging (MRI), bone islands are typically nonenhancing, homogenously hypointense, following the same signal as cortical bone on all pulse sequences. The signal intensity of the adjacent marrow is normal, helping to distinguish the lesion from a sclerotic metastasis [1].

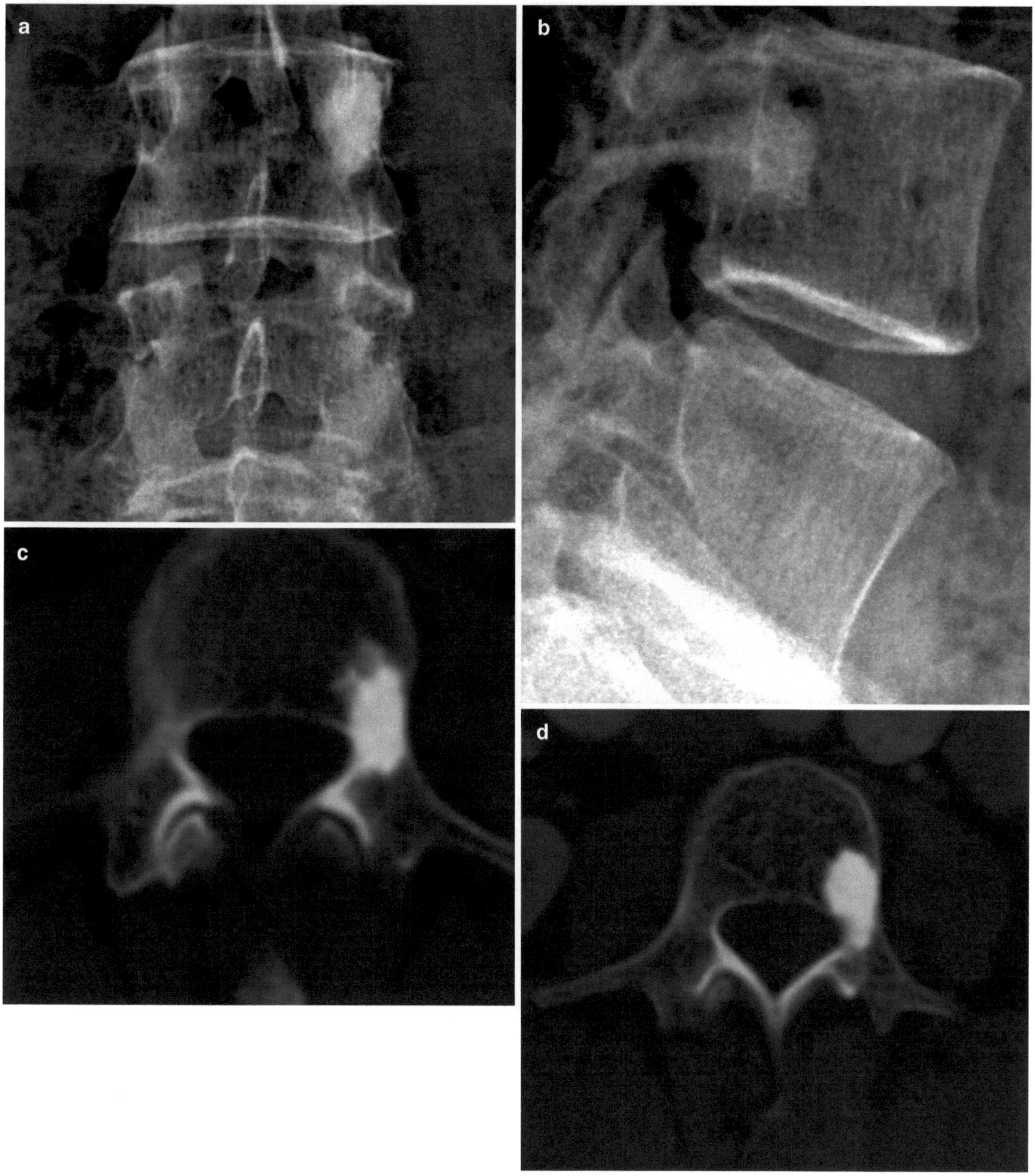

Fig. 4.1 Bone island. Anteroposterior (AP) and lateral conventional radiographs (**a** and **b**) of the lumbar spine demonstrate an ovoid, sclerotic lesion centered within the left pedicle of the L4 vertebral body. Given its nonspecific appearance further work-up is required to exclude an osteoblastic metastasis. Axial CT images (**c** and **d**) further delineate the margins of the lesion, which appear irregular and spiculated. Sagittal T1 (**e**), sagittal T2 (**f**), and axial T2 (**g**), MRI demonstrates the lesion to be homogeneously T1/T2 hypointense, following the same signal intensity as cortical bone, with well-defined, spiculated margins. MRI helps determine that the surrounding vertebral marrow is normal, thereby supporting a diagnosis of enostosis rather than osteoblastic metastasis. No enhancement was present following contrast administration

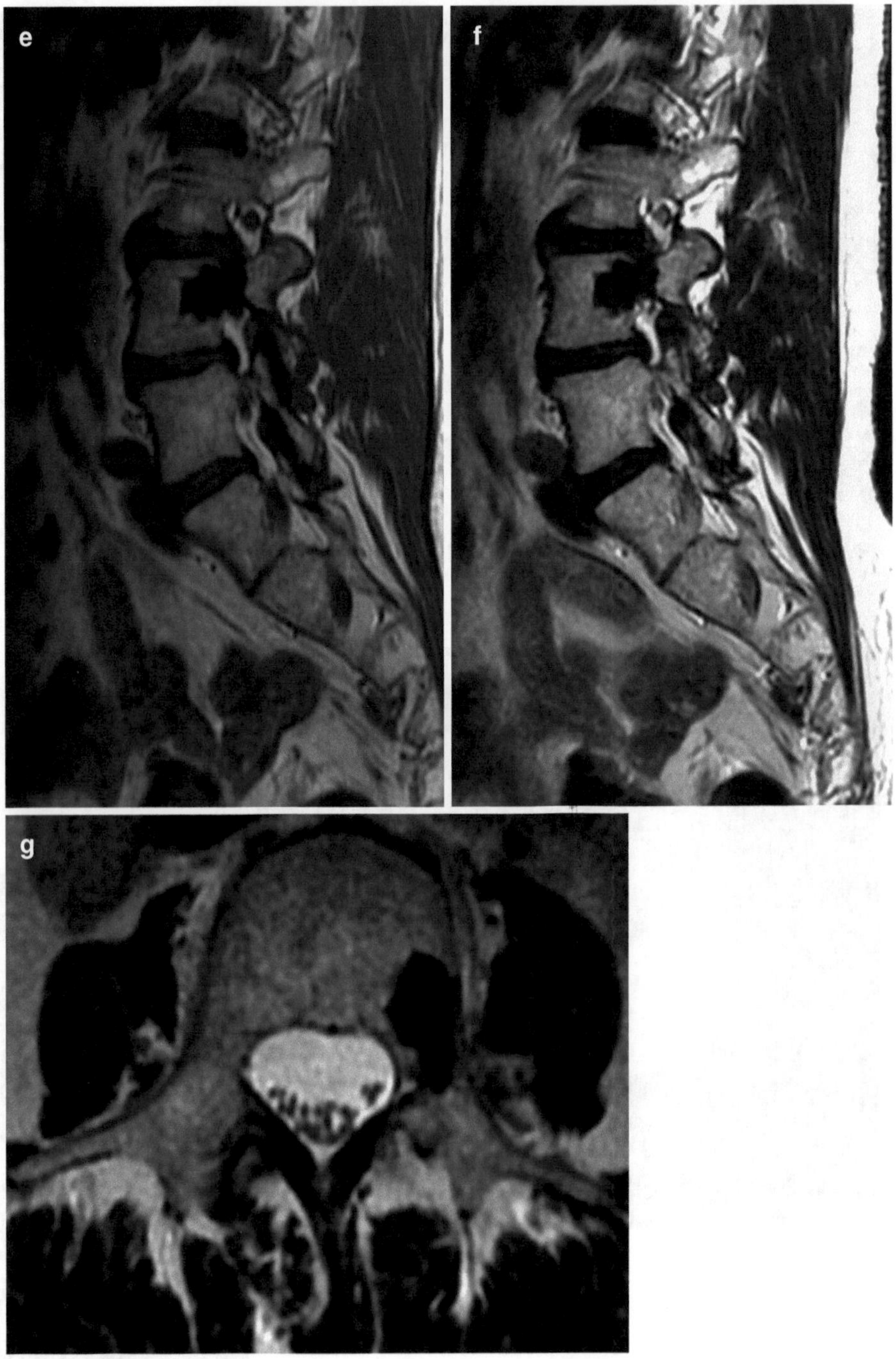

Fig. 4.1 (continued)

Hemangioma

Vertebral hemangiomas are benign, usually asymptomatic, incidental, vascular lesions with a slight female predilection and an increased incidence with age. They may be solitary or multiple and most commonly occur within the lower thoracic and upper lumbar spine [2]. In some cases they may exhibit aggressive features, extending beyond the confines of the vertebral body into the posterior elements, epidural space, and neural foramina, resulting in spinal cord or nerve root impingement. Vertebral hemangiomas are composed of endothelium-lined capillary and cavernous sinuses with interspersed vertical bony trabeculae and adipose tissue [3]. Due to infiltration of the medullary cavity, there is resultant compensatory thickening of the vertical trabeculae, making pathologic compression fracture a rare occurrence.

On computed tomography (CT), the thickened vertical trabeculae give the lesion its characteristic "corduroy" or "honeycomb" appearance when viewed in the sagittal plane and a "polka dot" appearance when viewed in the axial plane. On MRI, hemangiomas typically exhibit hyperintense T1 and T2 signal due to the presence of fatty stroma. The hyperintense T1 signal is the hallmark of this lesion. No other nonexostotic tumor except some melanoma metastases exhibits this particular feature [2]. Avid post-contrast enhancement is characteristic. Occasionally, hemangiomas with less adipose tissue will be iso- or hypointense on T1 and as a result may be difficult to distinguish from a metastasis, particularly when multiple. On short TI inversion recovery (STIR) or T2 fat-saturation imaging, hemangiomas containing higher adipose content will demonstrate hypointense signal whereas those with less adipose content may demonstrate hyperintense signal.

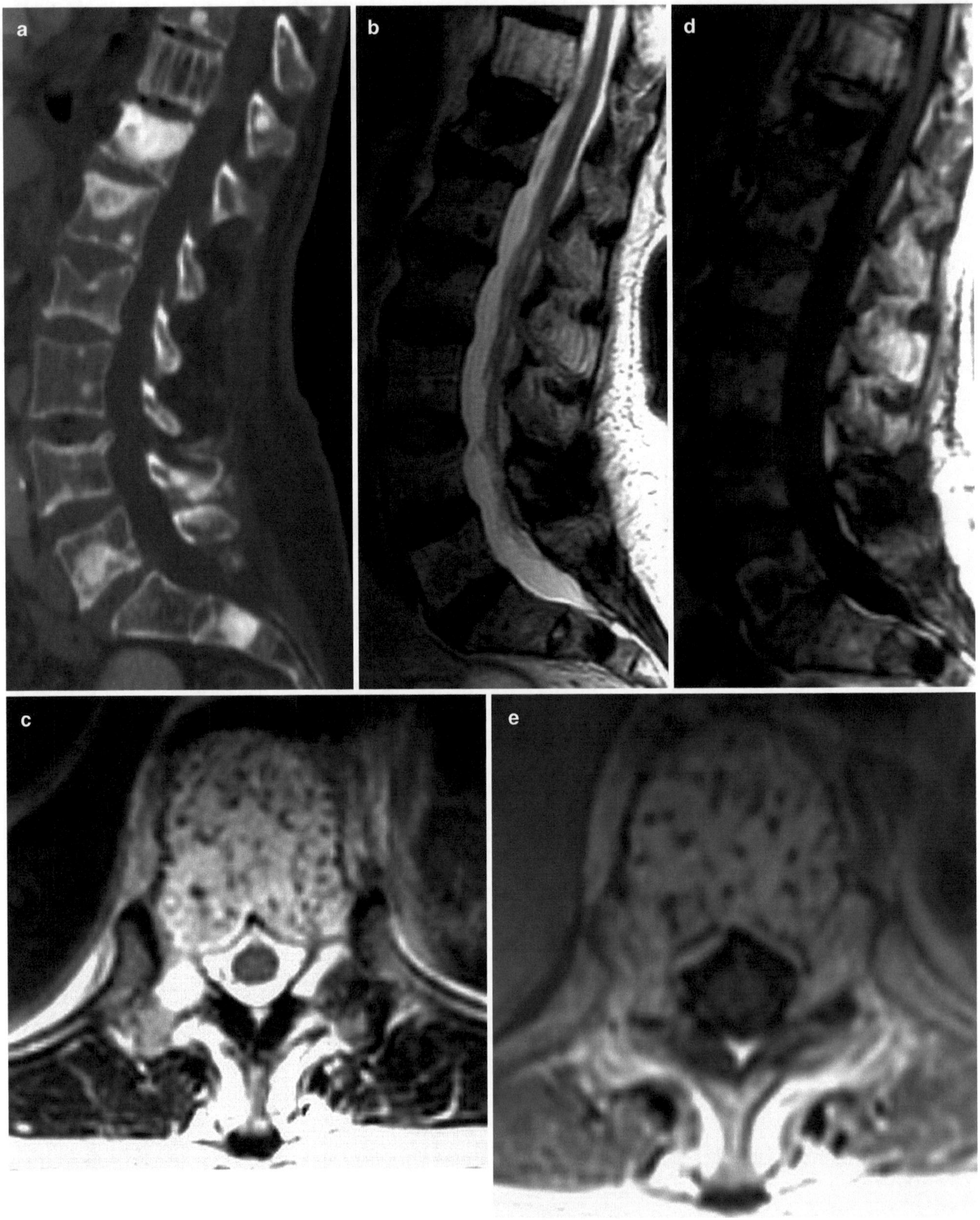

Fig. 4.2 Vertebral hemangioma. Sagittal reformatted CT image (**a**) demonstrates a slightly expansile lesion within the T11 vertebral body containing coarsened vertical trabeculae and interspersed areas of hypodense fatty attenuation producing a "corduroy" appearance characteristic of a vertebral hemangioma. Multilevel, multifocal, sclerotic vertebral metastases are also noted in this patient with known prostate carcinoma. Sagittal T2 (**b**), axial T2 (**c**) and sagittal T1 (**d**) weighted MRI depicts the lesion's characteristic T1/T2 hyperintense signal resulting from high adipose content. The axial T2 image further delineates the lesion's margins extending into the pedicles and ventral epidural space. The coarsened hypointense trabeculae produce the characteristic "polka dot" appearance on axial imaging. Axial contrast T1-weighted (**e**) MRI demonstrates enhancing, epidural, extraosseous extension, a feature that is less common and may sometimes produce cord impingement. In symptomatic cases surgical intervention, transarterial embolization or often times localized radiation therapy may be indicated. Radiation therapy alone may produce satisfactory results secondary to vessel obliteration and tumor shrinkage [3]

Aneurysmal Bone Cyst

Aneurysmal bone cysts (ABC) are pseudotumoral, hyperemic, hemorrhagic lesions of unknown etiology typically presenting before age 20 [4]. They are most commonly found within the long bones of the lower extremities, followed by those of the upper extremities [5]. Twelve to thirty percent of ABCs occur within the mobile spine, most commonly affecting the thoracic segments, followed by the lumbar and cervical spine [6]. They are usually centered within the posterior elements with frequent extension into the vertebral body. Sometimes they may extend into adjacent vertebral bodies, across intervertebral disc spaces, or into adjacent ribs or paraspinal soft tissues. ABCs are classified as primary if no underlying lesion is present or secondary if found in association with bone tumors such as giant cell tumor, osteoblastoma, chondroblastoma, or osteosarcoma. Pathologically, they are multiloculated blood-filled spaces that are not lined by endothelium. Solid components consisting of giant cells, fibrous tissue, and reactive bone may be found interspersed between the blood-filled cystic spaces. Rarely, ABCs may be predominantly solid, thereby referred to as solid variant ABCs, comprising approximately 5–7.5 % of cases, with an unusual predilection for the spine [1].

On CT, ABCs are expansile, lytic lesions lacking mineralized matrix contained by a thin periosteal layer. In approximately one third of cases, fluid levels consisting of hemorrhage with sedimentation may be observed [2]. MRI is more sensitive for detecting fluid levels that may sometimes be hyperintense on T1 due to the presence of methemoglobin. On T2-weighted MRI, ABCs are predominantly hyperintense, marginated by a low signal intensity rim of intact periosteum. Following contrast administration, enhancement is usually seen along the margins and septations separating the nonenhancing blood filled spaces.

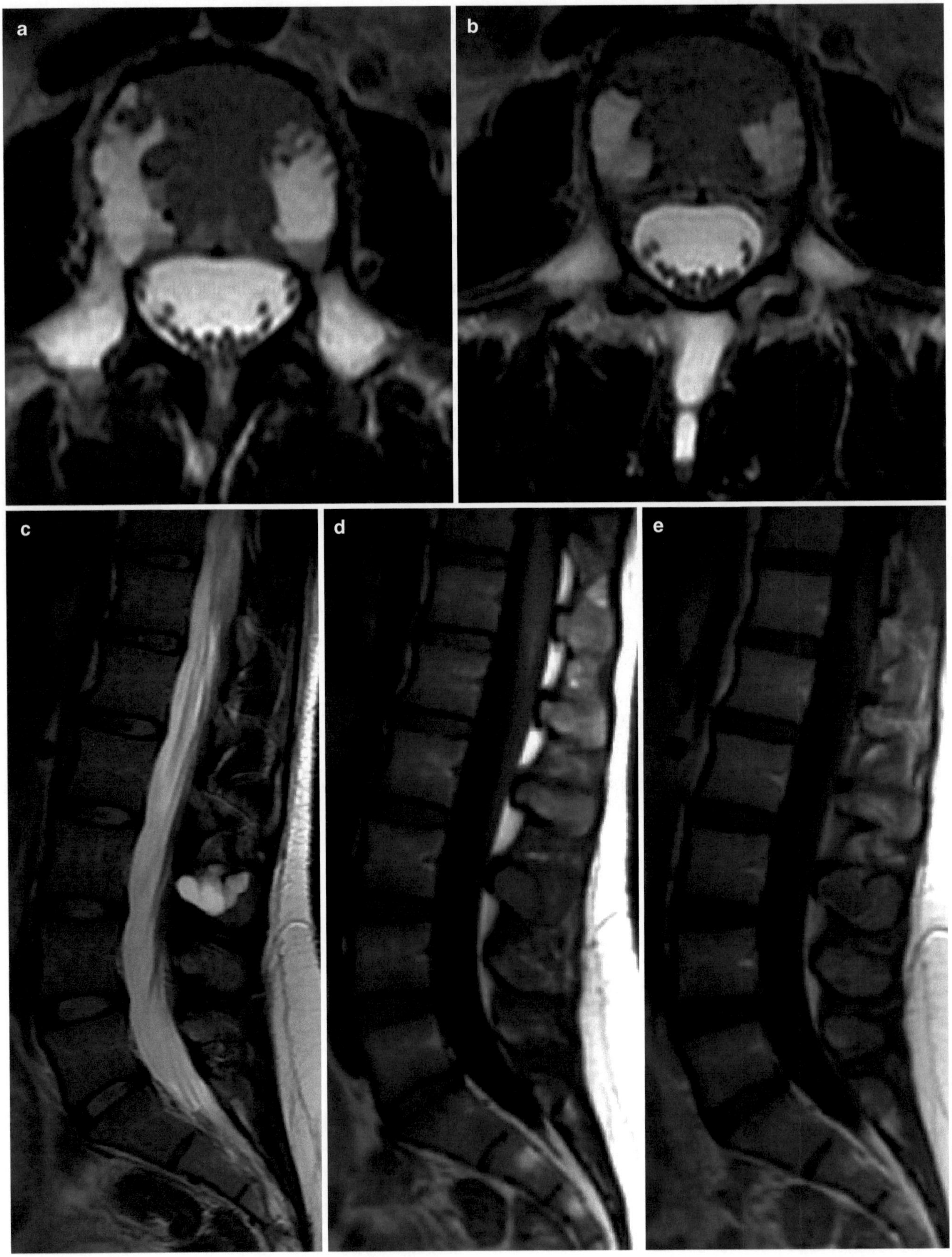

Fig. 4.3 Aneurysmal bone cyst. Axial T2- (**a** and **b**) and sagittal T2- (**c**) weighted MRI demonstrates a multicystic lesion expanding the L3 spinous process extending into the pedicles, transverse processes, and vertebral body. The lesion is largely T2 hyperintense and contains multiple lower signal intensity fluid levels. On sagittal T1 (**d**) and sagittal contrast T1 (**e**) weighted images, the lesion demonstrates predominantly low T1 signal characteristics with only marginal enhancement following gadolinium administration

Osteoid Osteoma

Osteoid osteomas are benign, primary, osteoblastic neoplasms typically affecting children between 10 and 20 years of age, with a male predominance ranging from 2:1 to 3:1 [1]. They are most often found within the lumbar spine (59 %), followed by the cervical (29 %) and thoracic spine (12 %) [1]. They commonly affect the posterior elements of the vertebra (pedicles, laminae, articular facets), and much less frequently involve the vertebral body [1]. Unlike osteoblastomas, osteoid osteomas are less than 1.5 cm in size and present with intense rather than dull back pain that exacerbates at night, but is relieved by aspirin [6]. Painful scoliosis may be present with convexity occurring opposite the side of the lesion. Osteoid osteomas consist of a nidus of vascular fibrous connective tissue surrounded by osteoid matrix.

Nuclear medicine bone scintigraphy is often utilized for initial localization of a suspected nidus, which appears as a focal region of avid radionuclide uptake. On CT, the nidus is typically hypodense with or without areas of central calcification surrounded by sclerotic reactive bone. On MRI, the lesions are usually heterogeneous in signal intensity. The calcified central nidus and peripheral reactive sclerosis is T1/T2 hypointense. The noncalcified portion of the nidus is T2 hyperintense and T1 isointense with associated enhancement following contrast administration. The peripheral sclerotic reactive marrow may also demonstrate enhancement.

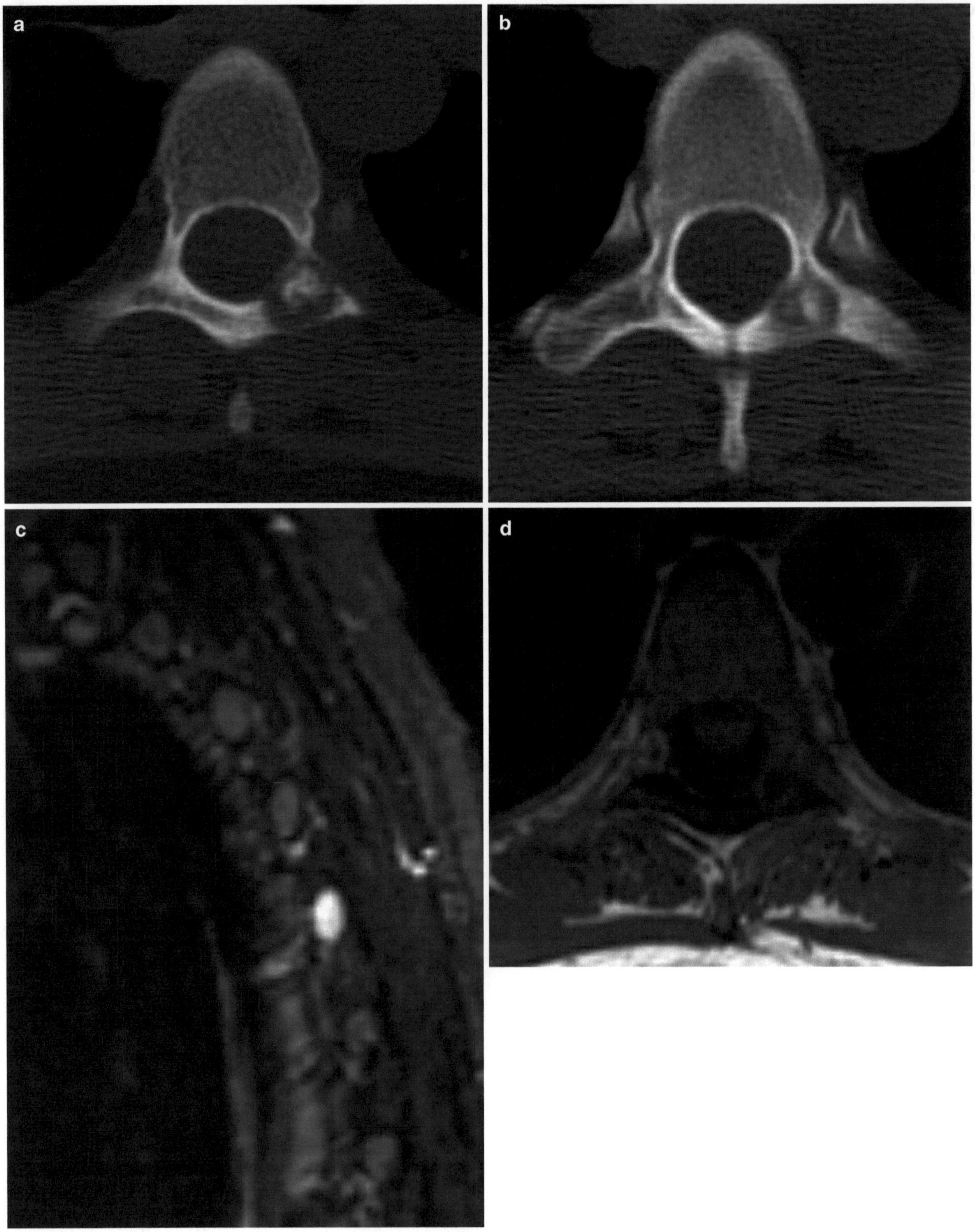

Fig. 4.4 Osteoid osteoma. Axial CT images (**a** and **b**) demonstrate a 1.5 cm peripherally hypodense lesion with central mineralized matrix within the left lamina of the T4 vertebral body. Reactive surrounding sclerosis is notable, particularly within the left lamina and transverse process. Sagittal STIR (**c**) and axial T1 (**d**) weighted MR images demonstrate the nidus to be markedly STIR hyperintense, peripherally T1 isointense and centrally T1 hypointense. Following contrast administration (**e**), the peripheral portion of the nidus enhances, whereas the mineralized central portion does not. On Tc99m MDP bone scintigraphy (**f** and **g**), the lesion is easily detected due to its characteristic intense focal radionuclide uptake

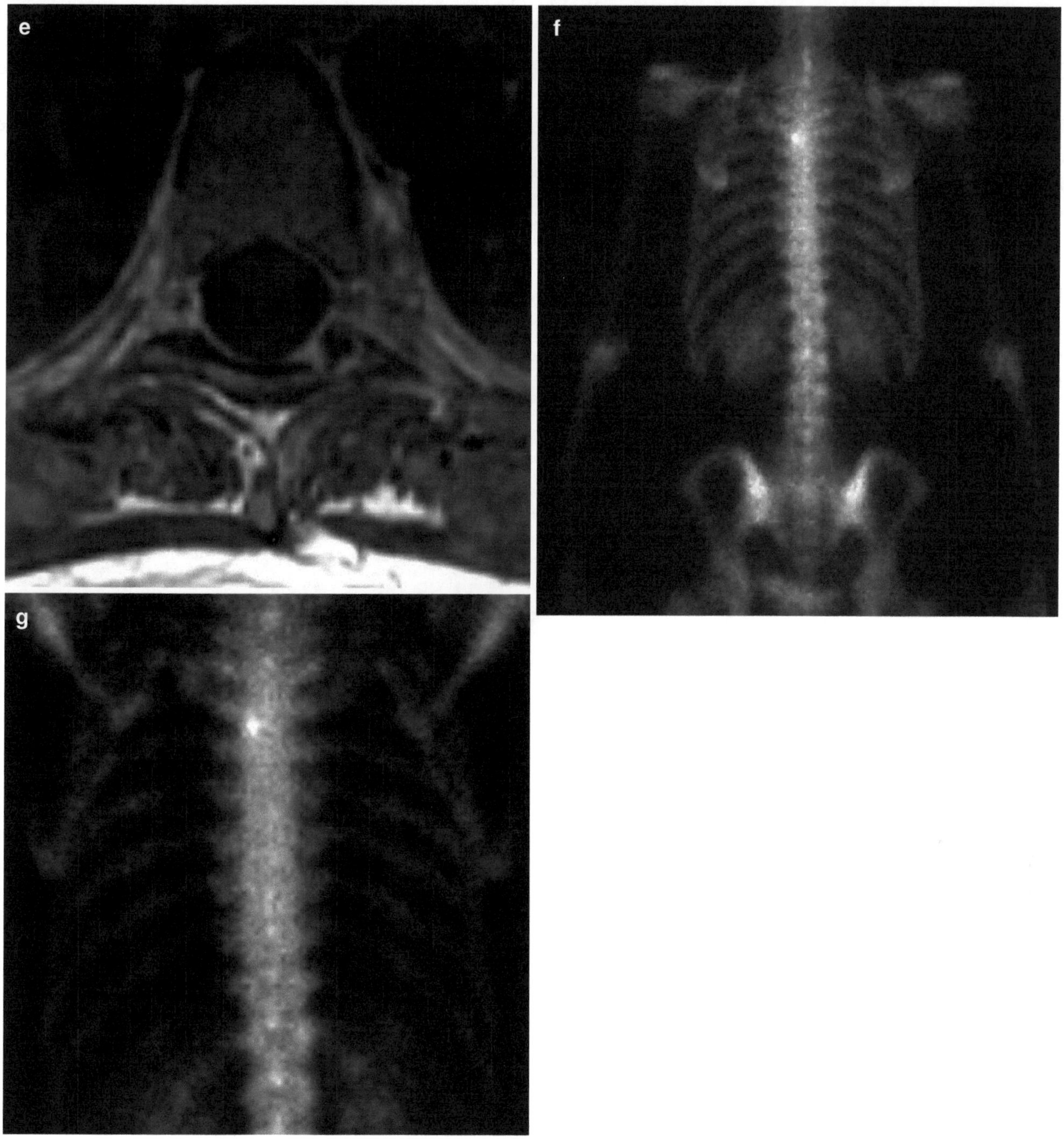

Fig. 4.4 (continued)

Osteoblastoma

Osteoblastomas are benign, primary, bone neoplasms, 90 % occurring in young adults in the second and third decades of life with a 2:1 male predominance [1, 6]. These lesions typically occur within the posterior elements but may extend into or occur within the vertebral body. They are histologically similar to an osteoid osteoma but are differentiated by their size and associated clinical symptoms. Osteoblastomas are usually greater than 1.5–2 cm and, unlike osteoid osteomas, produce dull localized pain and paresthesias, as opposed to intense night pain without neurologic symptoms [1, 7]. Like osteoid osteomas, they are also associated with scoliosis; however, the scoliotic convexity is typically toward the side of the tumor [1].

On CT or plain radiographs, the lesions are expansile with lucent and partially calcified centers often surrounded by a peripheral rim of sclerosis. They sometimes may have a more aggressive appearance with osseous destruction and infiltration of the surrounding soft tissues. MRI is ideal for assessing the extent of disease and any associated compromise of the thecal sac. On T2-weighted sequences, the lesions are typically hyperintense surrounded by a rim of T2 signal void corresponding to the peripheral sclerotic reaction. They are usually low to intermediate signal intensity on T1-weighted sequences with variable contrast enhancement that may be lobular, marginal, or septal [6].

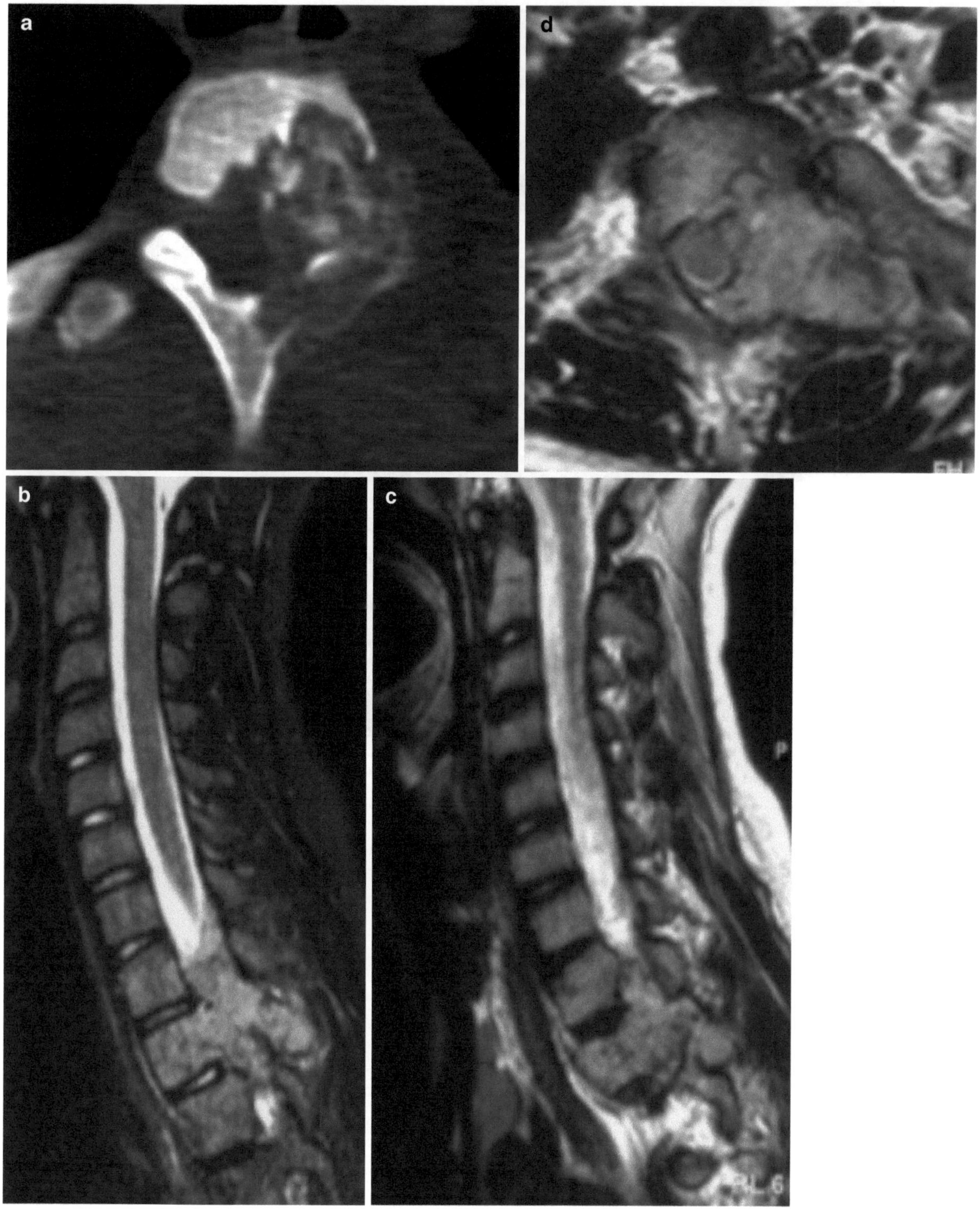

Fig. 4.5 Aggressive osteoblastoma. Axial CT imaging (**a**) demonstrates an aggressive, expansile, destructive, osseous lesion centered within the left T2 pedicle with extension into the vertebral body, left transverse process, lamina, and articular facets. Discrete foci of mineralized matrix are noted centrally and peripherally within the lesion. Sagittal STIR (**b**), as well as sagittal and axial T2 (**c** and **d**) and nonenhanced axial T1 (**e**) weighted MR images, demonstrates the lesion's T2 hyperintense, T1 hypointense signal and delineates its extension into the left paraspinal soft tissues, as well as the left ventral, lateral, and dorsal epidural space. There is resultant, near complete obliteration of the normal subarachnoid CSF space and mass effect on the spinal cord, which is displaced to the right of midline. The lesion demonstrates homogenous enhancement after the administration of intravenous contrast (**f**)

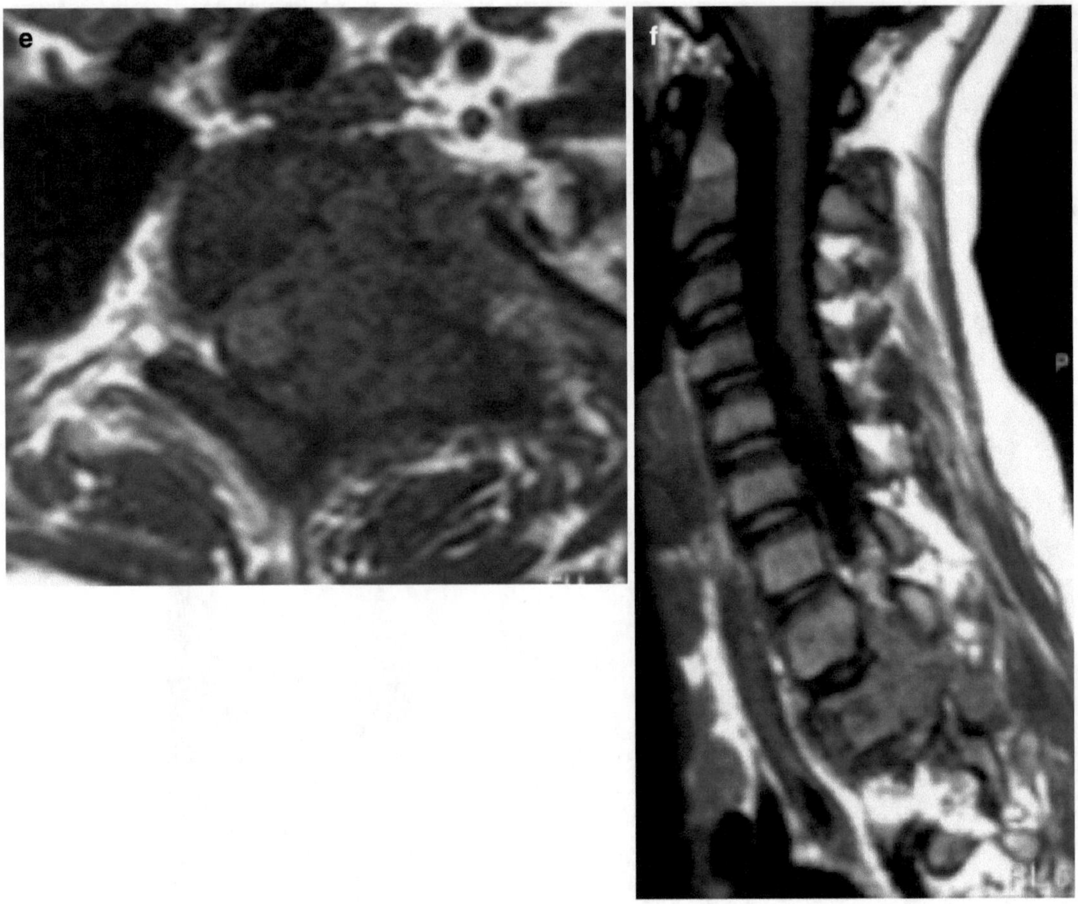

Fig. 4.5 (continued)

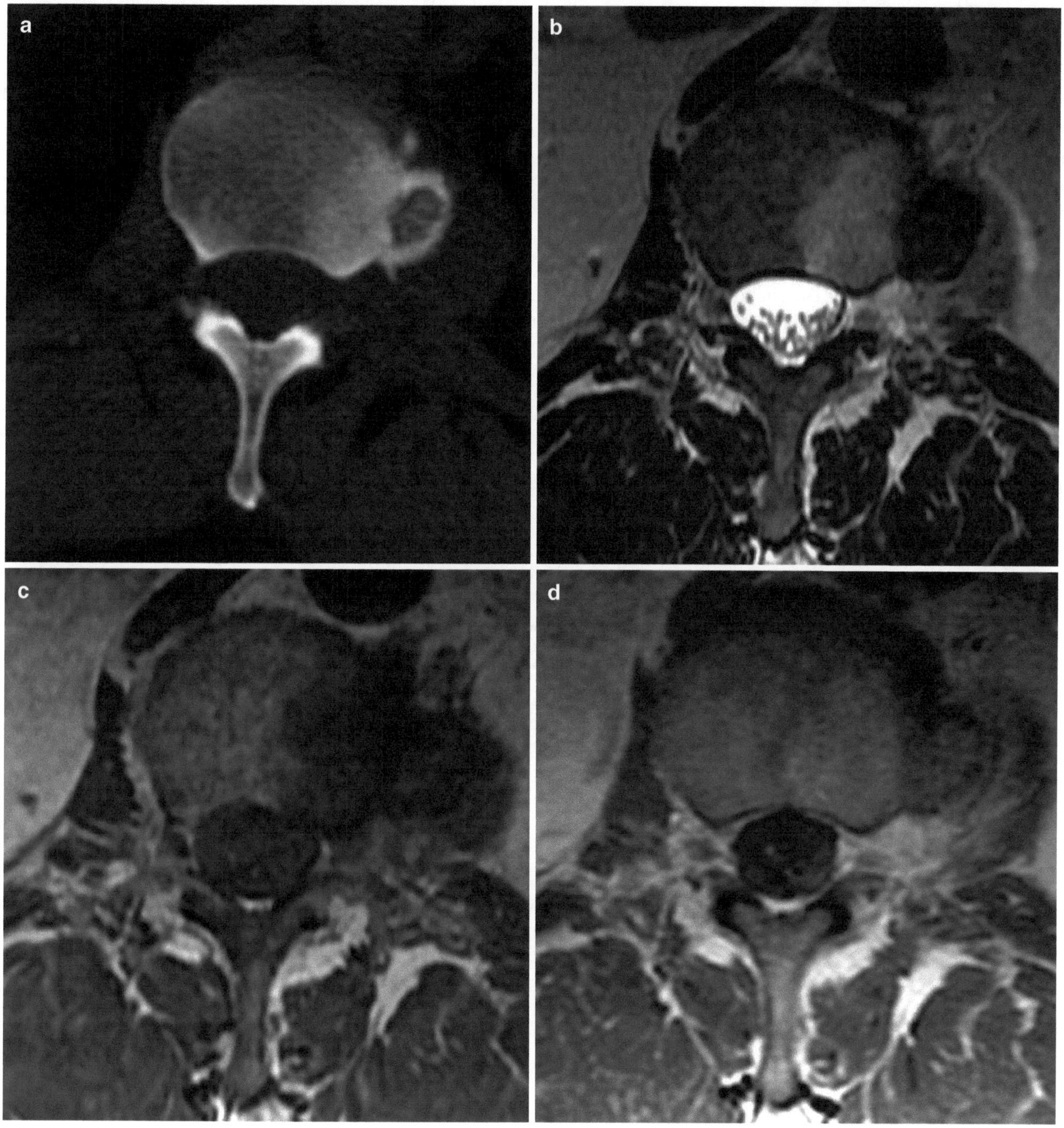

Fig. 4.6 Osteoblastoma. Axial CT (**a**) imaging demonstrates a lobular, exophytic, osseous lesion arising from the left lateral portion of the vertebral body. It contains associated dense peripheral and central mineralized matrix as well as surrounding reactive sclerosis. On Axial T2 (**b**) and axial T1 (**c**) weighted MRI, it is largely T2/T1 hypointense with associated infiltrative T2 hyperintense, T1 hypointense changes involving the left paravertebral soft tissues. Similar infiltrative signal changes are noted within the left portion of the vertebral body, likely representing reactive edema. Following the administration of intravenous gadolinium (**d**), there is diffuse enhancement of the exophytic component. There is also enhancement of the left portion of the vertebral body and left paravertebral soft tissues

Giant Cell Tumor

Giant cell tumors (GCTs) are aggressive, primary bone tumors with a slight female predilection, typically presenting during the second to fourth decades of life and rarely before adolescence or after age 50 [7]. Although they are most common within the appendicular skeleton at the metaphysis of long bones, up to 10 % of all GCTs occur within the spinal column, typically affecting the sacrum, followed by the thoracic, cervical, and lumbar vertebrae [1, 7]. Malignancy is rare but may develop in GCTs primarily or more often secondarily after surgery or radiation therapy, transforming into high-grade sarcomas with poor prognosis [8]. GCTs are typically expansile, osteolytic masses without mineralized matrix. Sacral GCTs tend to be large and expansile with associated destruction of the sacral foramina, as well as extension across both sides of midline and frequently across the sacroiliac joints. In contrast, GCTs of the long bones characteristically do not cross the articular cartilage into the joint space. GCTs of the mobile spine usually affect the vertebral body but may extend into the neural arch and paraspinal soft tissues.

On CT, giant cell tumors are typically nonmineralized, osteolytic masses that are isodense with respect to the paraspinal musculature. On MRI, they are heterogeneous regardless of the pulse sequence but predominantly low to intermediate signal intensity on T1 and low to isointense to the spinal cord on T2 [9]. This unusually low to isointense T2 signal appears to be the result of a combination of dense collagen matrix and hemosiderin serving as a helpful distinguishing feature of GCTs from other spinal neoplasms that are typically higher intensity on T2-weighted sequences [9]. Other helpful distinguishing features include: intralesional hemorrhage manifesting as areas of hyperintense T1 and T2 signal, and fluid-fluid levels within cysts similar to those seen in aneurysmal bone cysts [9]. Following the administration of intravenous contrast, enhancement is variable ranging from mild to marked, homogenous to heterogeneous enhancement.

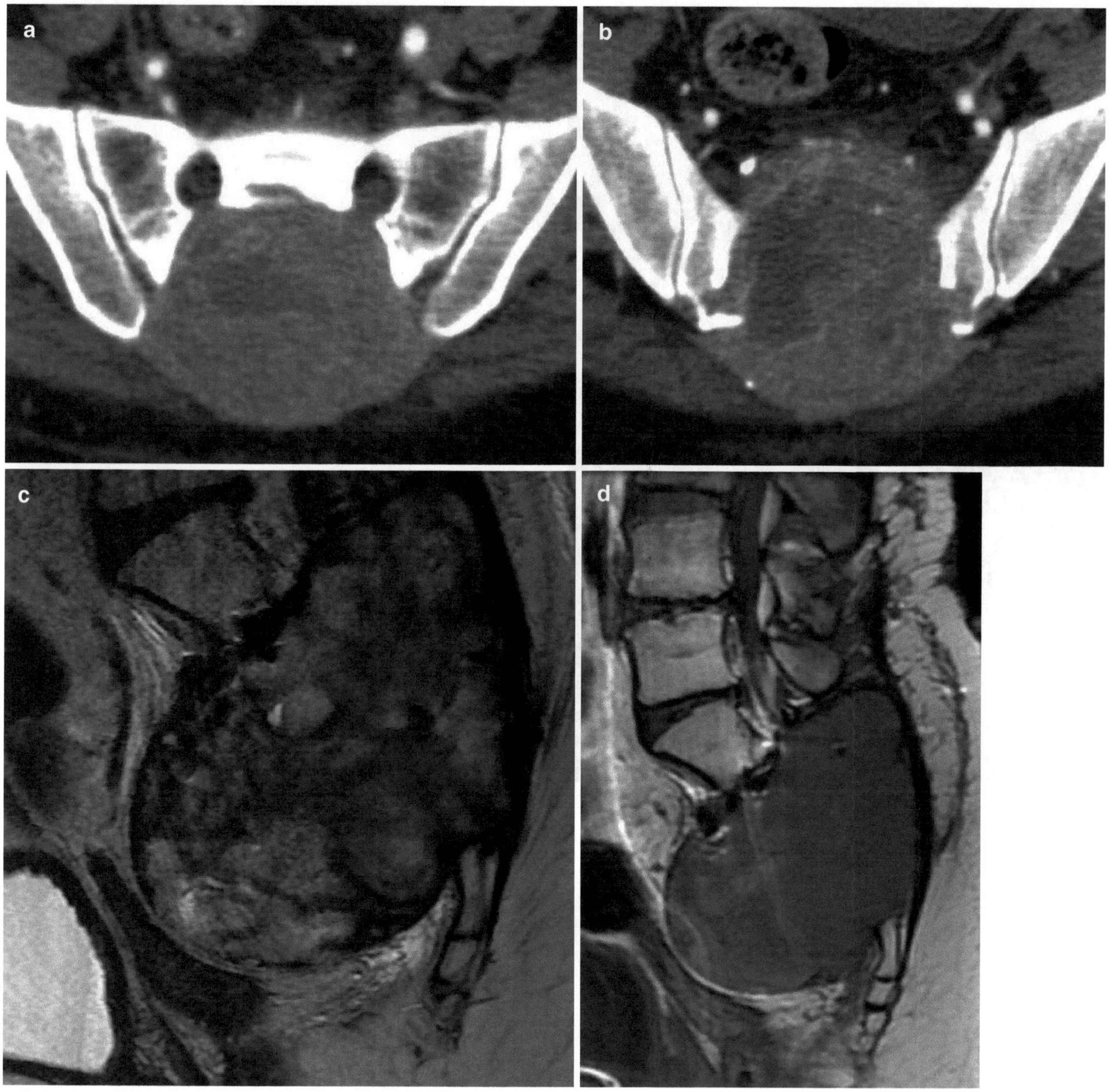

Fig. 4.7 Giant cell tumor of the sacrum. Axial CT (**a** and **b**) demonstrates a large, expansile, soft tissue mass causing bony destruction with extraosseous extension into the presacral and dorsal soft tissues. The mass appears nonmineralized and is predominantly isodense to muscle but contains areas of lower density suggesting cystic change. On MRI, the lesion demonstrates both hypointense and hyperintense T2 signal characteristics with areas of higher signal intensity corresponding to the cystic components (**c**). The lesion is homogeneously T1 hypointense (**d**) demonstrating heterogeneous enhancement with relative lack of enhancement of the cystic portions (**e**)

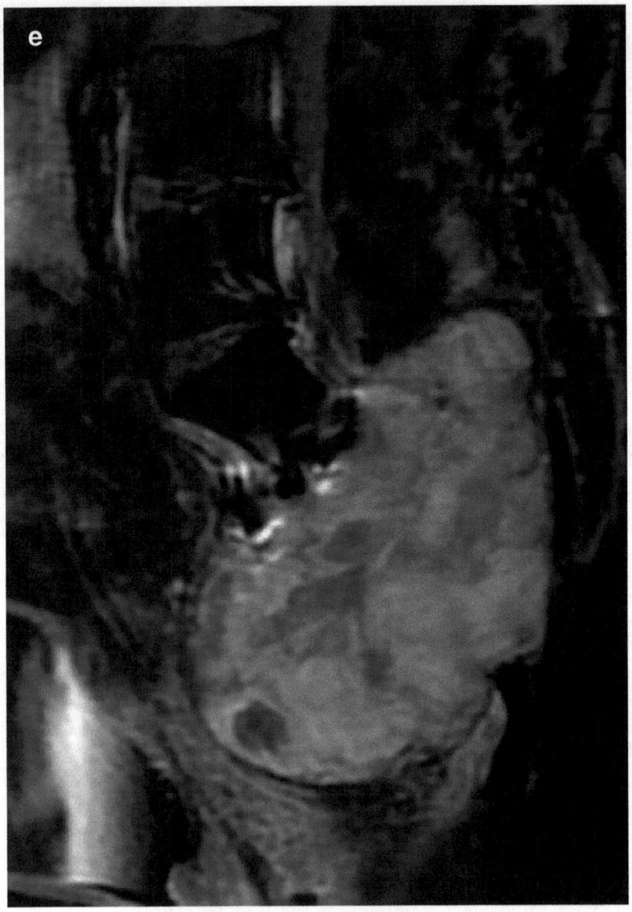

Fig. 4.7 (continued)

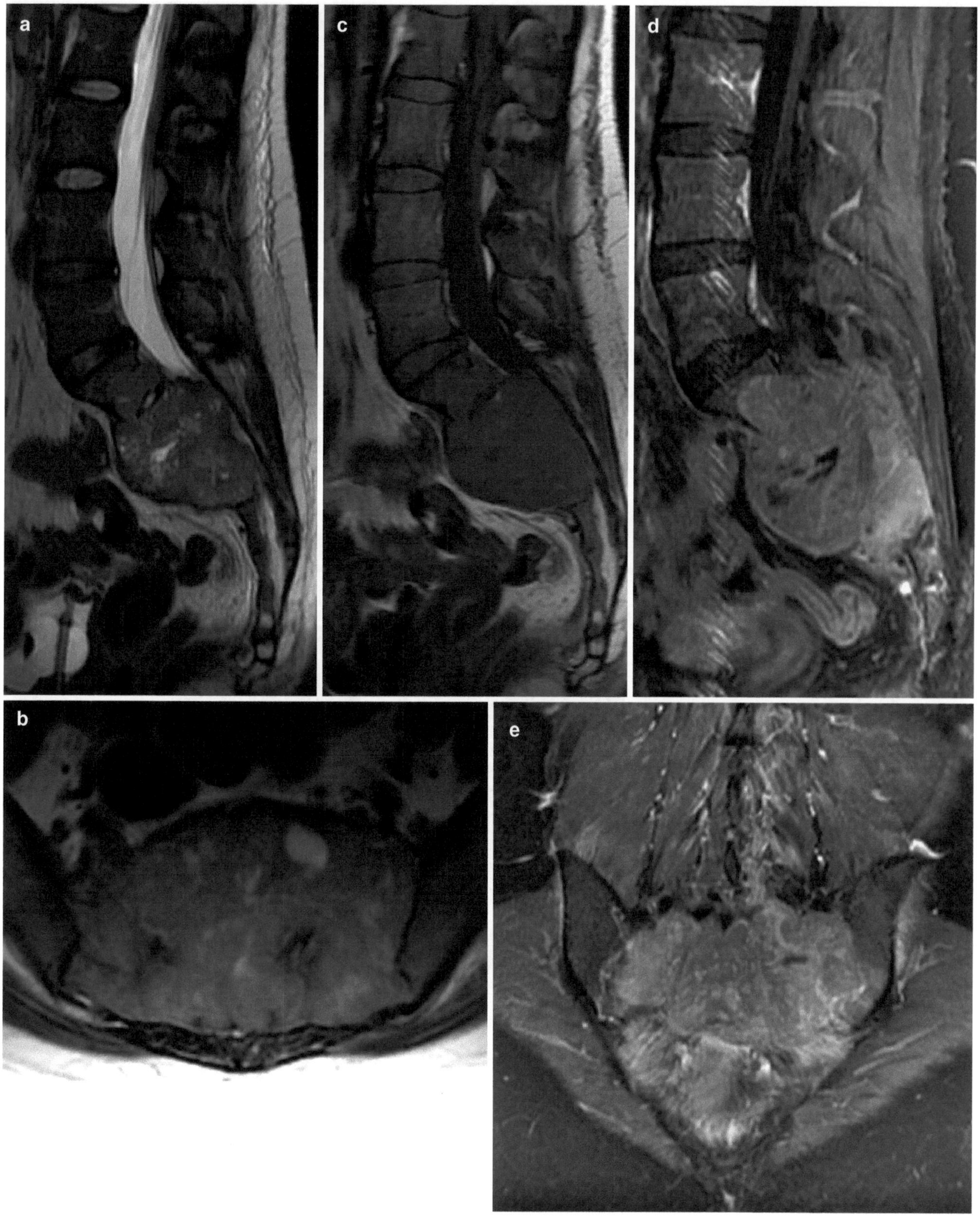

Fig. 4.8 Giant cell tumor of sacrum. Sagittal and axial T2-weighted MR images (**a** and **b**) demonstrate an expansile sacral mass with particularly low T2 signal characteristics intermixed with regions of higher signal, representing cystic change. Note a discrete fluid–fluid level within the largest cyst seen on the axial T2 image (**b**). On sagittal T1 imaging (**c**), the lesion is homogeneously T1 hypointense. Sagittal (**d**) and coronal (**e**) T1 fat-suppressed images after the administration of gadolinium contrast demonstrate avid heterogeneous enhancement and further delineate the margins of the mass that extend across the sacro-iliac joints into the iliac bones bilaterally

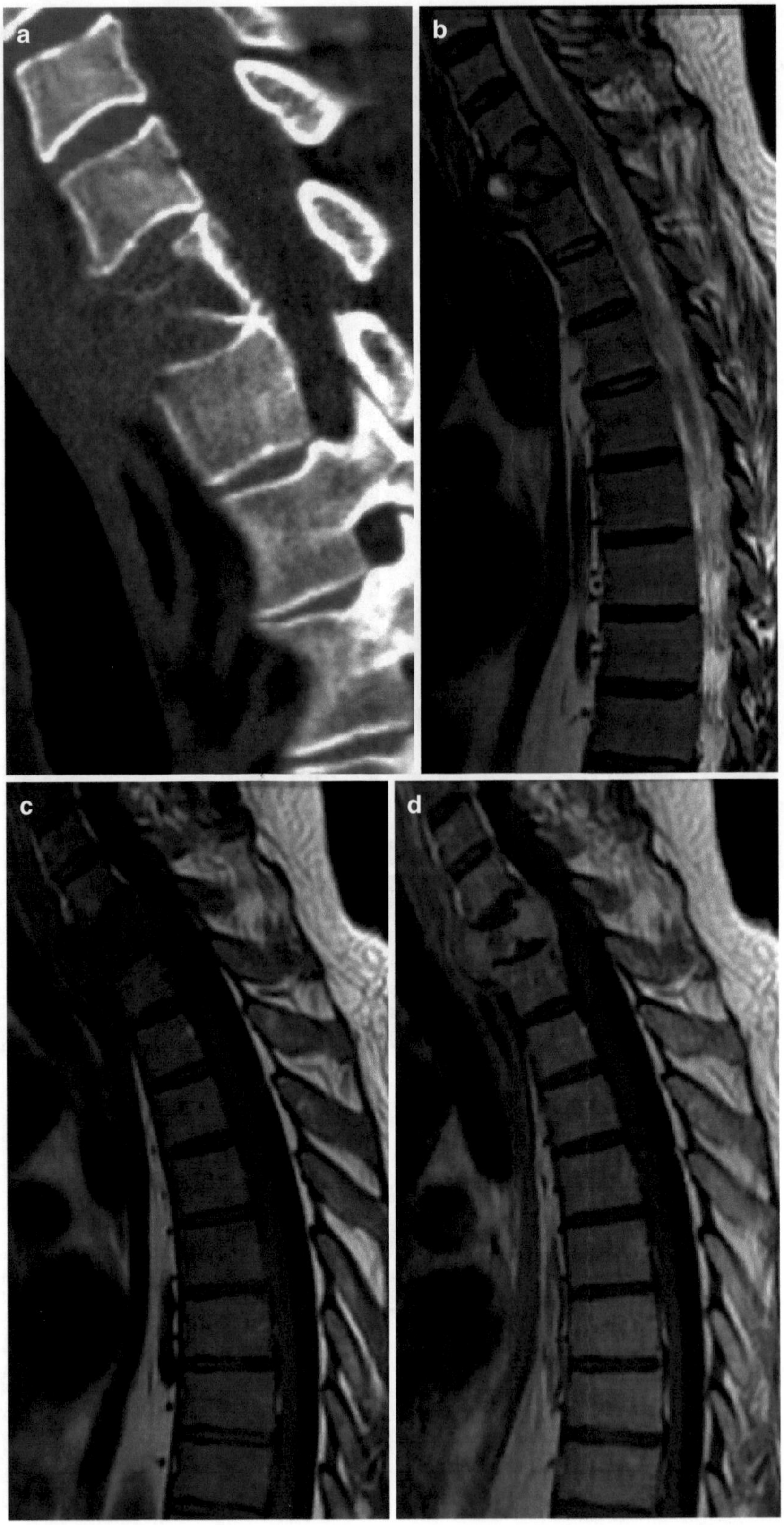

Fig. 4.9 Giant cell tumor of the T4 vertebra. Sagittal CT of the thoracic spine (**a**) demonstrates an expansile, lytic, nonmineralized, isodense mass centered within the T4 vertebral body with associated extraosseous extension into the prevertebral soft tissues and pathologic collapse deformity of the vertebra. On MRI, the mass is predominantly T2 hypointense with the exception of a T2 hyperintense, focal, cystic component involving the anterior portion of the vertebra (**b**). The mass is also predominantly T1 hypointense (**c**) demonstrating avid enhancement with the exception of the nonenhancing cystic component (**d**)

Chondrosarcoma

Chondrosarcomas are malignant neoplasms of cartilaginous origin presenting as primary tumors or as secondary tumors in the setting of preexisting cartilaginous lesions such as osteochondromas. They most commonly affect the pelvic bones, but may involve the spine and sacrum, originating within the vertebral body or posterior elements. The thoracic and lumbar spine is frequently affected, while involvement of the sacrum is rare [3]. Three percent to 12 % of all chondrosarcomas occur in the spine with a peak prevalence during 30–70 years and a mean age of presentation of 45 years [2, 3]. The clinical course is generally indolent as these tumors are usually lower grade, with slow but locally aggressive growth. Eleven percent of chondrosarcomas undergo anaplastic transformation, resulting in high-grade noncartilaginous sarcoma with more aggressive growth and even a propensity to metastasize [10].

Chondrosarcomas manifest as osteolytic lesions with a hallmark calcified chondroid matrix of "rings and arcs" configurations that may be best appreciated on CT [3]. On MRI, the mineralized components of the tumor will present as signal voids on both T1 and T2 whereas the nonmineralized portions will appear hypointense on T1 and hyperintense on T2 due to the high water content of hyaline cartilage [3]. Post gadolinium MRI typically reveals patchy enhancement of the lesion, sometimes with a ring and arc appearance.

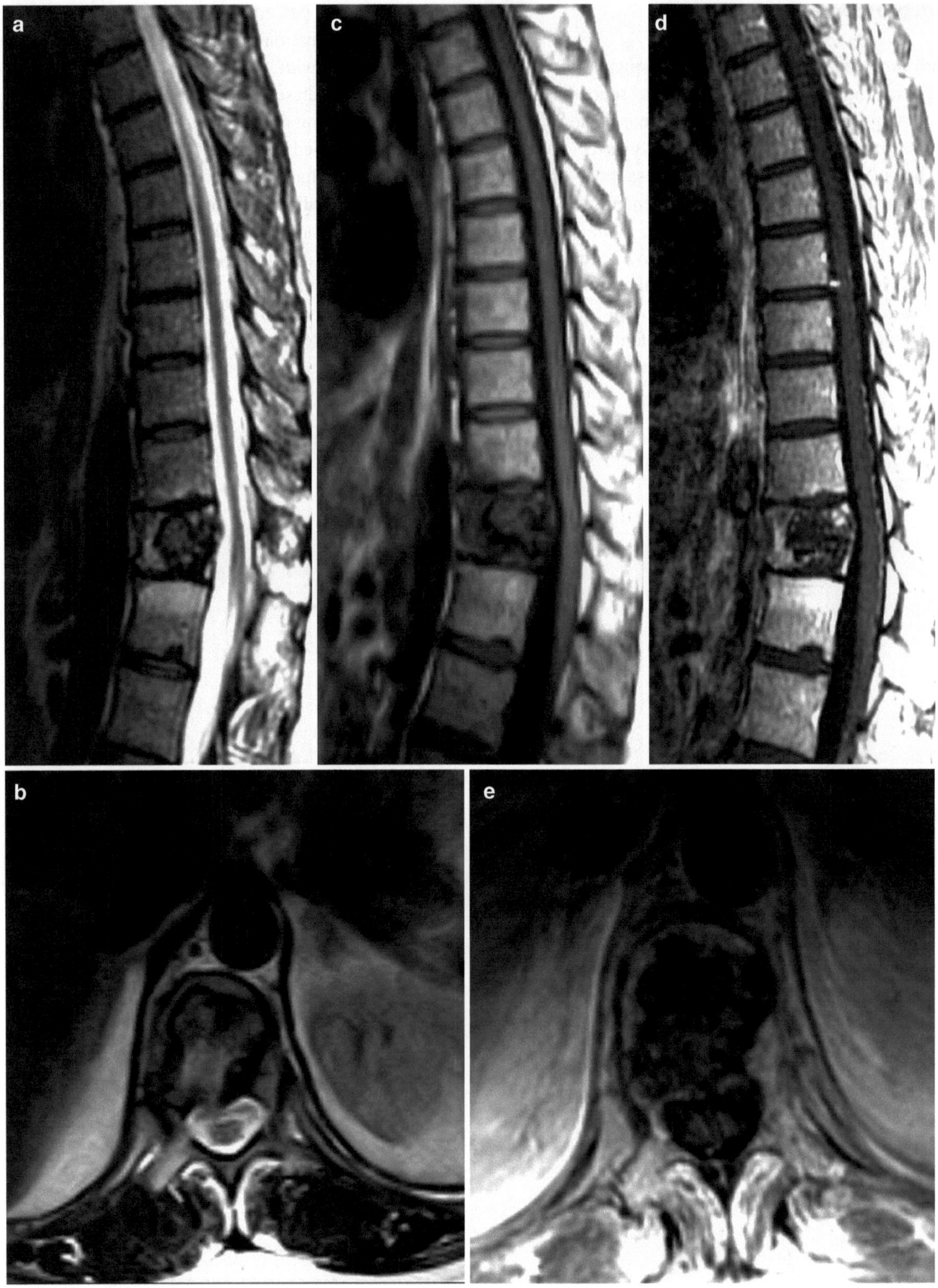

Fig. 4.10 Chondrosarcoma. Sagittal and axial T2 (**a** and **b**) and sagittal nonenhanced T1 (**c**) MRI demonstrates a heterogeneous, lobulated, slightly expansile lesion centered within the T10 vertebral body. The lesion contains curvilinear T1/T2 signal voids related to mineralized matrix, interspersed with foci of marked T2 hyperintensity related to hydrated hyaline cartilage. On sagittal and axial-enhanced T1 (**d** and **e**) MR imaging, the lesion demonstrates patchy somewhat stippled enhancement with a ring and arc configuration. Sagittal CT myelogram (**f**) in bone algorithm delineates the dense mineralized matrix at the periphery of the lesion and foci of less dense cartilaginous matrix centrally

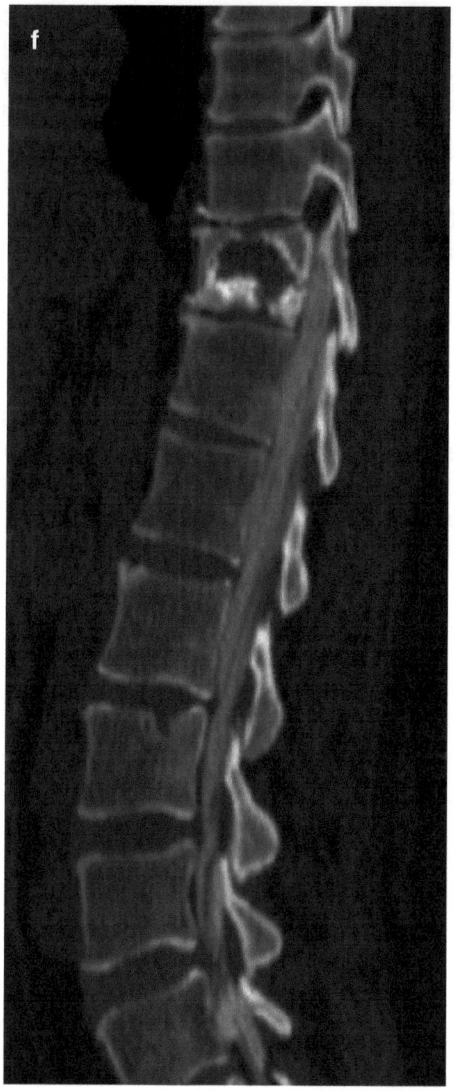

Fig. 4.10 (continued)

Chordoma

Chordomas are midline, lobular, slow-growing, locally aggressive, malignant tumors that arise from notochord remnants. Although they may occur anywhere along the course of the notochord, they are most prevalent within the sacrococcygeal (50–60 %) or sphenooccipital regions (20–40 %), and to a lesser extent within the cervical vertebrae, followed by the other spinal segments [11]. Chordomas occur in late middle age, with a peak incidence during the fifth and sixth decades of life [11]. Lesions involving the vertebrae typically spare the posterior elements and are more likely to metastasize than those affecting the sacrum and clivus [3, 12]. The presence of an associated soft tissue mass spanning several vertebral levels is considered highly characteristic of chordomas and may occur ventrally, laterally, or dorsally within the epidural space. In cases of cervical chordoma, encasement of the vertebral arteries is common [12].

On CT, chordomas are typically well-defined masses that are isodense to muscle and sometimes contain amorphous calcification. On MRI, they are typically T1 iso- to hypointense and markedly T2 hyperintense. This characteristic, strikingly hyperintense T2 signal is the result of highly vacuolated cells, as well as the production of intracellular and extracellular mucin [11]. The gelatinous mucoid material is typically separated by hypointense fibrous septations best appreciated on T2-weighted MRI [3]. Focal areas of hemorrhage and high protein content may also be present, manifesting as foci of increased signal on T1-weighted images [11]. Enhancement is variable including heterogeneous, homogeneous, total, or peripheral septal enhancement [13].

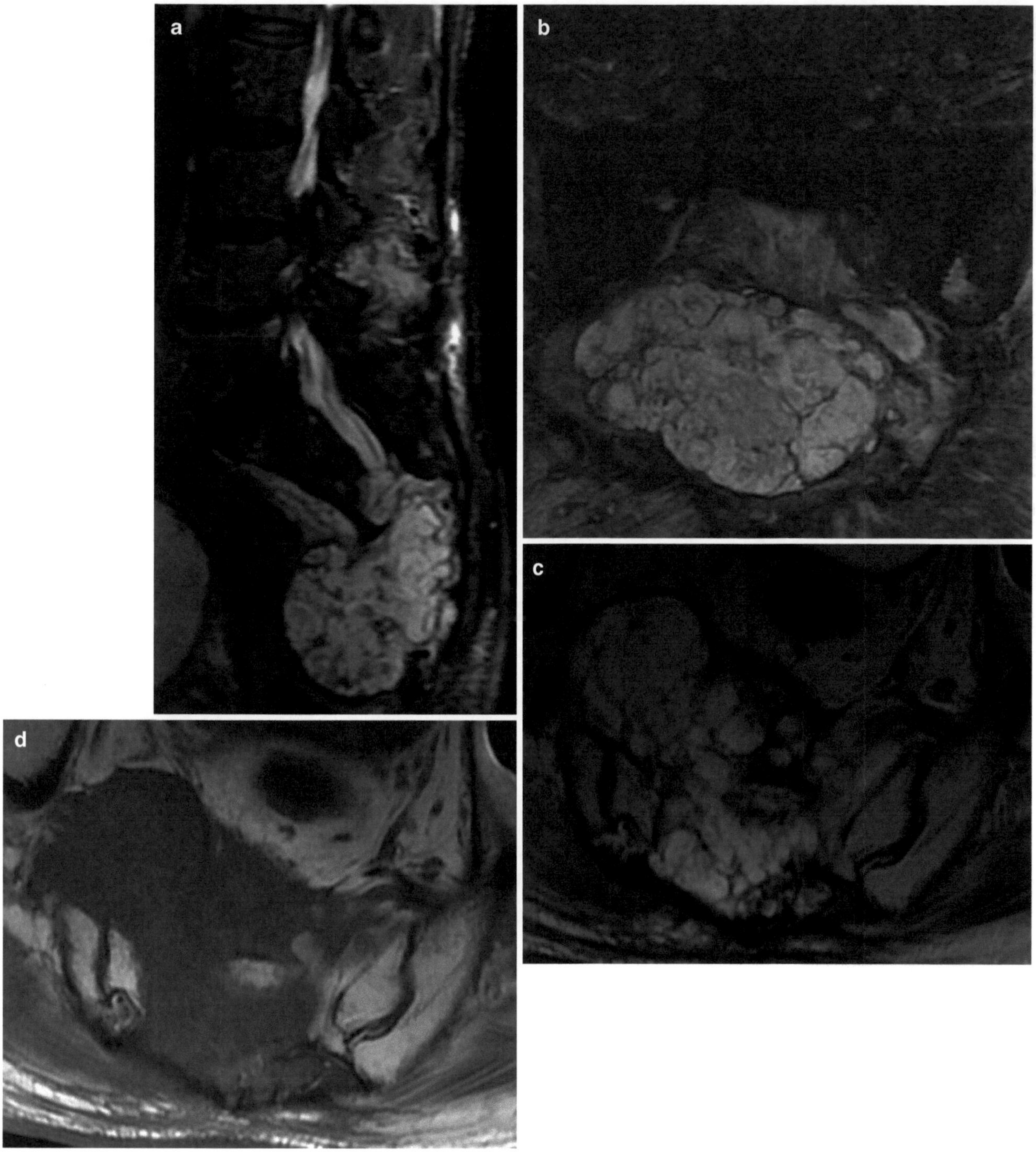

Fig. 4.11 Sacral chordoma. Sagittal (**a**) and coronal (**b**) STIR as well as axial T2 (**c**) weighted MR images demonstrate an expansile, multilobulated, markedly T2 hyperintense sacral mass associated with T2 hypointense septations extending into the presacral soft tissues. The mass is largely T1 hypointense (**d**) and demonstrates heterogeneous enhancement following the administration of intravenous gadolinium (**e**)

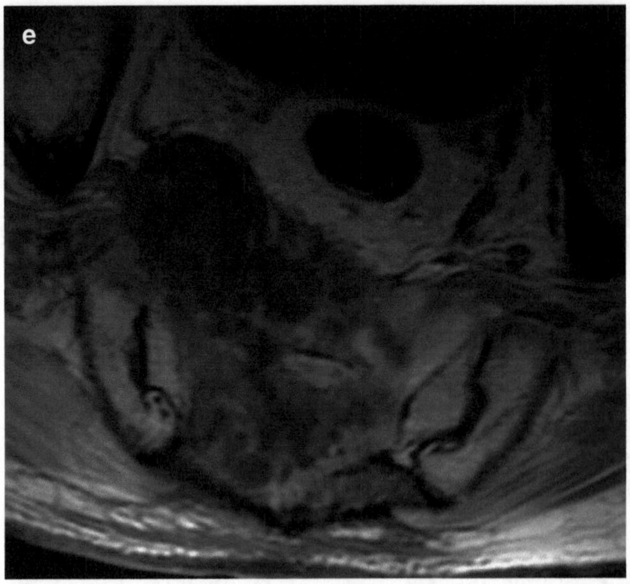

Fig. 4.11 (continued)

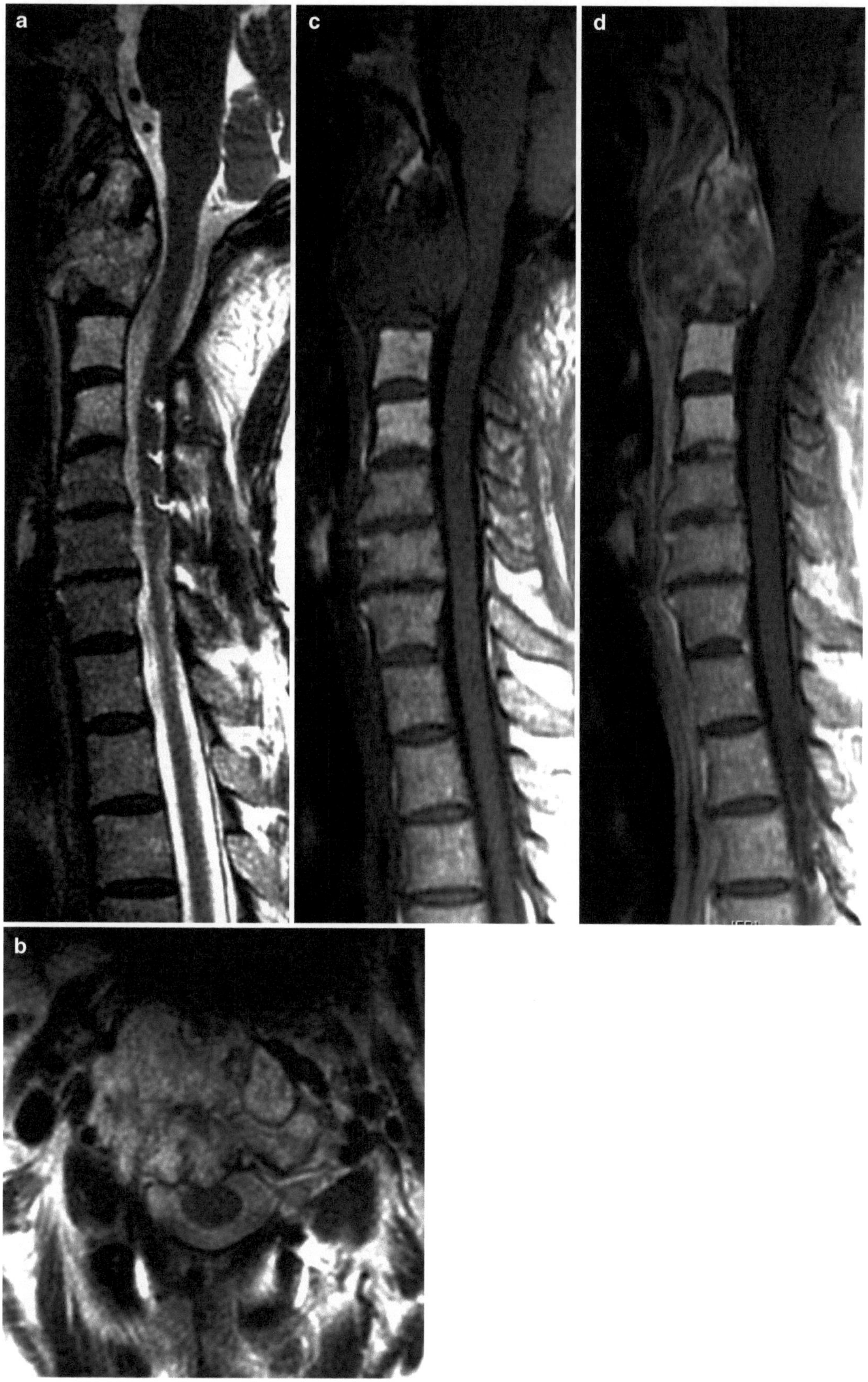

Fig. 4.12 Cervical chordoma. Sagittal (**a**) and axial (**b**) T2-weighted MR images demonstrate an expansile, lobular mass involving the C2 vertebrae with characteristic hyperintense T2 signal changes and numerous T2 hypointense septations. There is associated extraosseous extension into the prevertebral soft tissues and ventral epidural space abutting the ventral spinal cord. The lesion appears T1 hypointense (**c**) and demonstrates heterogeneous enhancement (**d**)

Benign Notochordal Cell Tumor

Benign notochordal cell tumors (BNCT) are now increasingly accepted as benign intraosseous lesions of notochordal cell origin with the same distribution as chordomas, typically occurring within the clivus and sacrum followed by the mobile spine. At autopsy, they are identified in approximately 20 % of adult cadavers and are increasingly being detected on CT and MRI [14]. BNCT are histologically distinct from chordomas; however, the distinction is sometimes overlooked and imaging features play a large role in making the proper diagnosis, ultimately avoiding unnecessary surgical management.

The most helpful imaging features discriminating BNCTs from chordomas are the absence of bone destruction on CT, as well as the absence of extraosseous extension and lack of contrast enhancement on MRI [14]. On CT, they are typically sclerotic, centrally located within the vertebral body, extending partly to the cortex but without associated cortical disruption or bone destruction [15]. On MRI, the lesions are homogeneously T1 hypointense and T2 intermediate to hyperintense in signal. Unlike chordomas, they characteristically do not demonstrate enhancement following contrast administration [14, 15].

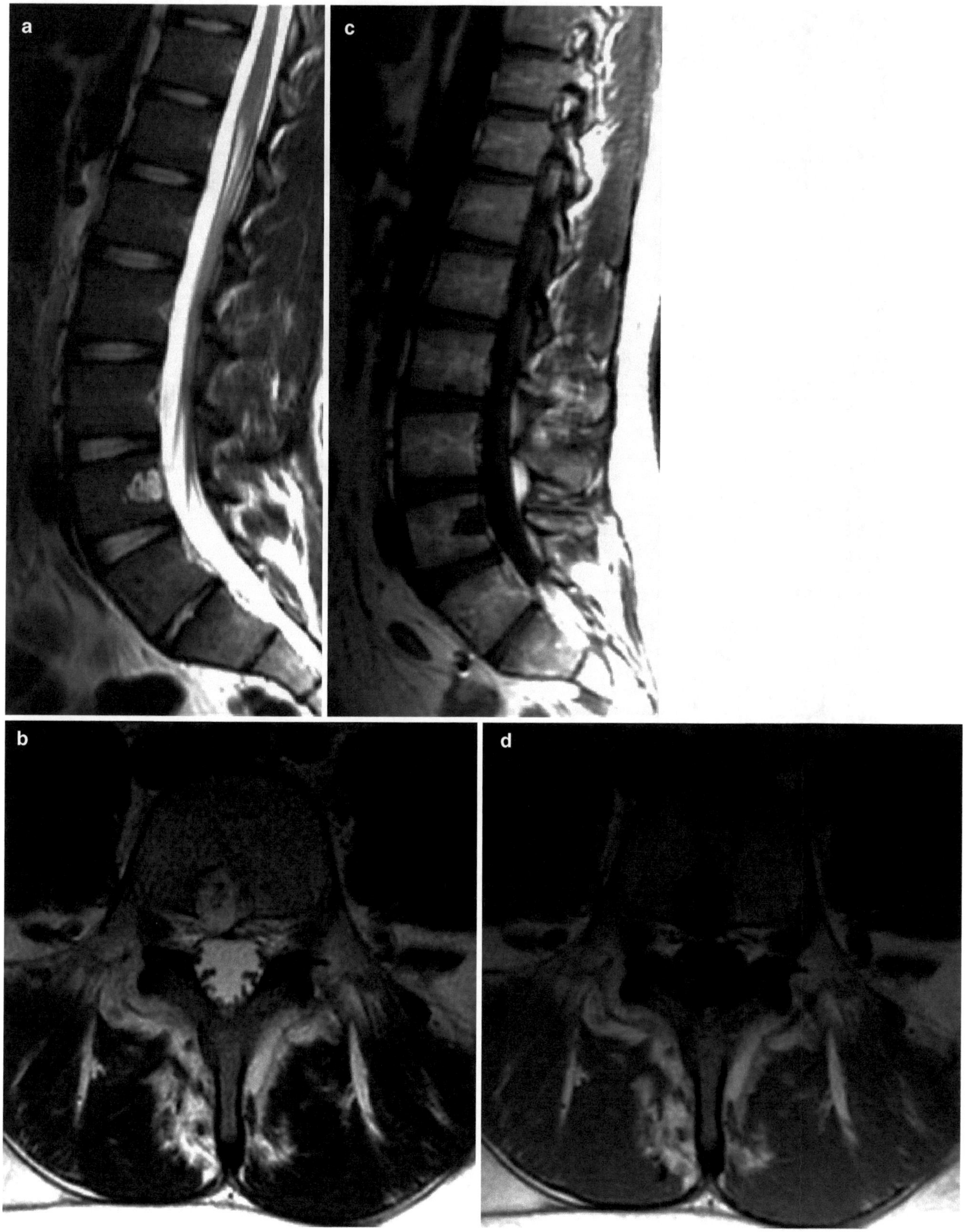

Fig. 4.13 Benign notochordal cell tumor. Sagittal and axial T2 (**a** and **b**) as well as nonenhanced sagittal and axial T1-weighted images (**c** and **d**) demonstrate a well-circumscribed, T2 hyperintense, T1 hypointense, midline, dorsally located lesion within the L4 vertebral body. There is no associated enhancement on the sagittal and axial T1 post-contrast images (**e** and **f**), helping to distinguish it from a chordoma

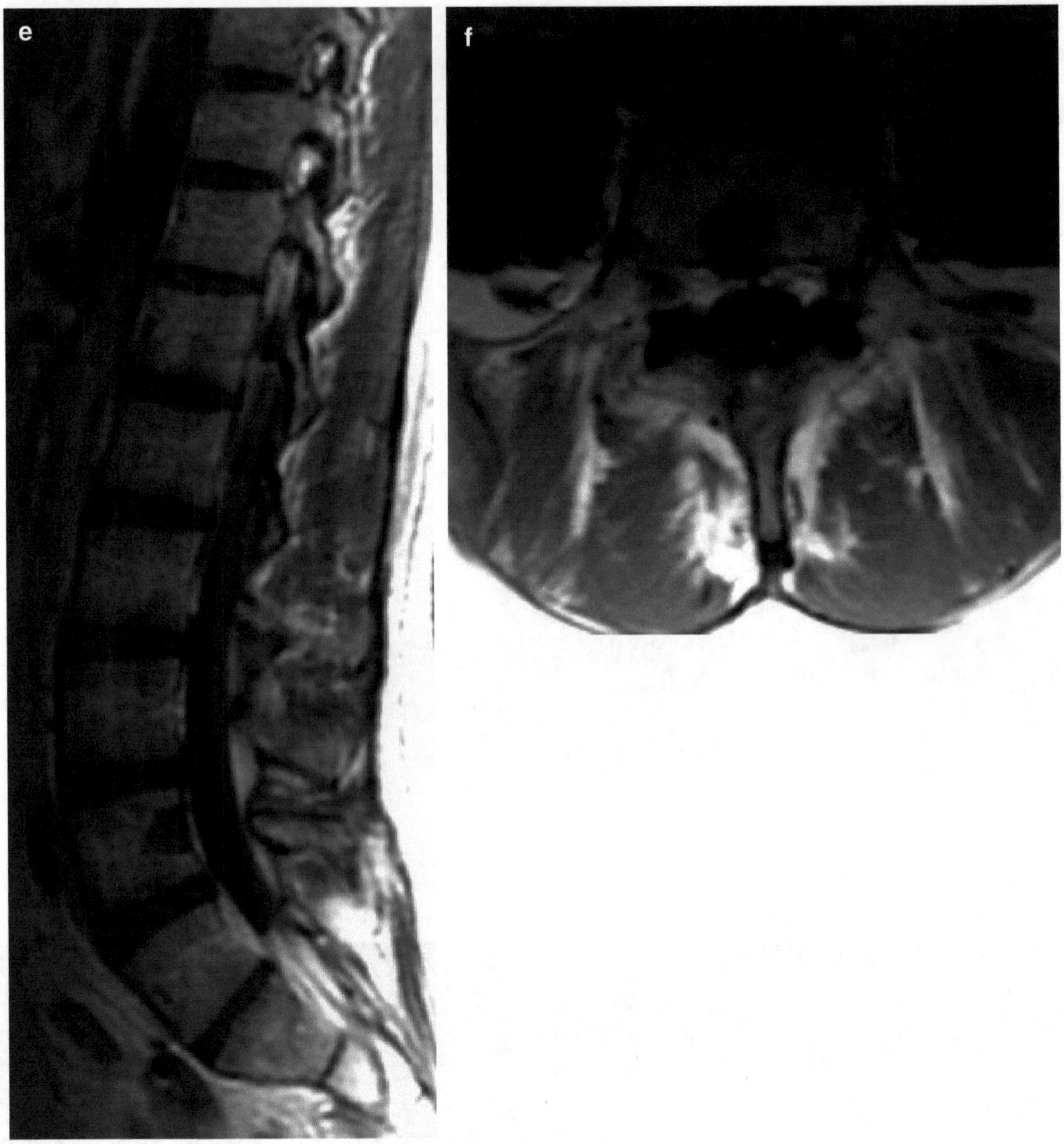

Fig. 4.13 (continued)

Neuroblastoma, Ganglioneuroma, Ganglioneuroblastoma

Neuroblastomas, ganglioneuroblastomas, and ganglioneuromas are neoplasms originating from primordial neural crest cells, typically within the paravertebral sympathetic chain but also within the adrenal medulla. Despite originating from the same cell lineage, ganglioneuromas are typically benign, well-differentiated lesions composed of mature ganglion cells. In contrast, neuroblastomas and ganglioneuroblastomas are less differentiated malignant neoplasms with a propensity to metastasize. All three present during early childhood; however, neuroblastomas tend to present before age 5, whereas ganglioneuromas and ganglioneuroblastomas usually present later between the ages of 5 and 8 [8]. Morphologically, they are often oblong masses, spanning 3–5 vertebral bodies, anterior and lateral to the spinal column [16]. They may often extend into the adjacent neural foramina and epidural compartment compromising the spinal cord and exiting nerve roots.

On T1-weighted MR imaging, all three neoplasms are typically homogenously hypointense. In contrast, they tend to be heterogeneous on T2 with areas of hyperintense and hypointense signal. Foci of interspersed hyperintense T1/T2 signal that suppress on fat saturation imaging have also been described with ganglioneuromas suggesting intratumoral adipose tissue. When present, this finding may serve as a helpful distinguishing feature of ganglioneuromas [16]. Enhancement following contrast administration is typical, with or without areas of nonenhancing intralesional necrosis or hemorrhage which may sometimes be present.

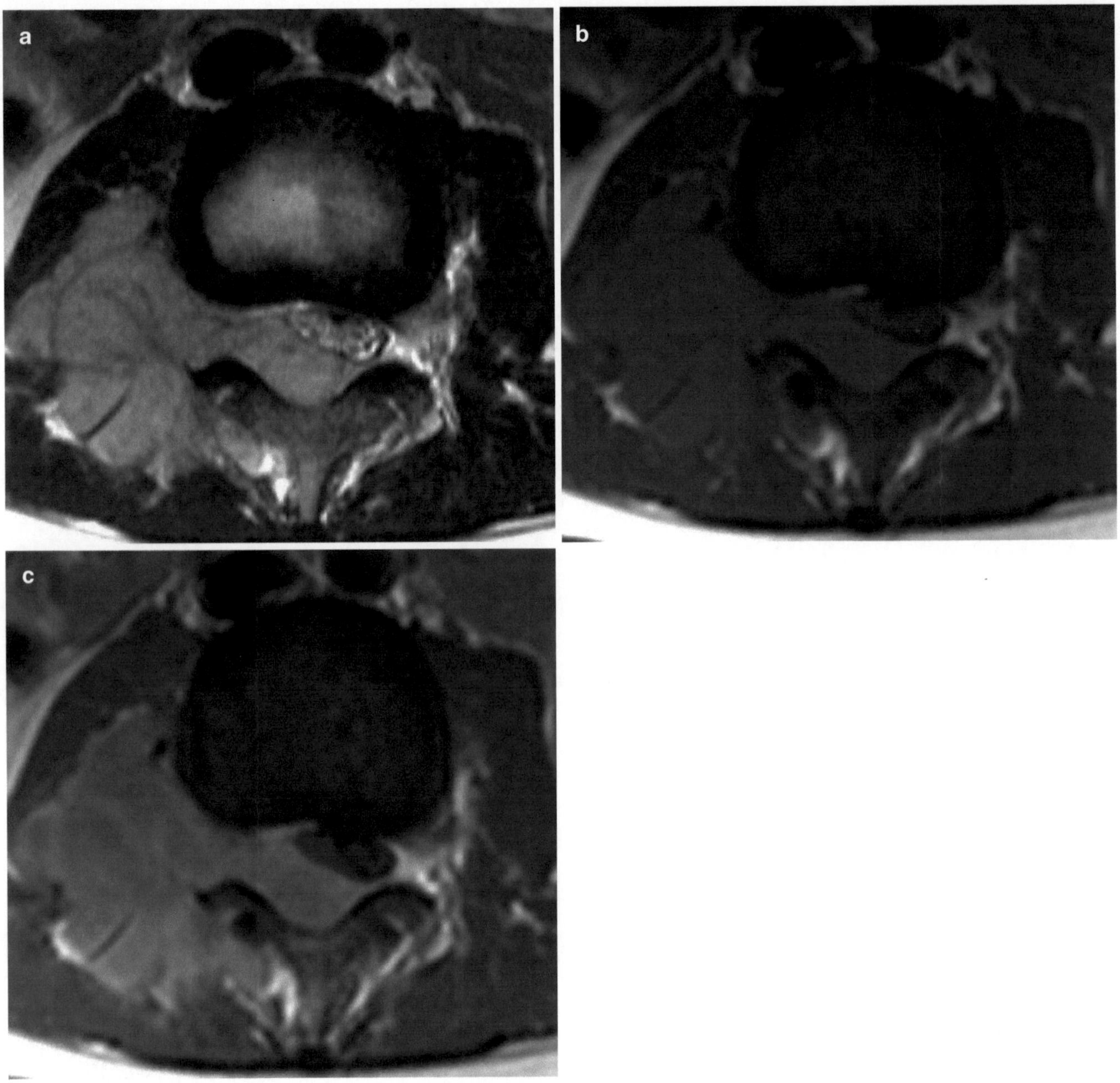

Fig. 4.14 Neuroblastoma. Axial T2 (**a**), axial T1 (**b**), and axial contrast T1 (**c**) weighted images demonstrates a T2 hyperintense, T1 hypointense, homogeneously enhancing right paravertebral mass extending into the spinal canal via the right L2/L3 neural foramen. There is resultant partial effacement of the thecal sac and compromise of the exiting right L2 nerve root

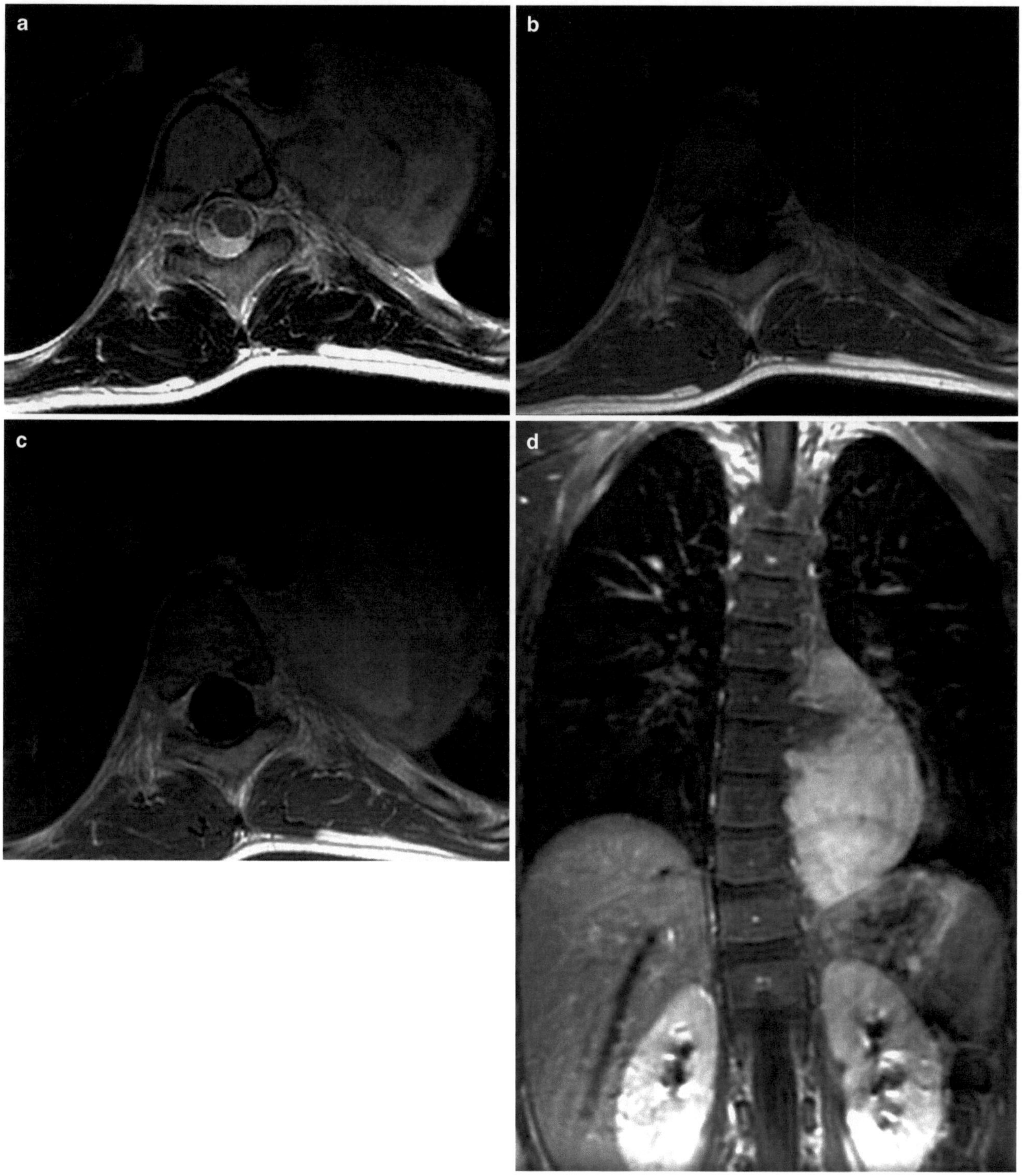

Fig. 4.15 Ganglioneuroma. Axial T2 (**a**), axial T1 (**b**), axial contrast T1 (**c**), and coronal contrast T1 fat-suppressed (**d**) MRI images demonstrate a heterogeneously T2 hyperintense lesion within the left anterolateral paravertebral region in the expected location of the sympathetic chain. The lesion demonstrates homogenous pre-contrast T1 hypointense signal and avid homogeneous contrast enhancement

Bone Metastases

The spine is the third most common site for metastatic disease, following the lung and liver, and the most common osseous site [17]. Sixty to seventy percent of patients with systemic cancer develop spine metastases [17]. Tumors with high rates of metastases to bone include prostate, breast, lung, thyroid, and renal cell carcinoma [17].

The typical MRI appearance of osseous spine metastases include focal, often numerous, infiltrative, osteolytic lesions that are T1 hypointense and T2 hyperintense relative to the normal surrounding non-infiltrated marrow. Exceptions to this include osteoblastic metastases or melanoma metastases. Osteoblastic metastases usually manifest as focal, low signal intensity lesions on all pulse sequences, whereas melanoma metastases often present as well circumscribed, T1 hyperintense lesions due to the presence of melanin and/or hemorrhage [18]. Cancers that may commonly produce osteoblastic metastases include prostate, breast, lymphoma, carcinoid, medulloblastoma, osteosarcoma, and non–small cell lung carcinoma.

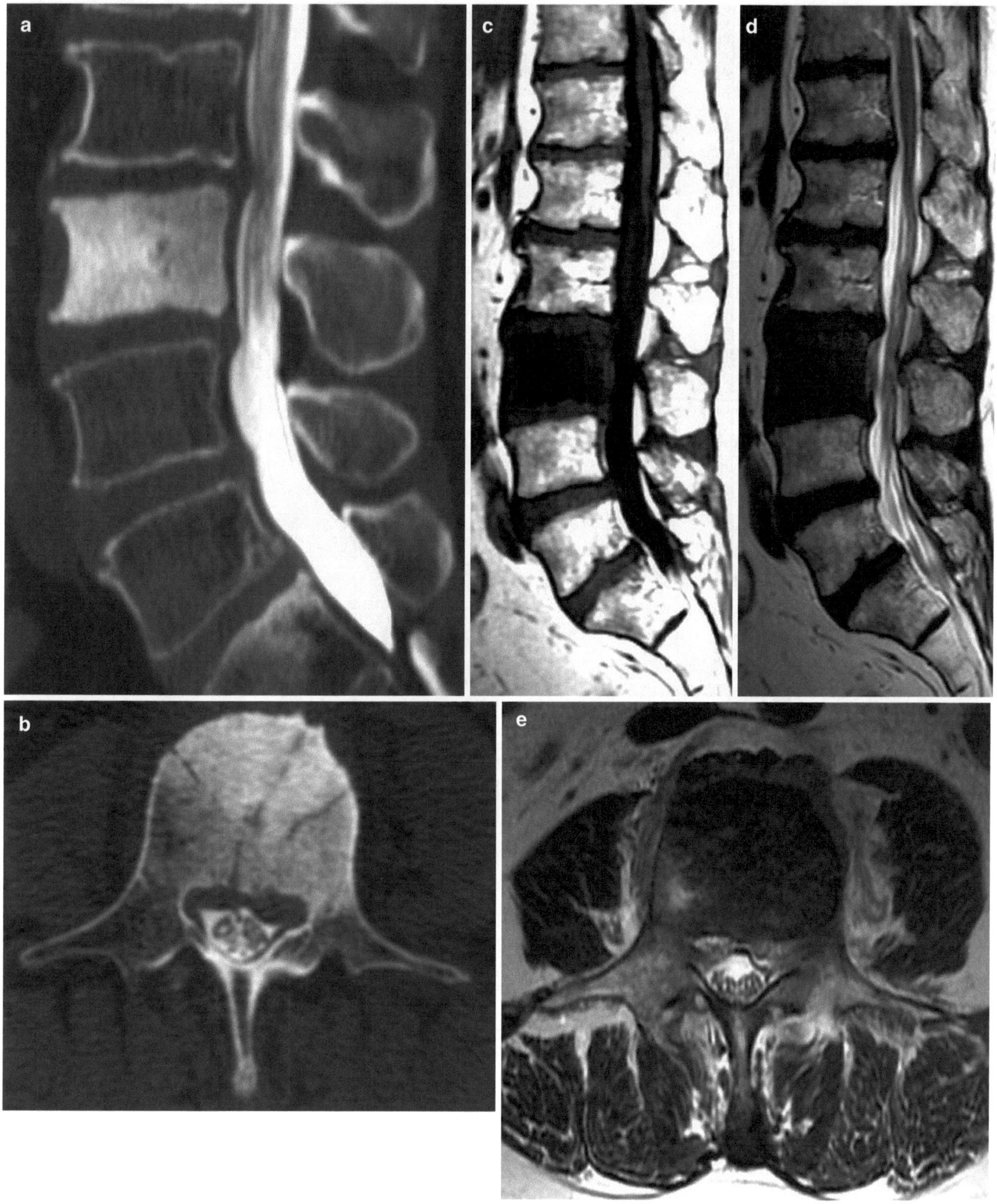

Fig. 4.16 Prostate metastasis. Sagittal (**a**) and axial (**b**) images from a CT myelogram demonstrate an osteoblastic L3 vertebral metastasis with associated extraosseous extension of disease into the prevertebral and ventral epidural spaces without associated spinal canal compromise. On sagittal T1 (**c**) as well as sagittal and axial T2 (**d** and **e**) weighted MR imaging, the lesion is markedly T1/T2 hypointense related to osseous sclerosis

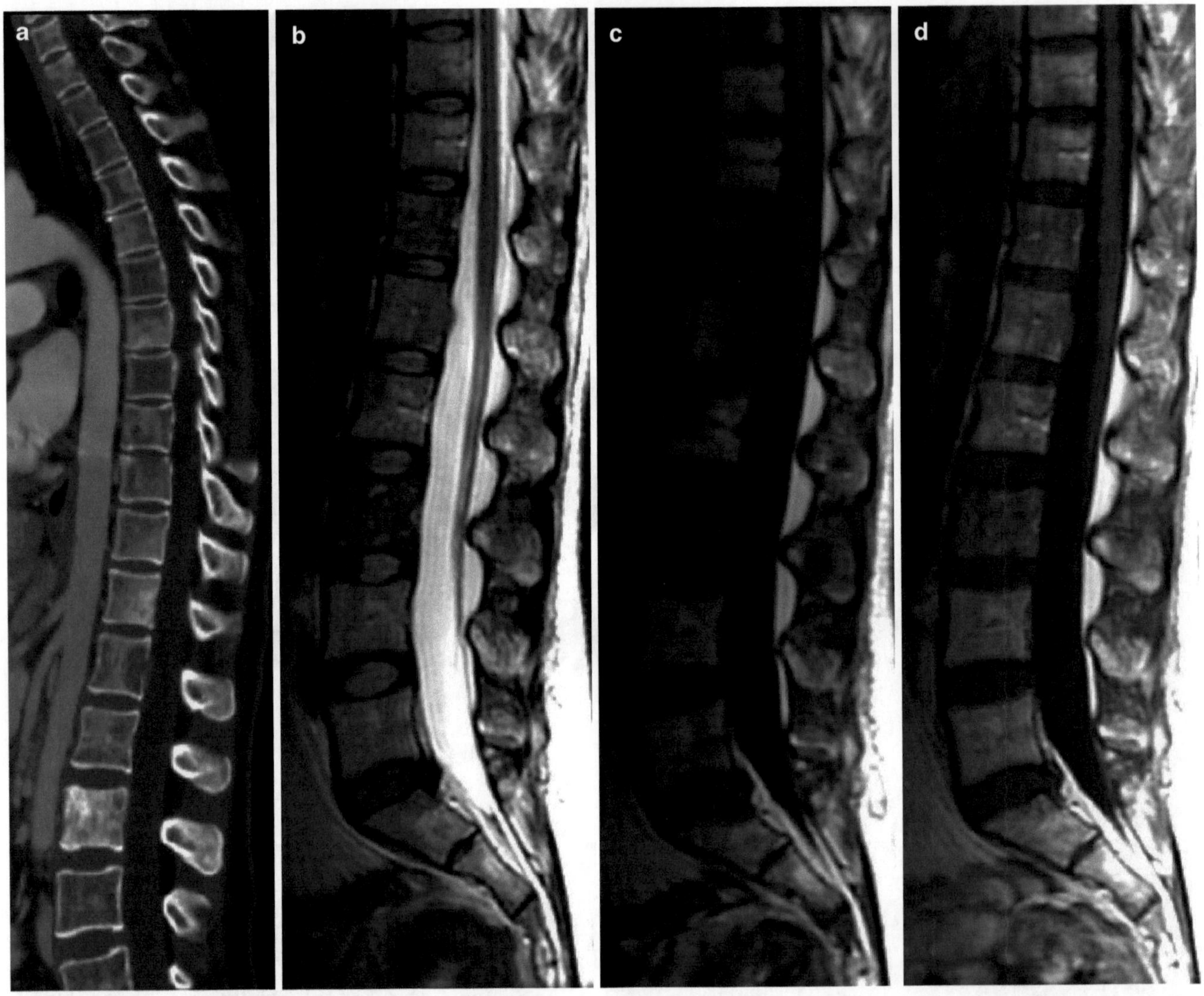

Fig. 4.17 Breast metastases. Sagittal CT image in bone algorithm (**a**) demonstrates a mixed pattern of both hyperdense osteoblastic and hypodense osteolytic metastases in this patient with known breast carcinoma. Sagittal T2 (**b**) and sagittal T1 (**c**) weighted MRI of the same patient demonstrates the expected signal characteristics of T1/T2 hypointense osteosclerotic metastases involving the T12 and L3 vertebra, as well as T1 hypointense, T2 hyperintense osteolytic metastases involving the L1 and L2 vertebra. Heterogeneous enhancement is noted following contrast administration (**d**). Minimal enhancing ventral epidural disease is also noted at the L1 vertebral level

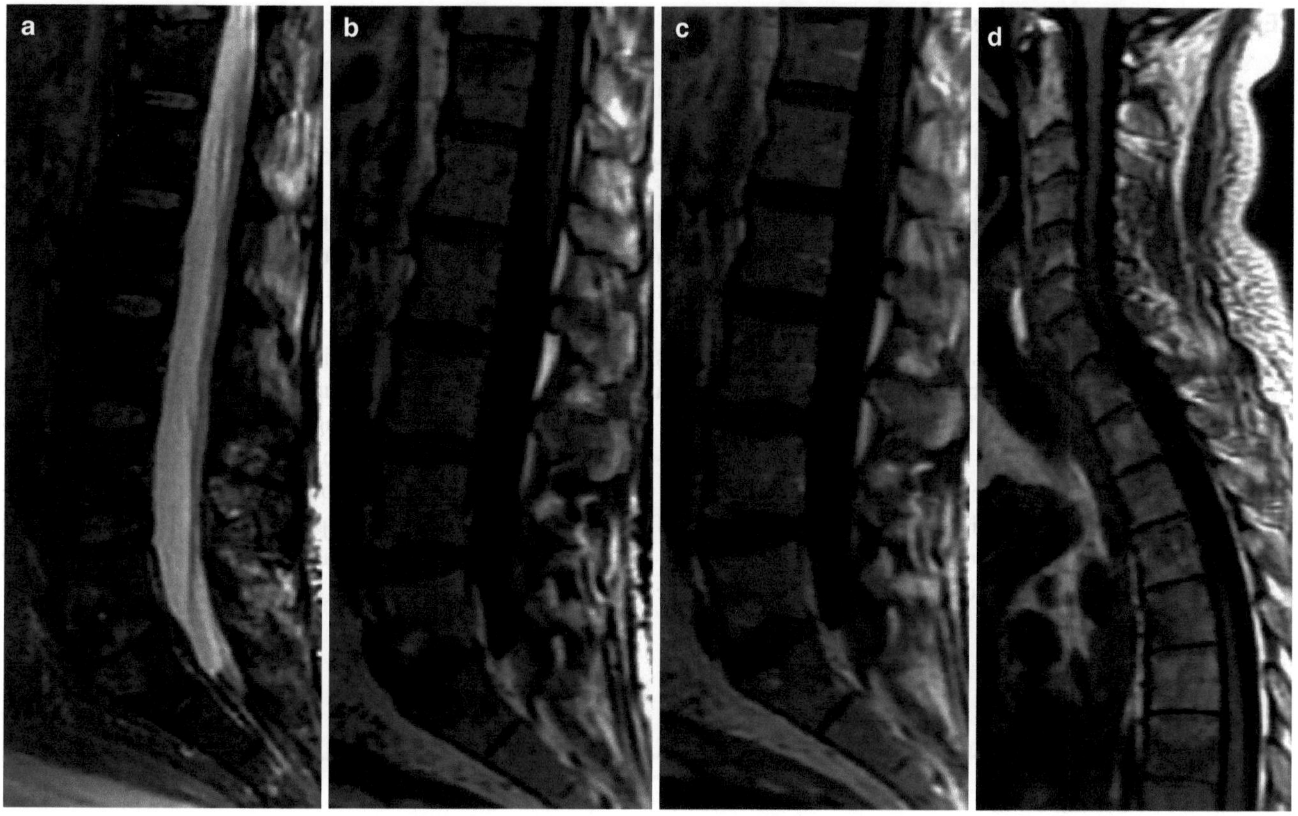

Fig. 4.18 Melanoma metastases. Sagittal STIR (**a**), sagittal T1 (**b**), and sagittal contrast T1 (**c**) weighted images of the lumbar spine demonstrate STIR hyperintense lesions within the anterior portions of the L5 and S1 segments consistent with metastases in this patient with known malignant melanoma. The L5 lesion demonstrates central T1 pre-contrast hyperintensity, presumably related to melanin or hemorrhage. Following contrast administration, both lesions mildly enhance. Sagittal T1 (**d**) imaging of the rest of the spine demonstrates an additional T1 hyperintense metastasis within the T2 vertebra

Epidural Metastatic Disease

Epidural metastases are most commonly indirect from an initial hematogenous metastasis to the vertebral body gradually growing and spreading into the epidural compartment [19]. A less common route of spread occurs from growth of paravertebral tumor directly into the spinal canal via a neural foramen, as is often seen with lymphoma and neuroblastoma [19]. Rarely, pure epidural metastases may occur from direct hematogenous seeding.

Metastatic epidural disease often produces severe mass effect on the spinal cord with ensuing cord compression, a common complication of malignancy affecting almost 5 % of patients [19]. Tumors with the greatest incidence and propensity to metastasize to bone include breast, lung, and prostate carcinoma, each accounting for 15–20 % of all cases of metastatic epidural spinal cord compression [19, 20]. Non-Hodgkin lymphoma, renal cell carcinoma, and multiple myeloma account for 5–10 %, and the remainder of cases are a result of colorectal cancers, sarcomas, and unknown primary tumors [19].

The first line of treatment for most patients with metastatic epidural spinal cord compression is corticosteroids, followed by external beam radiotherapy which remains the standard of treatment. In selected patients, recent randomized trials have shown that the combination of radical surgery and radiation therapy is superior to radiation therapy alone [1].

MRI is the method of choice for diagnosing and quantifying the severity of epidural metastases. As a result, MRI is particularly useful for guiding radiotherapy, playing a major role in determining the size of the radiation field used. Other techniques such as conventional myelography with or without CT are often used when patients are not able to undergo MRI evaluation due to various reasons such as the presence of metallic implants.

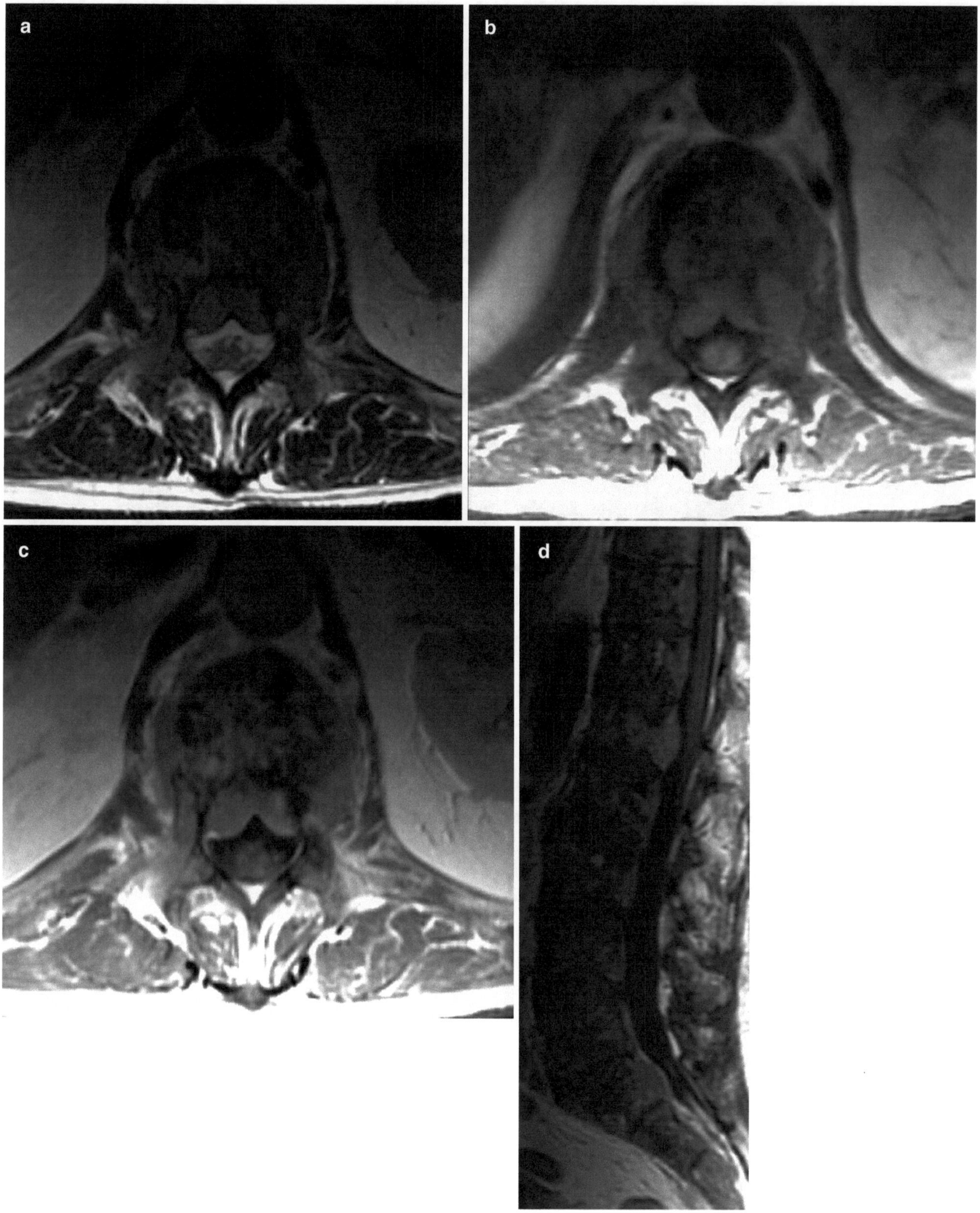

Fig. 4.19 Breast carcinoma metastases. Axial T2 (**a**), axial T1 (**b**), as well as axial and sagittal contrast T1 (**c** and **d**) weighted images demonstrate multilevel, multifocal, heterogeneously enhancing vertebral body metastases with T1/T2 isointense homogeneously enhancing ventral epidural disease. Notice the bilobed ventral configuration bound posteriorly by a T2 hypointense band representing the posterior longitudinal ligament and dural thickening that have been displaced dorsally into the thecal sac. The bilobed appearance with characteristic central depression is due to the presence of the median sagittal septum

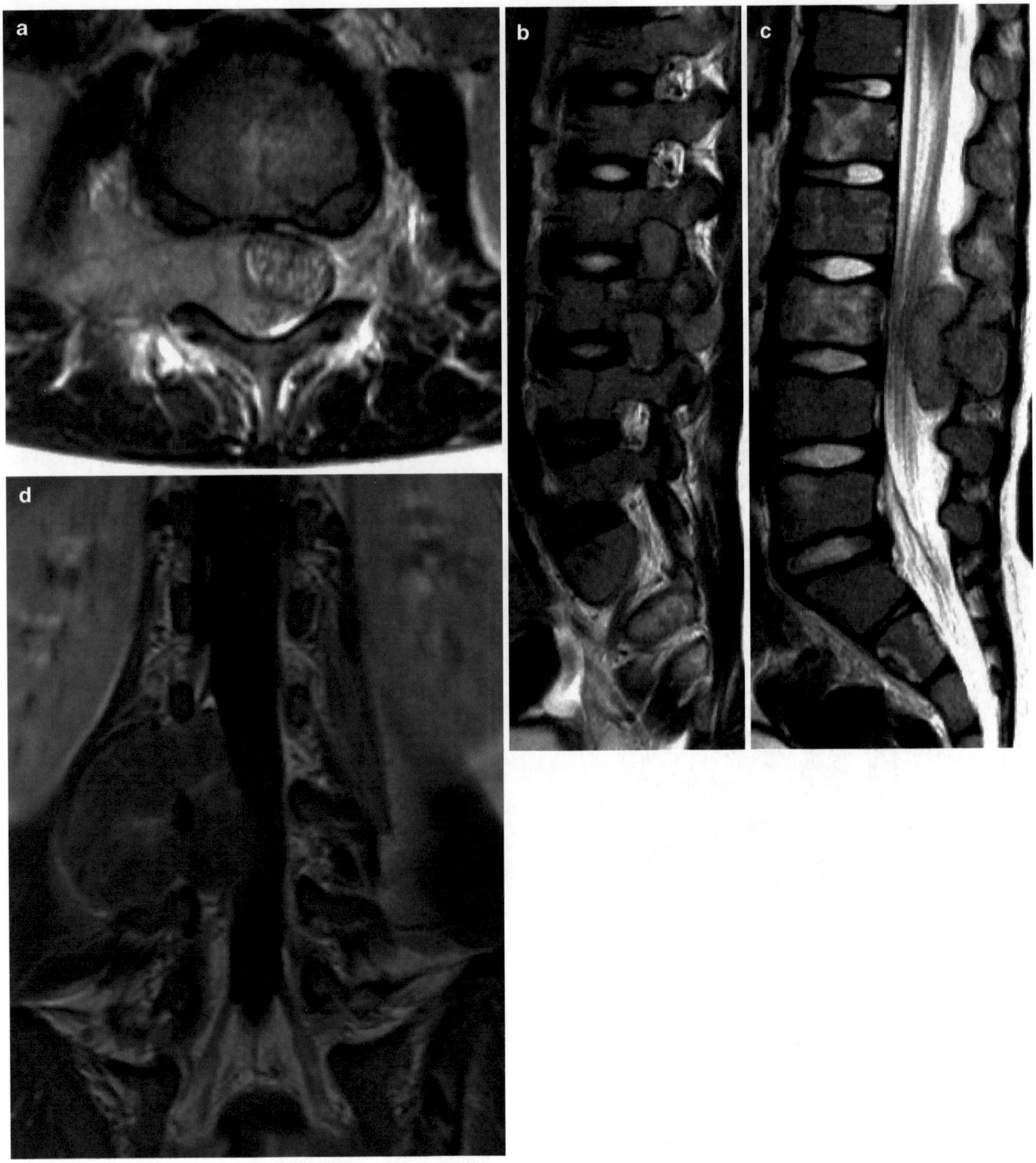

Fig. 4.20 Neuroblastoma. Axial T2 (**a**) and sagittal T2 (**b** and **c**) weighted MR images demonstrate a lobular T2 hyperintense right paravertebral mass spreading into the right lateral and dorsal epidural space via direct extension through the right L1–L2 and L2–L3 neural foramina. There is associated mass effect on the thecal sac, which is mildly displaced ventrally and to the left of midline. Coronal contrast T1 (**d**) weighted MRI further delineates the margins of the mass and its route of spread into the central canal via contiguous lumbar neural foramina

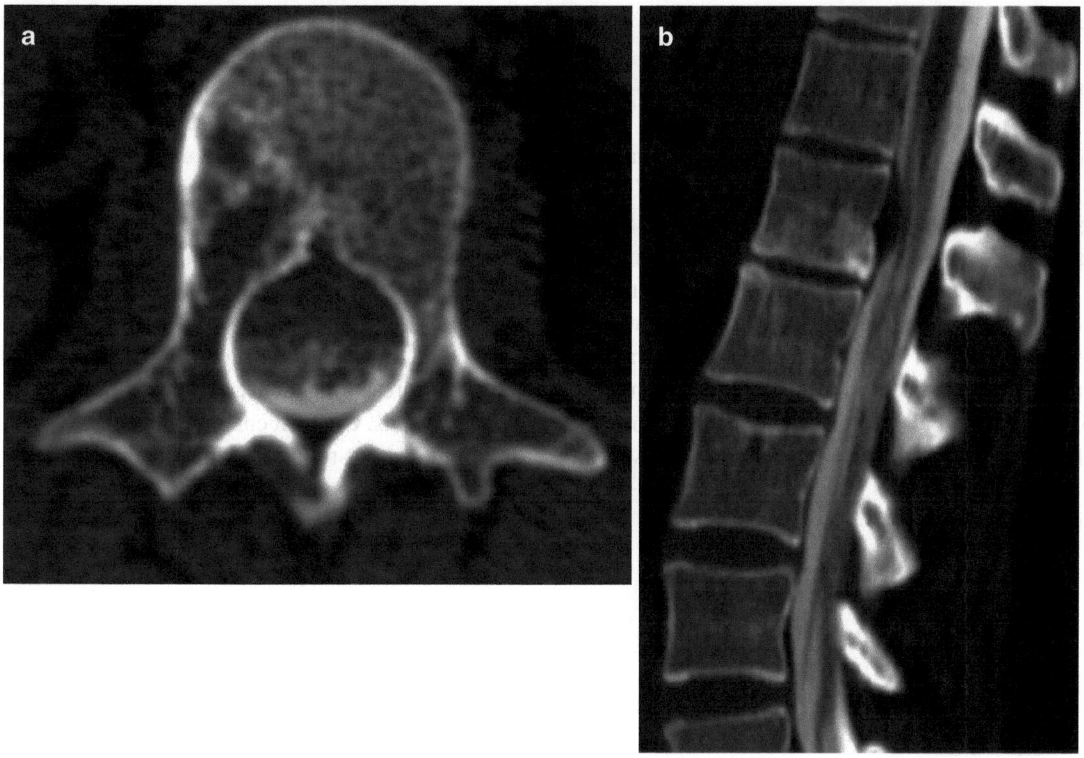

Fig. 4.21 Breast carcinoma metastasis. Axial (**a**) and sagittal (**b**) images from a CT myelogram in bone algorithm demonstrate an osteolytic metastasis involving the right portion of the L1 vertebral body and pedicle in this patient with known breast carcinoma. There is associated moderate degree of ventral epidural disease at the L1 level that is well delineated by the presence of intrathecal contrast. Effacement of the ventral thecal sac and mild mass effect on the cauda equina nerve roots is also evident

Intradural Extramedullary Neoplasms

Schwannoma

Schwannomas are the most common intradural extramedullary spinal neoplasm followed by meningiomas [20]. They are benign World Health Organization (WHO) grade I tumors with a high incidence in patients with neurofibromatosis type II (NF2) [20]. Seventy percent of schwannomas are intradural whereas 30 % are extradural [20]. Lesions that extend out of the neural foramen tend to be located both intradurally and extradurally. Unlike neurofibromas, schwannomas arise from a single focus typically along the dorsal sensory nerve roots of the cervical and lumbar spine; rather than enveloping the nerve, they displace it to the side. As a result, schwannomas have a lobular rather than a fusiform morphology. They are composed of Schwann cells and other elements of the peripheral nerve sheath such as fibroblasts. Fatty degeneration may occur; however, malignant transformation is almost never seen, except in patients with NF2 where the risk of transformation is much higher. Cystic formation is common whereas calcification and gross hemorrhage are not.

On MRI, schwannomas are usually T1 isointense and markedly T2 hyperintense secondary to their high water content. Often times, they will contain central foci of T2 hypointensity, representing denser areas of packed collagen and Schwann cells. Contrast enhancement may vary from intense and homogenous to faint peripheral enhancement.

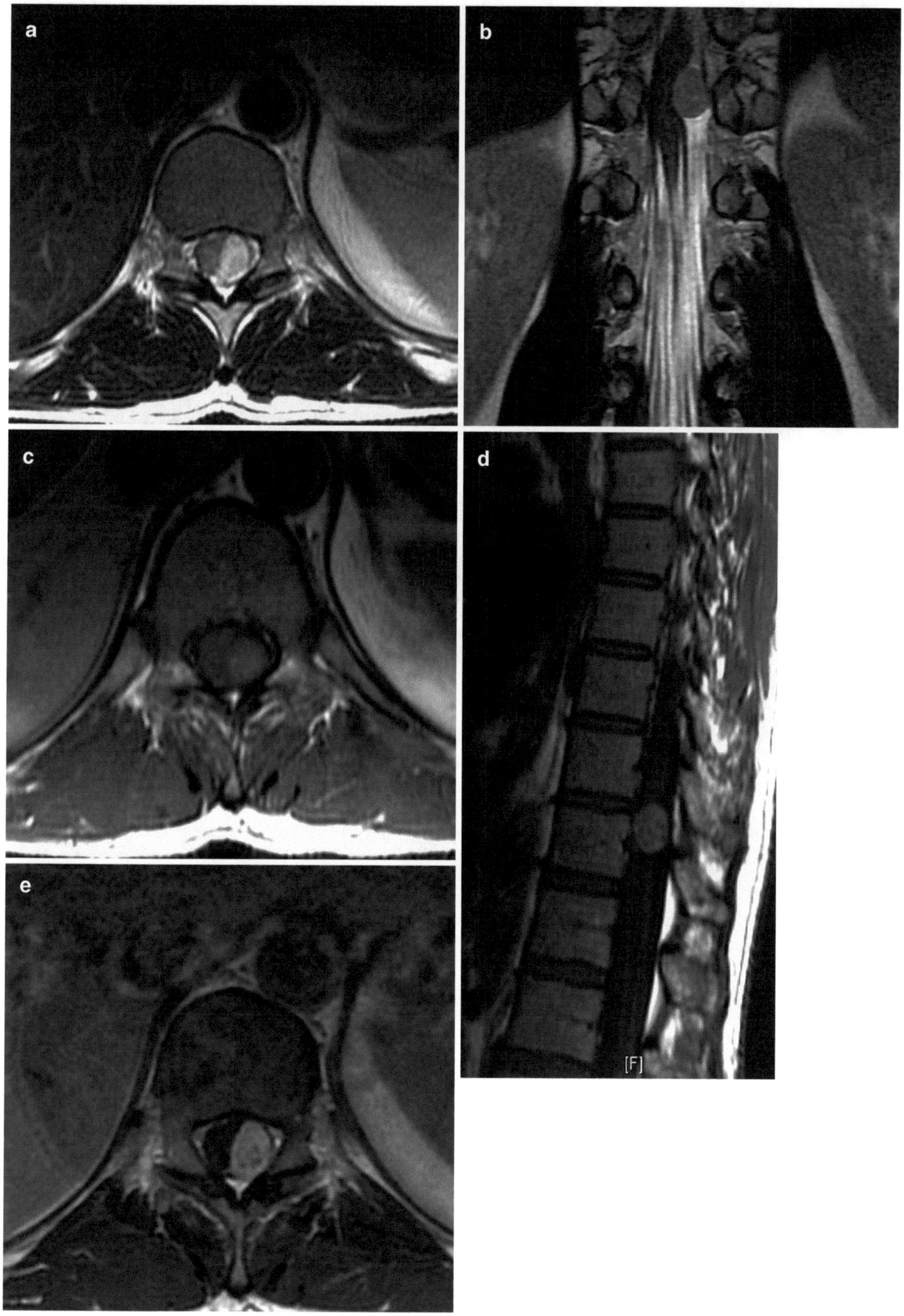

Fig. 4.22 Schwannoma. Axial and coronal T2 (**a** and **b**) as well as axial and sagittal T1-weighted MR images (**c** and **d**) demonstrate a well-circumscribed intradural, extramedullary lesion displacing the conus medullaris and cauda equina nerve roots to the right of midline. Contrast-enhanced axial, sagittal, and coronal T1-weighted images (**e–g**) demonstrate avid mildly heterogeneous enhancement of the lesion

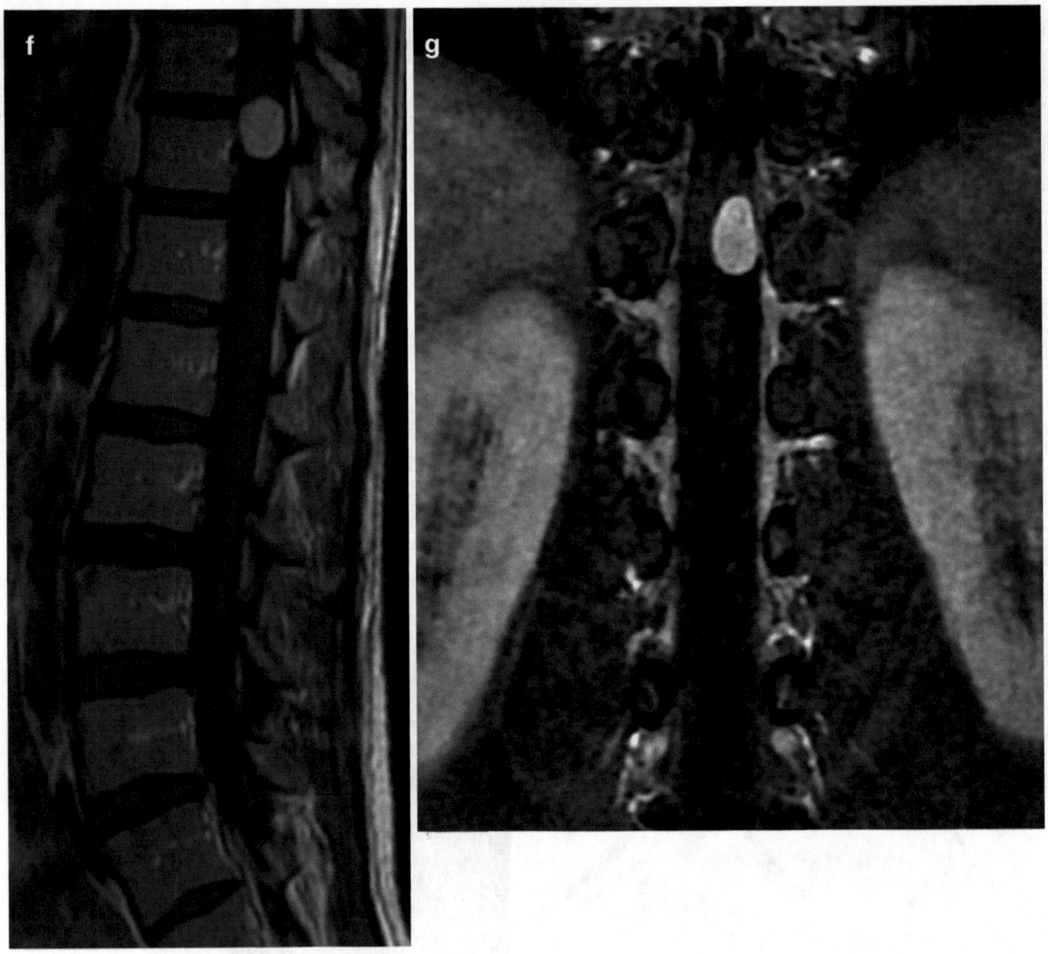

Fig. 4.22 (continued)

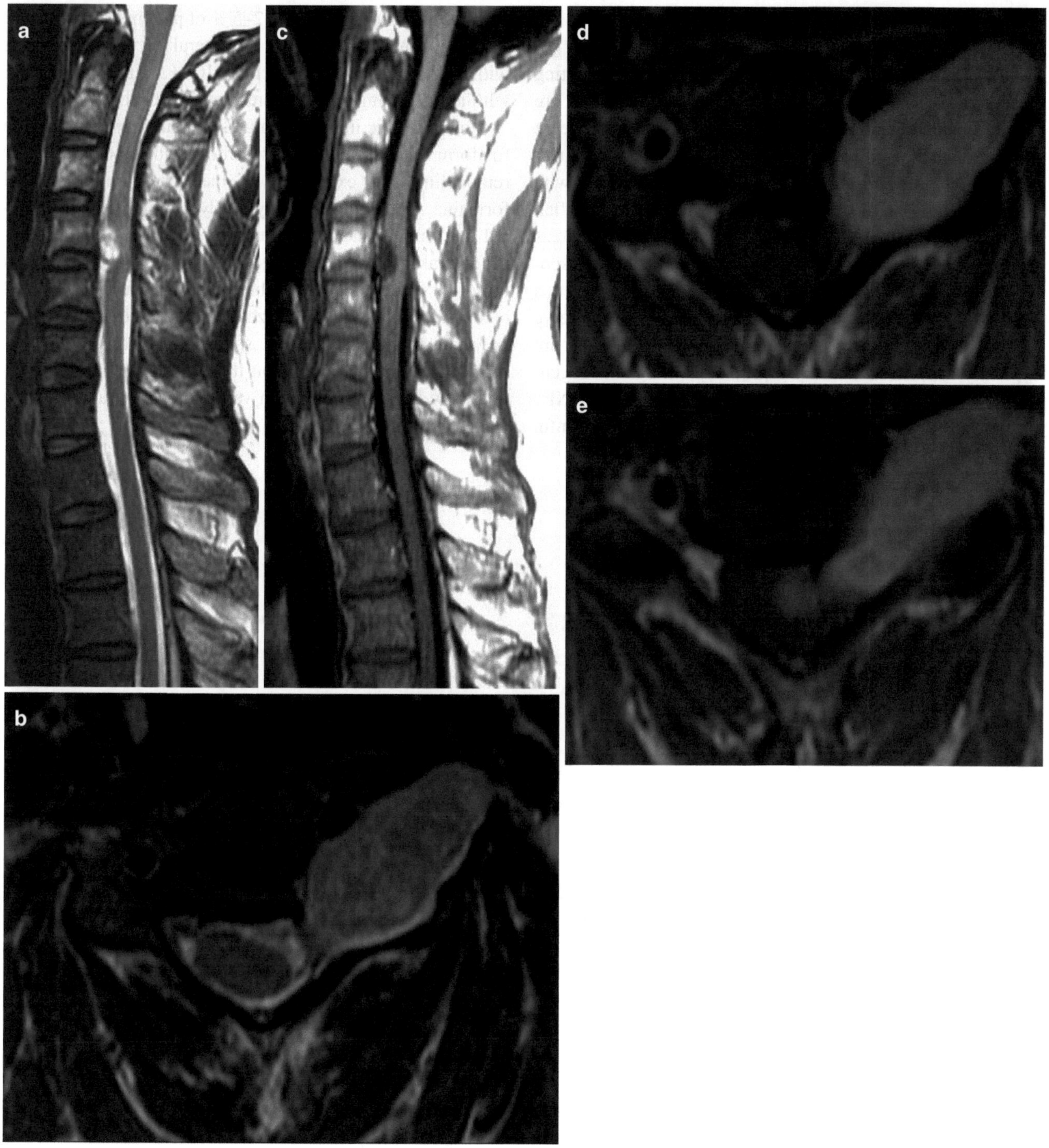

Fig. 4.23 Schwannoma. Sagittal and axial T2 (**a** and **b**) as well as sagittal T1 (**c**) MR images demonstrate a heterogeneous but predominantly T2 hyperintense, T1 hypointense, well-circumscribed, "dumbbell"-shaped mass with both an intradural component causing mass effect on the ventral spinal cord as well as an extradural component extending through the left C4–C5 neural foramen into the left lateral paravertebral space. There is associated bony remodeling and expansion of the left C4–C5 neural foramen. There is also asymmetric ventral displacement of the left vertebral artery without arterial thrombosis, likely owing to the slow growth and indolent nature of the lesion. Intense homogeneous enhancement is noted on the axial contrast T1-weighted images (**d** and **e**)

Neurofibroma

Neurofibromas are benign WHO grade I tumors affecting peripheral nerves. Unlike schwannomas, neurofibromas are not encapsulated and envelop rather than displace the nerve causing it to expand in a radial fashion [21]. They are usually entirely extradural in location or extramedullary with both intradural and extradural components. They are often multiple, particularly in patients with neurofibromatosis type I (NF1); however, they may also be solitary and sporadic. Lesions having a multinodular appearance likened to a "bag of worms" often involving several branches of a nerve plexus have been accordingly termed "plexiform" and are typically associated with NF1 [20, 21]. Malignant degeneration is uncommon but may occur more frequently in NF1 and may be distinguished by their rapid growth and painful presentation. Approximately 2–5 % of patients with NF1 are reported to have a malignant peripheral nerve sheath tumor with a lifetime risk approaching 10 %, usually occurring within preexisting neurofibromas rather than de novo [22].

Characteristic imaging features of neurofibromas include fusiform enlargement of nerve roots with associated bony remodeling and expansion of the corresponding neural formaina. The tumors are typically isointense to the spinal cord on T1 and hyperintense on T2 with a characteristic central hypointense focus producing a "target sign" on long TR sequences. Neurofibromas often have a dumbbell configuration as they squeeze out of the neural foramen; however, this finding is not specific and other benign or malignant tumors may exhibit this feature. Enhancement is relatively homogeneous with variable degree ranging from mild to moderate.

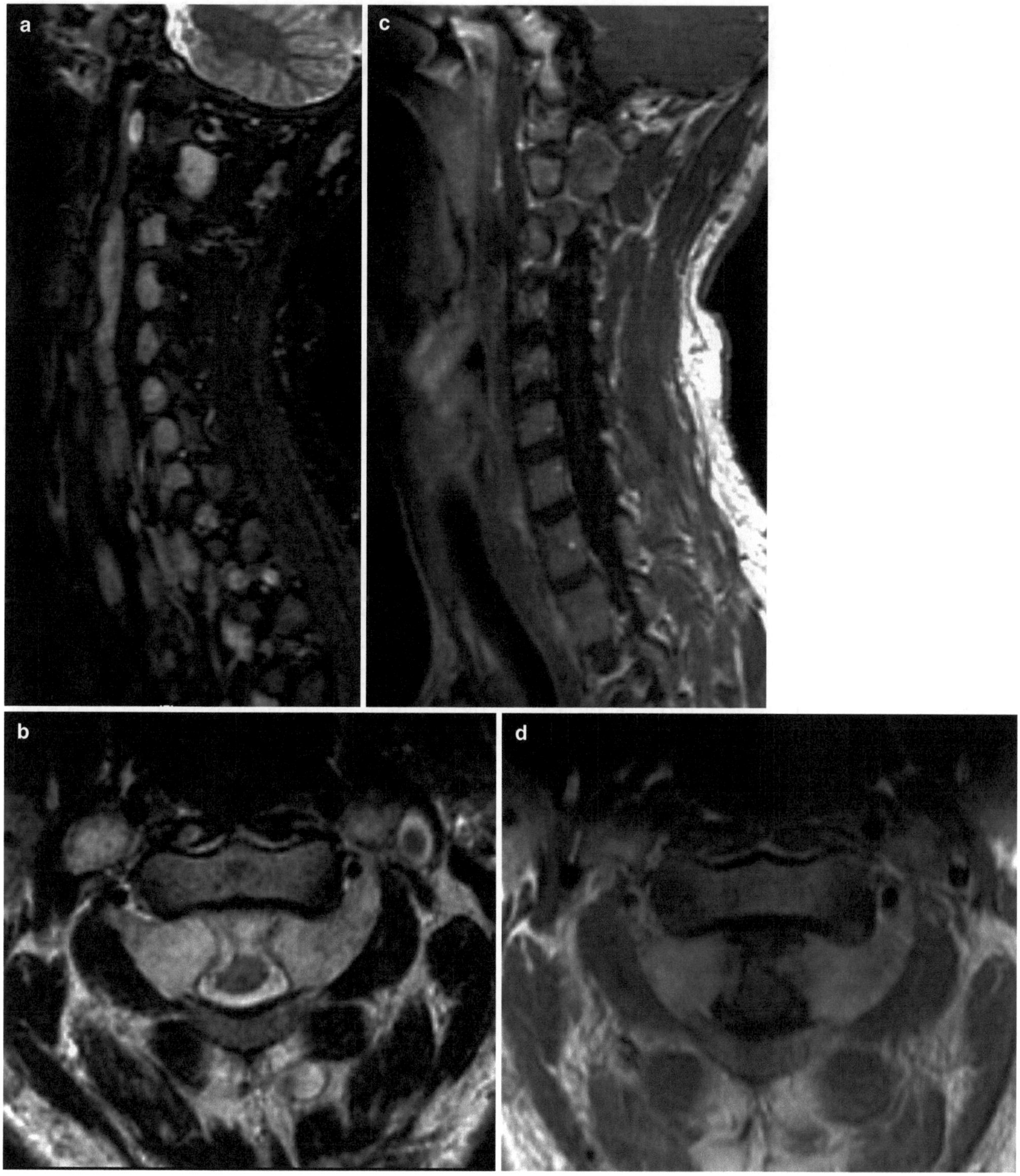

Fig. 4.24 Neurofibromas in NF1. Sagittal STIR (**a**) MRI demonstrates multilevel STIR hyperintense masses centered within the neural foramina which appear scalloped and expanded. Axial T2-weighted MRI (**b**) demonstrates the lesions to be bilateral bulging into the central spinal canal but confined to the extradural space as evidenced by T2 hypointense dura mater draped over the medial margins of the lesions. Following the administration of intravenous contrast, the lesions demonstrate relatively homogeneous enhancement (**c** and **d**)

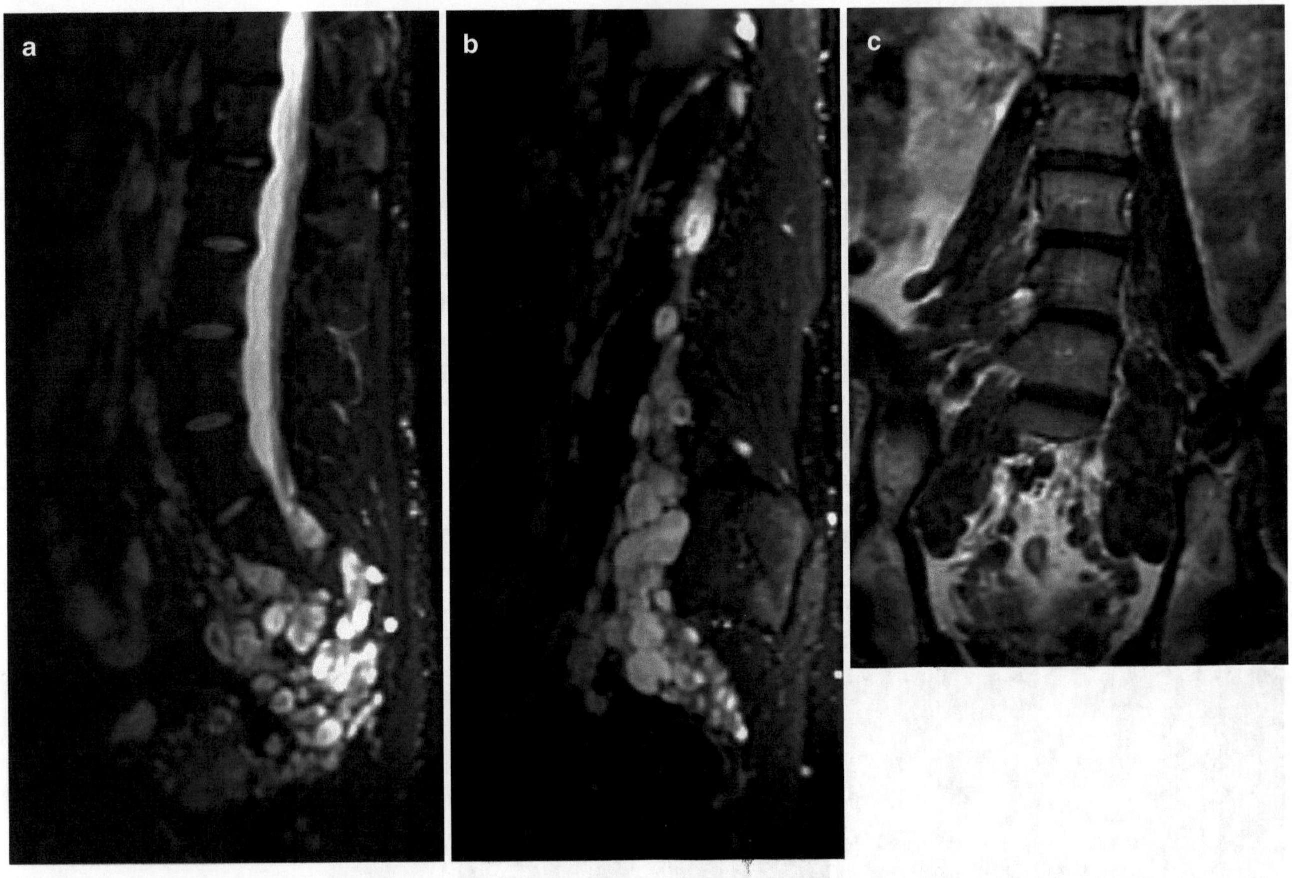

Fig. 4.25 Neurofibromas in NF1. Sagittal STIR (**a** and **b**) MR images demonstrate multilobulated T2 hyperintense lesions extending along the course of the lumbosacral plexus with a characteristic "bag of worms" morphology. Many of the lesions demonstrate a central area of STIR hypointensity producing the classic "target sign." Following contrast administration, mild slightly heterogeneous enhancement is evident (**c**)

Meningioma

Meningiomas are typically benign, intradural, extramedullary neoplasms arising from arachnoid cap cell rests that rarely may be extradural in location. They have a greater than 80 % female predilection and most commonly arise within the thoracic spinal canal (>70 %), followed by the cervical and lumbar spinal canal [23]. They are commonly seen in patients with neurofibromatosis type 2 or in patients with prior radiation exposure. Morphologically, they are well circumscribed, slow growing, dural based tumors that displace and compress adjacent structures. They are most often solid, highly cellular lesions although rarely they may be cystic.

On MRI, meningiomas are characteristically isointense to the spinal cord on T1 and iso to mildly hyperintense on T2. They may sometimes become densely calcified manifesting as markedly hypointense on both T1 and T2 weighted imaging. Homogeneous post contrast enhancement is typical, often associated with an enhancing, broad dural tail.

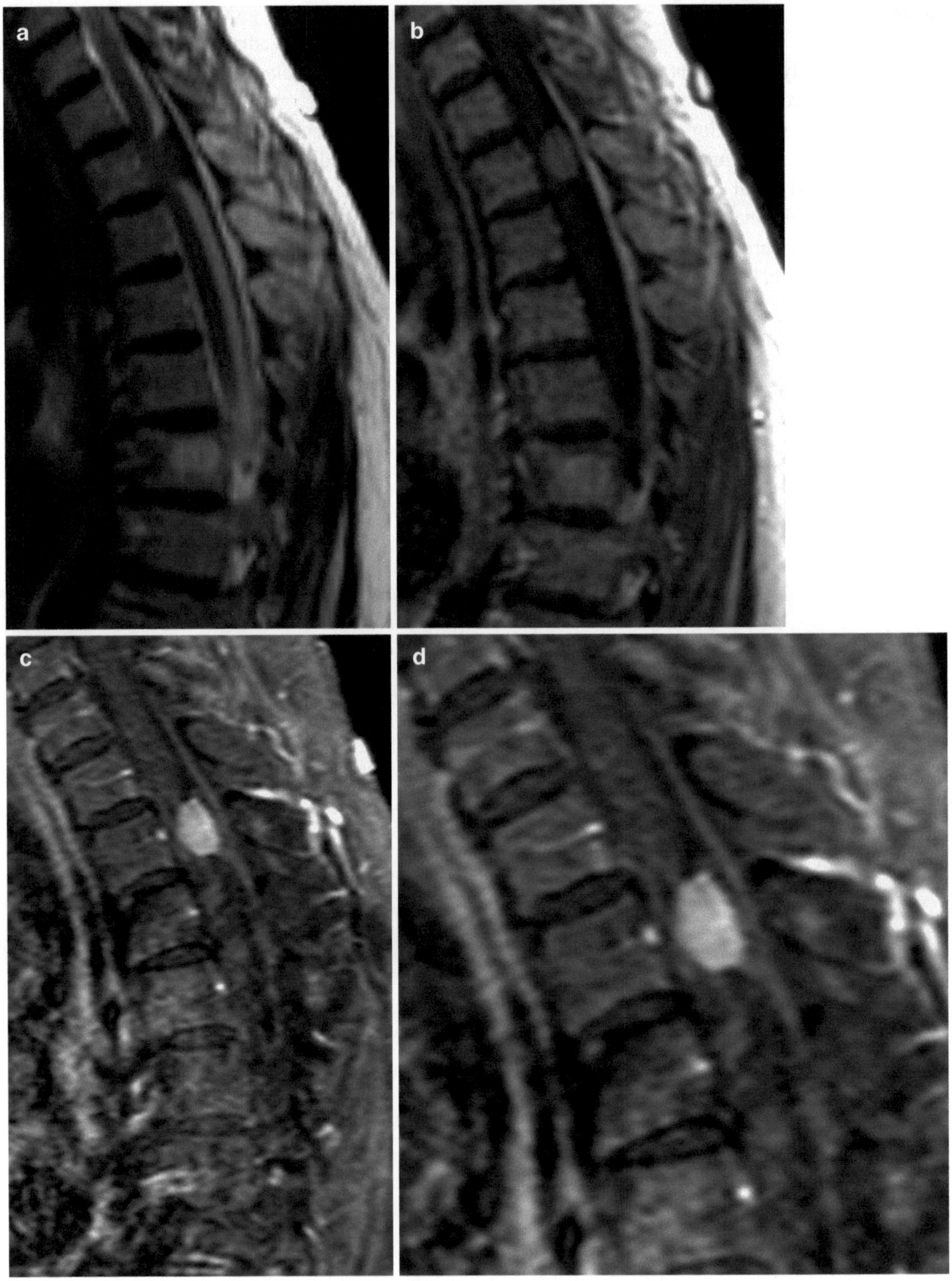

Fig. 4.26 Meningioma. Sagittal T2 (**a**), sagittal T1 (**b**), and sagittal contrast T1 fat-suppressed (**c** and **d**) MR images demonstrate a well-circumscribed, intradural, extramedullary mass that appears homogeneously T2 isointense to the spinal cord. The lesion has an associated broad-based T2 hypointense attachment to the dura which appears significantly thickened and probably partially calcified. There is mass effect on the dorsal surface of the spinal cord, which is compressed and ventrally displaced, resulting in widening of the ipsilateral dorsal subarachnoid space. Avid homogeneous contrast enhancement is characteristic. Incidentally noted is a circumscribed T1/T2 hyperintense lesion with coarsened, hypointense, vertical trabeculae within the T8 vertebral body consistent with a hemangioma

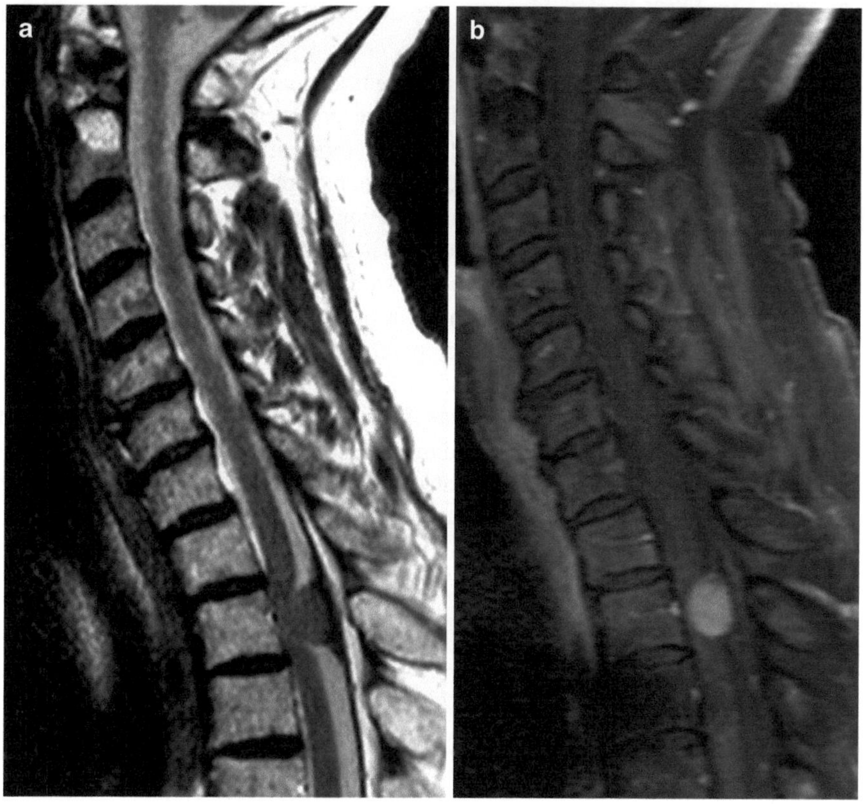

Fig. 4.27 Meningioma. Sagittal T2 (**a**) and sagittal contrast T1 fat-suppressed (**b**) MR images demonstrate a similar T2 isointense intradural extramedullary lesion compressing the spinal cord with marked associated T2 hypointense dural thickening. The lesion avidly enhances except for its dural attachment, which is partially calcified. Incidentally noted is a hemangioma involving the odontoid process of the C2 vertebra

Paraganglioma

Paragangliomas are benign neoplasms of neuroendocrine origin arising from accessory organelles of the peripheral nervous system termed paraganglia. They are most often located within the adrenal gland where they are named pheochromocytomas. Common extra-adrenal locations include the carotid bifurcation, jugular foramen, or in immediate proximity to the vagus nerve. They are rare within the central nervous system but may be found within the pineal region, sella turcica, petrous ridge, and spinal canal where they usually involve the conus medullaris, cauda equina and filum terminale [24]. Spinal paragangliomas are intradural extramedullary, soft, encapsulated masses, sometimes slightly hemorrhagic and often associated with prominent feeding arteries. The lesions sometimes form a pedicular attachment to nearby nerve roots or the filum terminale [25]. They may be locally aggressive; however, distant metastases are uncommon [25].

On MRI, paragangliomas are typically well-circumscribed masses that are T1 isointense relative to the spinal cord and iso- to hyperintense on T2. They tend to avidly enhance owing to their dense vascularity, often manifesting as serpentine flow voids within or along the surface of the tumor. Hemorrhage is common and as a result a low signal intensity hemosiderin rim or "cap sign" is often seen on T2-weighted imaging [20]. The "salt and pepper" appearance that is characteristic of neck and skull base paragangliomas has also been described in lesions arising within the cauda equina [26].

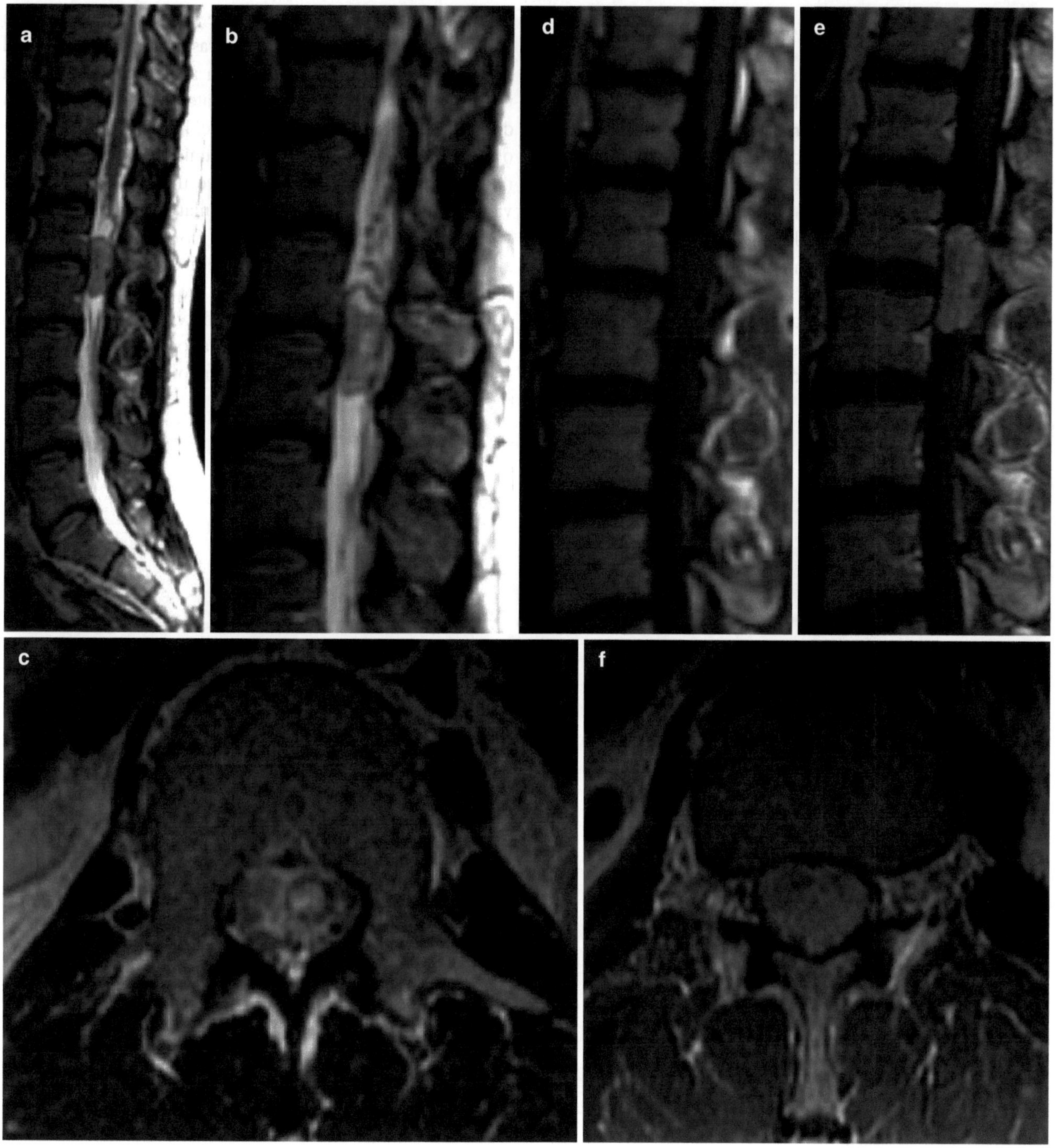

Fig. 4.28 Paraganglioma. Sagittal and axial T2-weighted MR images (**a–c**) demonstrate a well-circumscribed, predominantly T2 hyperintense intradural, extramedullary lesion within the lumbar spinal canal intimately associated with the cauda equine nerve roots. The lesion contains a low signal intensity hemosiderin cap suggesting repetitive hemorrhage and is also associated with numerous serpentine flow voids predominating along its superior surface. The lesion appears isointense to the spinal cord on the sagittal T1-weighted image (**d**) and demonstrates intense mildly heterogeneous enhancement on the sagittal and axial contrast T1-weighted images (**e** and **f**)

Arachnoid Cyst

Arachnoid cysts are benign, extramedullary lesions that may be intradural or extradural in location. They are usually well circumscribed and cause characteristic mass effect and displacement of the spinal cord and nerve roots, sometimes resulting in syringohydromyelia and myelopathy. Intradural arachnoid cysts are more commonly associated with mass effect and compressive myelopathy than those within the extradural space, which often extend out of the confines of the spinal canal through adjacent neural foramina. Although arachnoid cysts may occur at any level within the spinal canal, they are most frequently found within the thoracic region [27]. Intradural arachnoid cysts are thought to originate from a diverticulum of the arachnoid mater, which splits to form the cyst walls. In contrast, extradural arachnoid cysts are thought to originate from a diverticulum of dura mater or possibly from arachnoid mater protruding through a dural defect into the extradural space. In either case, they are often associated with a direct communication with the arachnoid space through a narrow orifice that can act as a ball valve mechanism resulting in cyst enlargement.

On MRI, arachnoid cysts are of CSF signal intensity on all pulse sequences. They may sometimes be of higher signal intensity than CSF on T2-weighted sequences with or without internal signal voids related to flow phenomenon within the cyst. Following the administration of contrast, there should be no associated enhancement of these lesions.

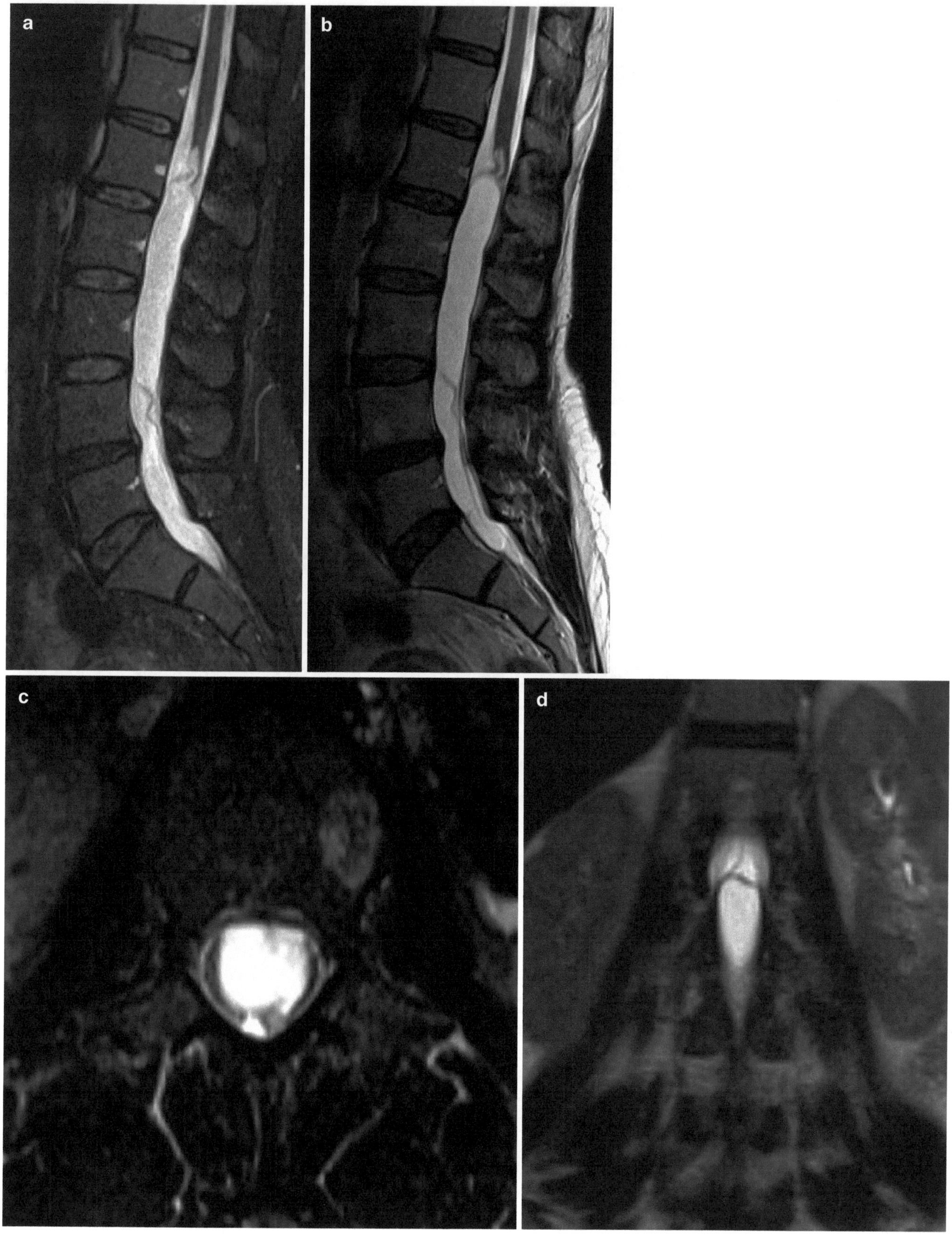

Fig. 4.29 Arachnoid cyst. Sagittal STIR (**a**), sagittal (**b**), axial (**c**), and coronal T2 (**d**) as well as sagittal T1 (**e**) weighted MR images demonstrate an oblong, intradural extramedullary, well-circumscribed, cystic lesion, following CSF signal intensity on all pulse sequences, displacing the conus medullaris and cauda equina nerve roots. The nerve roots are draped along the periphery of the cyst, thereby delineating its contours. There is no evidence for enhancement on the sagittal contrast T1-weighted image (**f**)

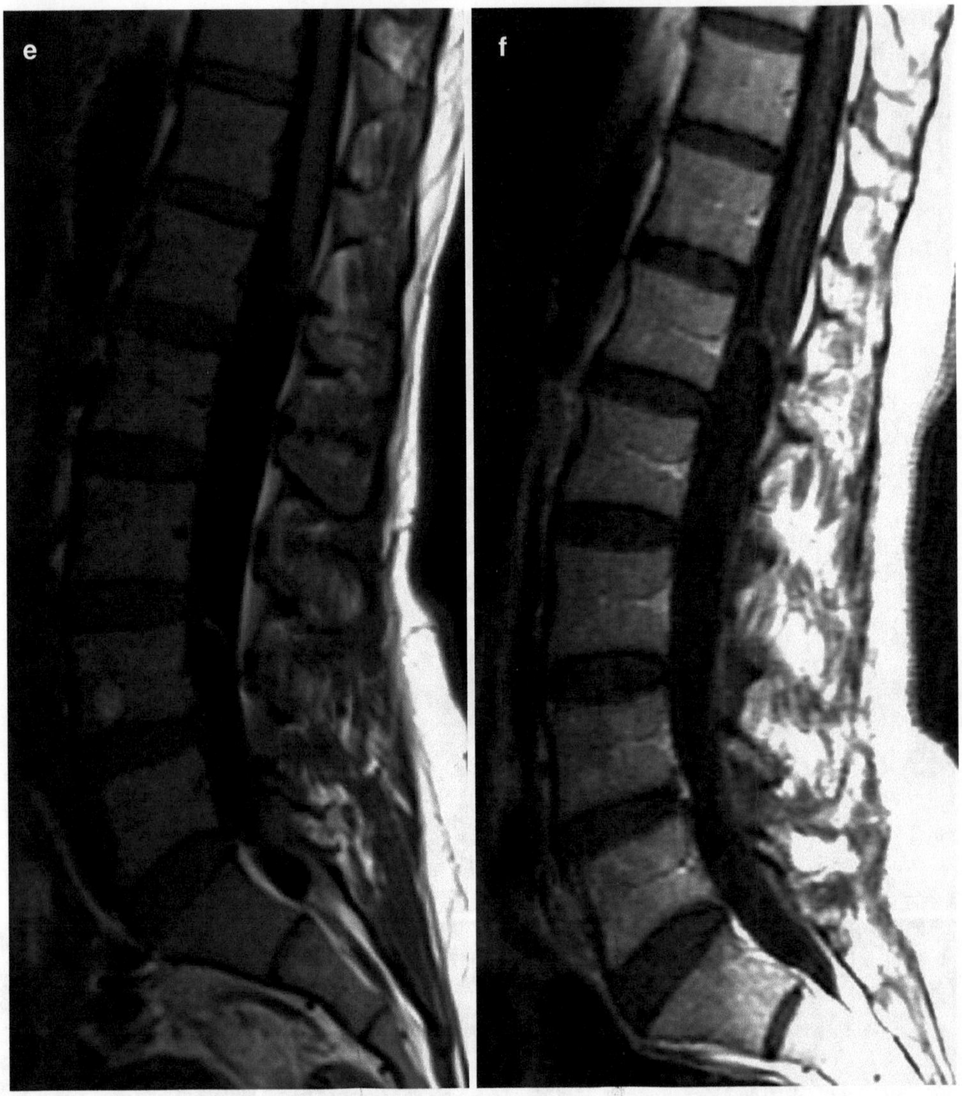

Fig. 4.29 (continued)

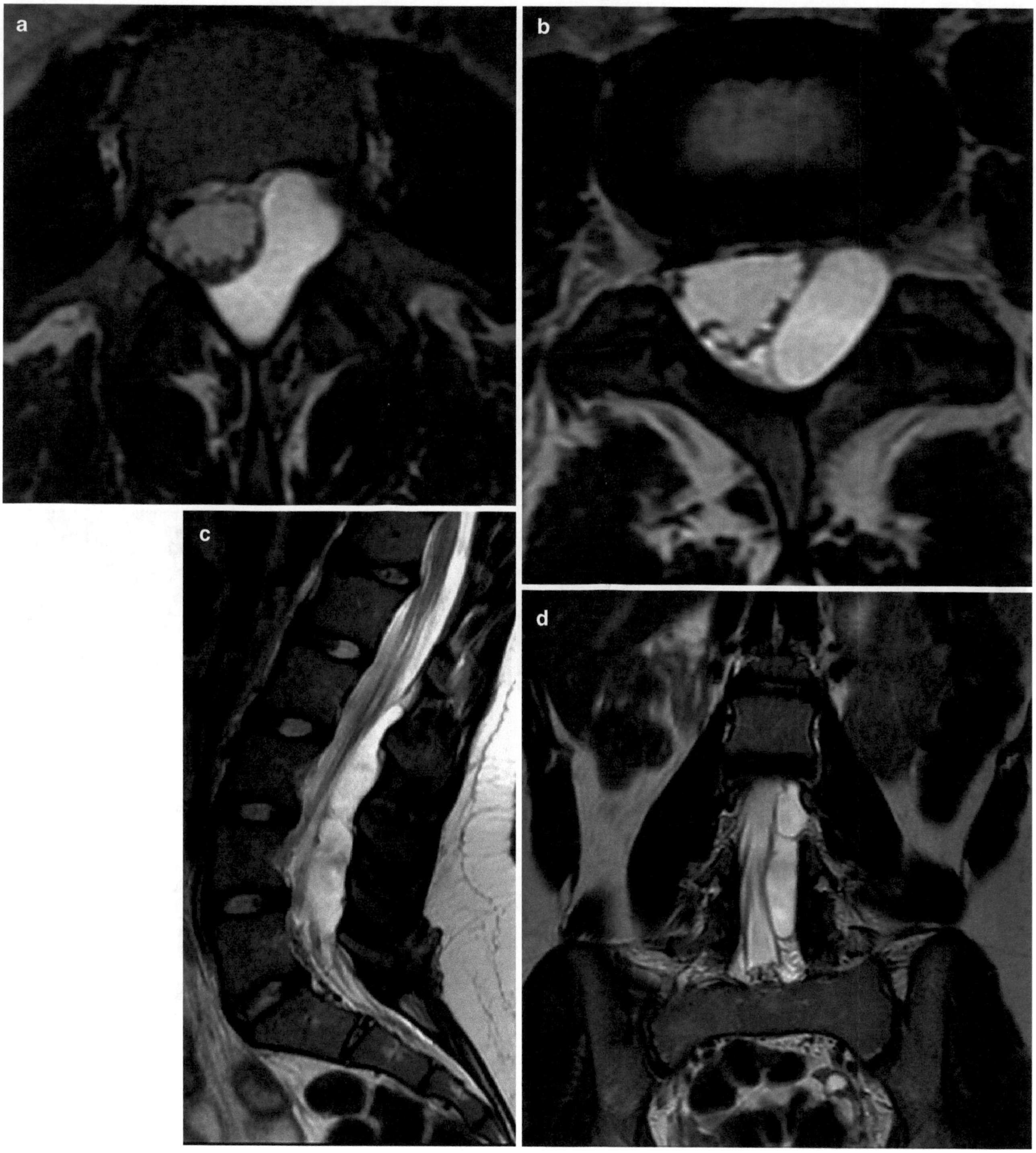

Fig. 4.30 Arachnoid cyst. Axial T2 (**a** and **b**) as well as sagittal and coronal T2-weighted MR images (**c**–**e**) demonstrate an extramedullary, extradural arachnoid cyst of CSF signal intensity located within the left dorsolateral spinal canal causing mild mass effect on the thecal sac, which is slightly displaced to the right of midline. Axial images from a CT myelogram (**f** and **g**) confirm the location of the lesion within the extradural space and demonstrate a discrete point of communication between the cyst, which is opacified with intrathecal contrast, and the intradural CSF space, which is likewise opacified with contrast

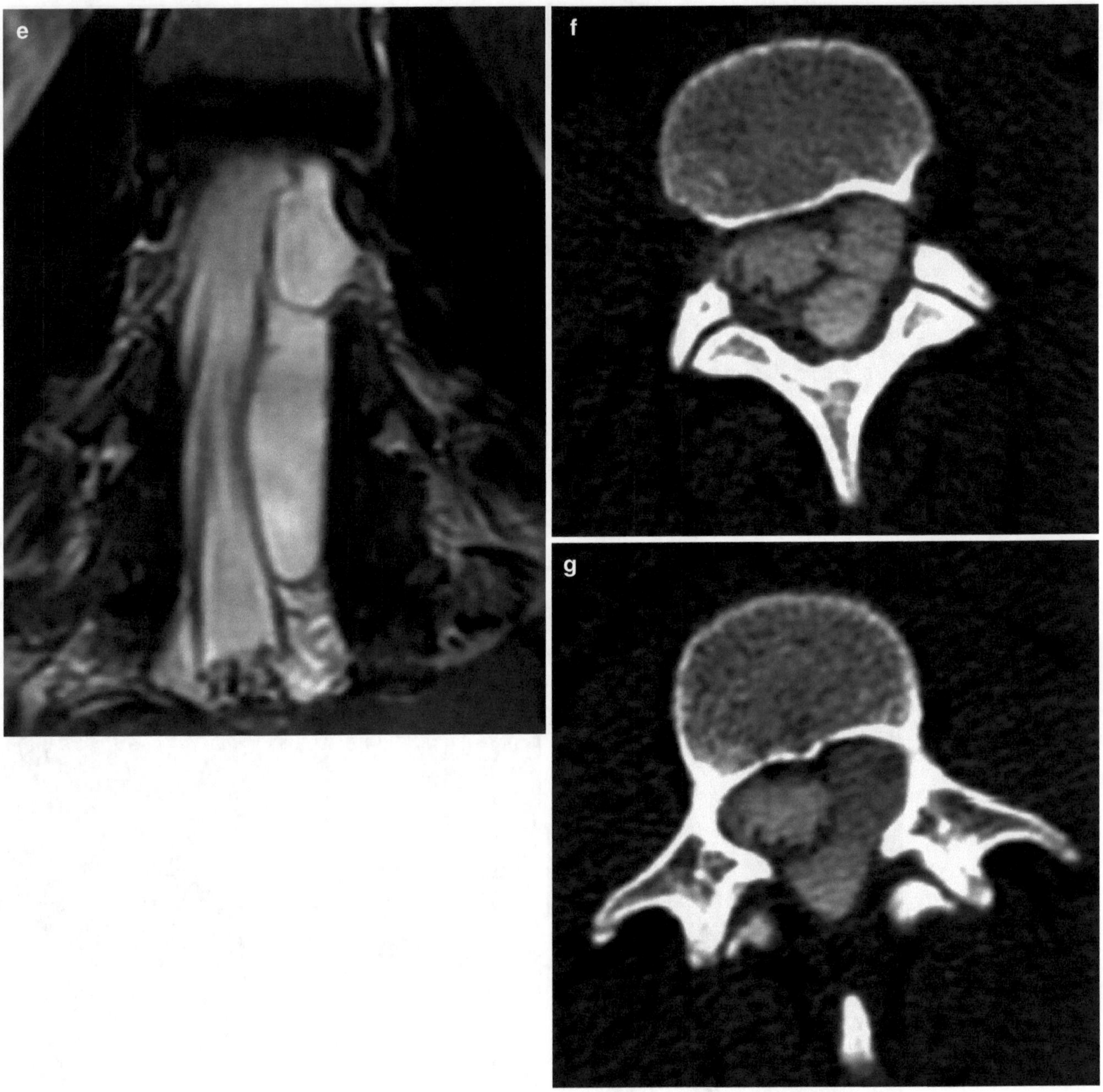

Fig. 4.30 (continued)

Epidermoid Cyst

Spinal epidermoid cysts are rare, benign, slow-growing inclusion cysts that comprise between 0.5 and 1.0 % of all spinal tumors typically presenting within the lumbosacral canal but also occurring throughout the cervical and thoracic levels [28, 29]. They are most commonly intradural extramedullary in location, although rarely may be intramedullary. Epidermoid cysts are usually congenital caused by inclusion of epidermal cells during the third or fourth week of gestation when the neural tube closes. They may also be acquired and have been described in patients with a history of repeated lumbar punctures where ectopic epidermal elements are introduced into the spinal canal. Despite their benign nature, spinal epidermoid cysts are usually treated surgically to avoid the risk of rupture and resultant chemical meningitis, as well as superimposed infection when a connecting dorsal-dermal sinus tract exists [30].

On MRI, the signal intensity of these lesions is highly variable. As a result, distinguishing them from other neoplasms may be difficult. They are most commonly homogenous or heterogeneously T1 hypointense and T2 hyperintense; however, atypical signal intensity changes have been reported including hyperintense signal on T1 and hypointense signal on T2 [31]. Generally these lesions do not demonstrate contrast enhancement, although a thin peripheral rim of enhancement has been reported [31]. Much like their intracranial counterparts, spinal epidermoid cysts may follow CSF signal intensity on all pulse sequences. As a result, they may be indistinguishable from spinal arachnoid cysts on conventional MR sequences. Diffusion-weighted imaging (DWI) has emerged as a helpful distinguishing tool because unlike arachnoid cysts, epidermoid cysts typically demonstrate restricted diffusion with hyperintense signal on DWI and corresponding hypointense signal on apparent diffusion coefficient (ADC) images. Distinguishing these two entities becomes important for preoperative planning. Arachnoid cysts may be fenestrated or drained percutaneously, whereas epidermoid cysts typically require traditional laminectomy and gross resection [30].

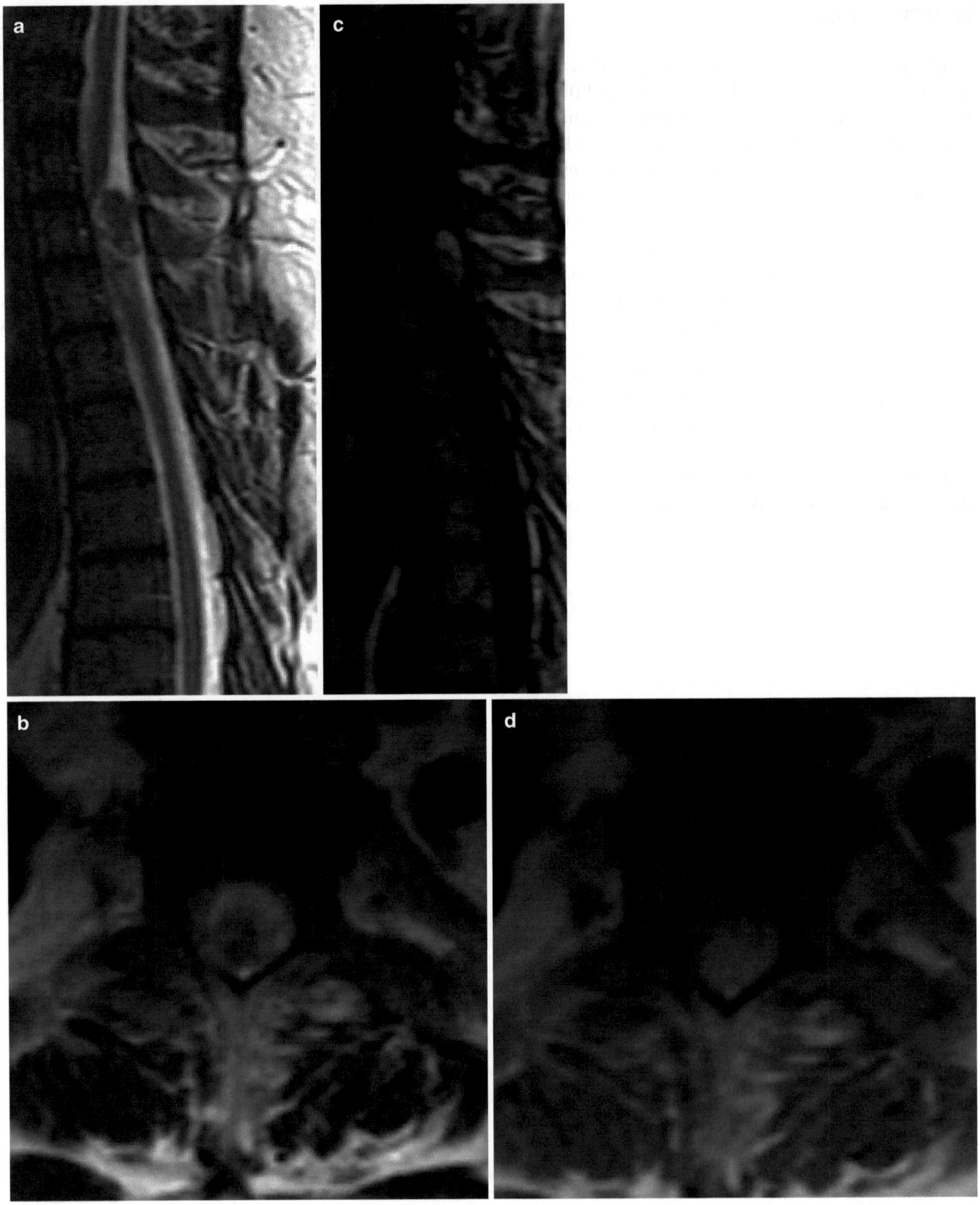

Fig. 4.31 Epidermoid cyst. Sagittal and axial T2-weighted MR images (**a** and **b**) depict an ovoid intradural extramedullary lesion within the thoracic spinal canal with mixed T2 signal intensities including a central T2 hypointense component and a peripheral T2 hyperintense portion. On nonenhanced T1 sagittal and axial imaging (**c** and **d**), the lesion appears heterogeneously hyperintense to the spinal cord. Sagittal and axial contrast T1-weighted images (**e** and **f**) demonstrate only minimal peripheral enhancement of the anterior inferior portion of this surgically proven epidermoid cyst

Fig. 4.31 (continued)

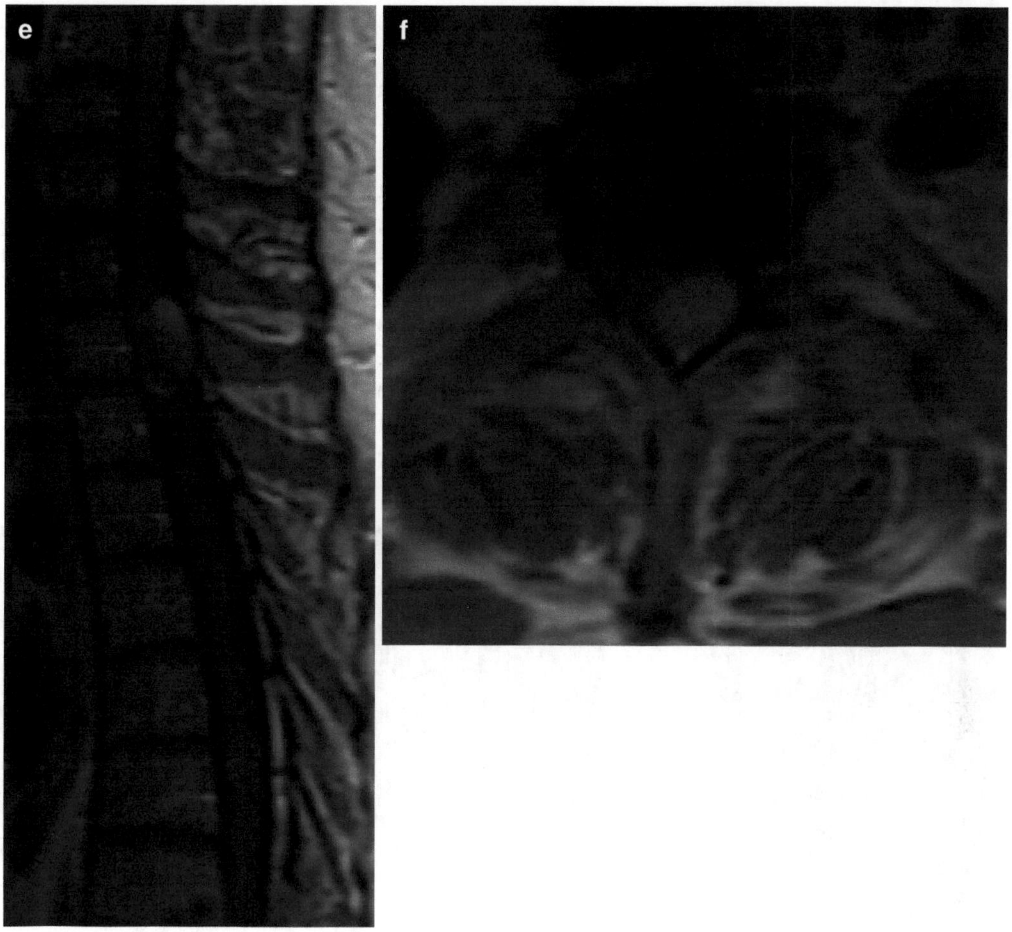

Leptomeningeal Metastasis

Leptomeningeal disease may be a result of drop metastases from primary CNS neoplasms or hematogenous or lymphatic spread of disease, as well as seeding via direct extension or via the choroid plexus. Primary CNS neoplasms that tend to spread to the leptomeninges include glioblastoma, medulloblastoma, high-grade astrocytoma, oligodendroglioma, retinoblastoma, and pineoblastoma. Secondary neoplasms that commonly spread to the leptomeninges include breast, lung, colon, and malignant melanoma. Leptomeningeal spread of disease has a predilection for the lumbosacral region, which is thought to be a direct result of the effects of gravity whereby tumor cells tend to aggregate in the lower spinal canal [8]. There also seems to be a predilection for the dorsal spinal canal, which is felt to be a result of the natural flow of CSF traveling from the base of the brain dorsal to the spinal cord and returning ventral to the cord [8].

On MRI, leptomeningeal deposits may manifest as linear or nodular plaque-like foci along the surface of the spinal cord and cauda equina nerve roots. Often times leptomeningeal deposits are so small and granular that they appear to "sugar coat" the surfaces of the leptomeninges. They are usually T1 isointense and T2 iso to hyperintense but often difficult to discern without the aid of intravenous contrast. Avid homogenous enhancement is typical following intravenous contrast administration.

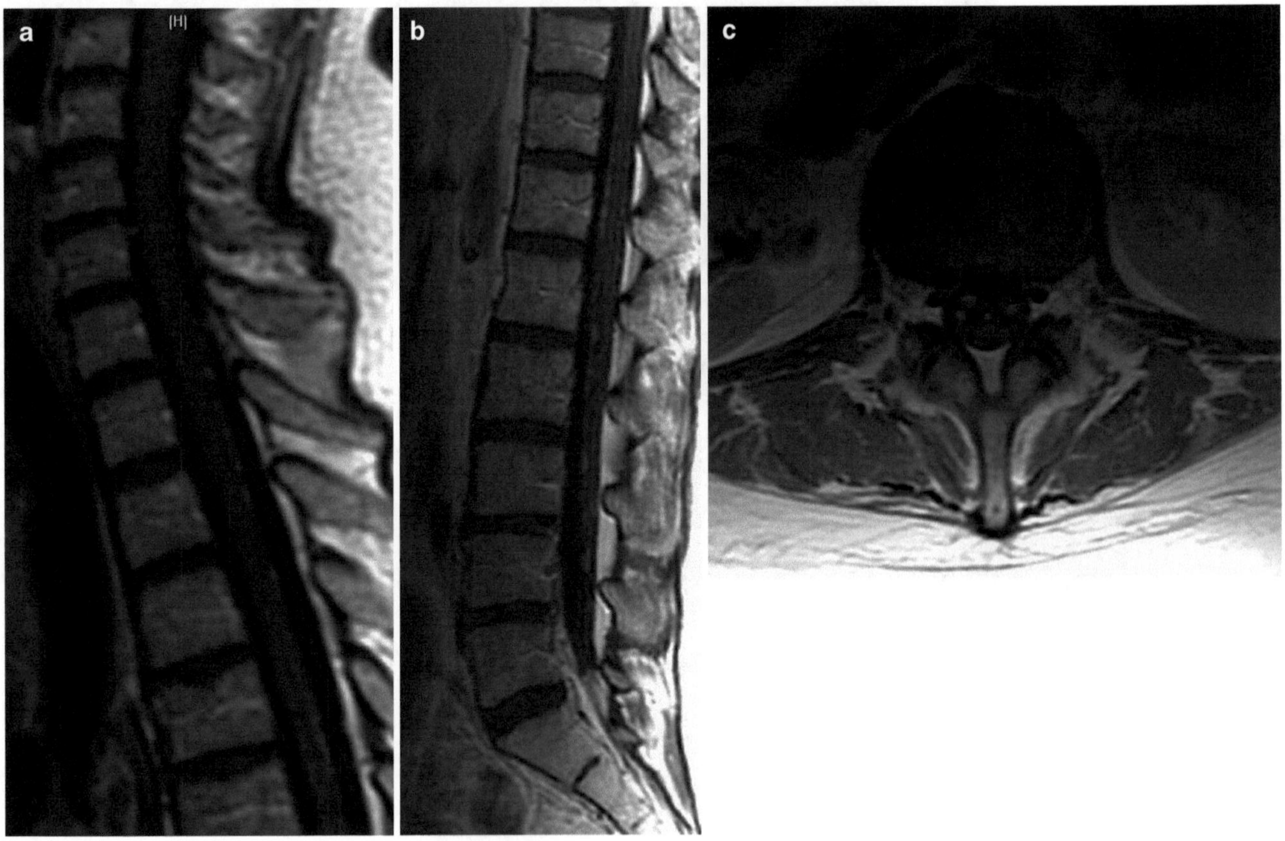

Fig. 4.32 Leptomeningeal metastases. Sagittal (**a** and **b**) and axial (**c**) contrast T1-weighted MR images of the cervical and lumbar spine demonstrate fine, linear, plaque-like and nodular foci of enhancement "sugar coating" the surfaces of the spinal cord and cauda equina nerve roots consistent with leptomeningeal metastases in a patient with known history of malignant melanoma

Fig. 4.33 Leptomeningeal metastases. Sagittal T2 (**a**) MRI of the lumbar spine in a patient with lung carcinoma demonstrates nodular T2 isointense leptomeningeal deposits with a caudal predilection along the cauda equine nerve roots. Nodular enhancement is noted following contrast administration (**b**)

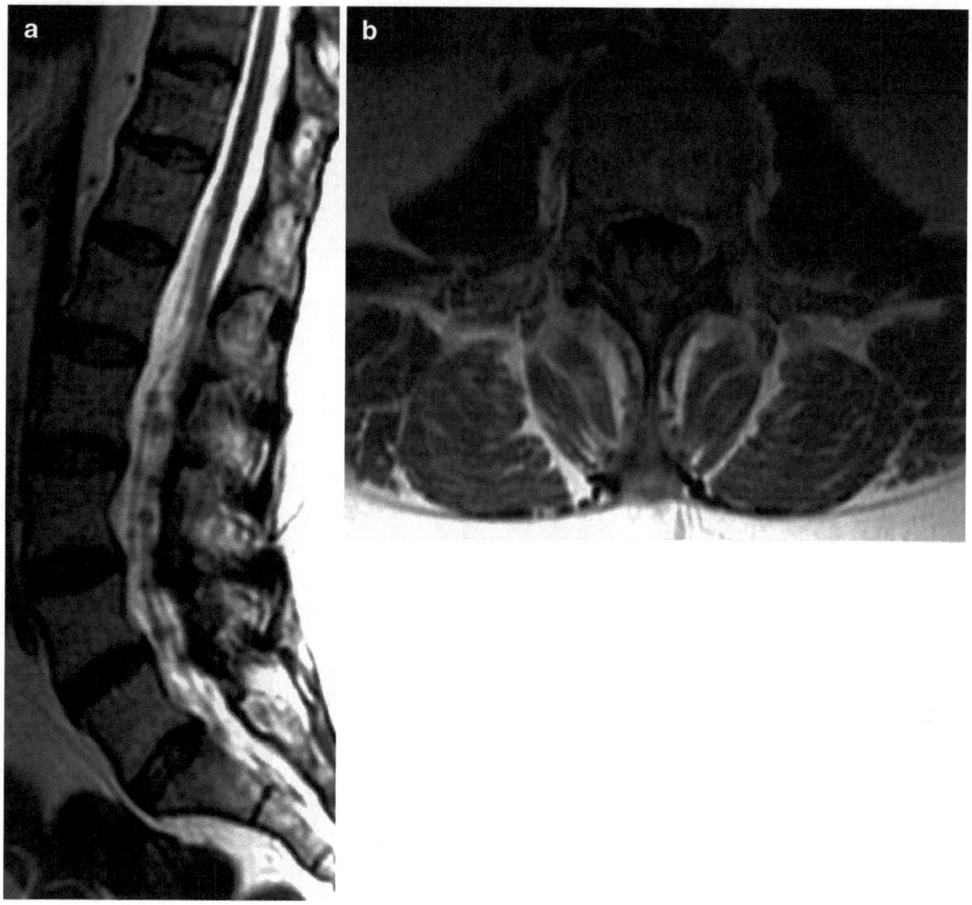

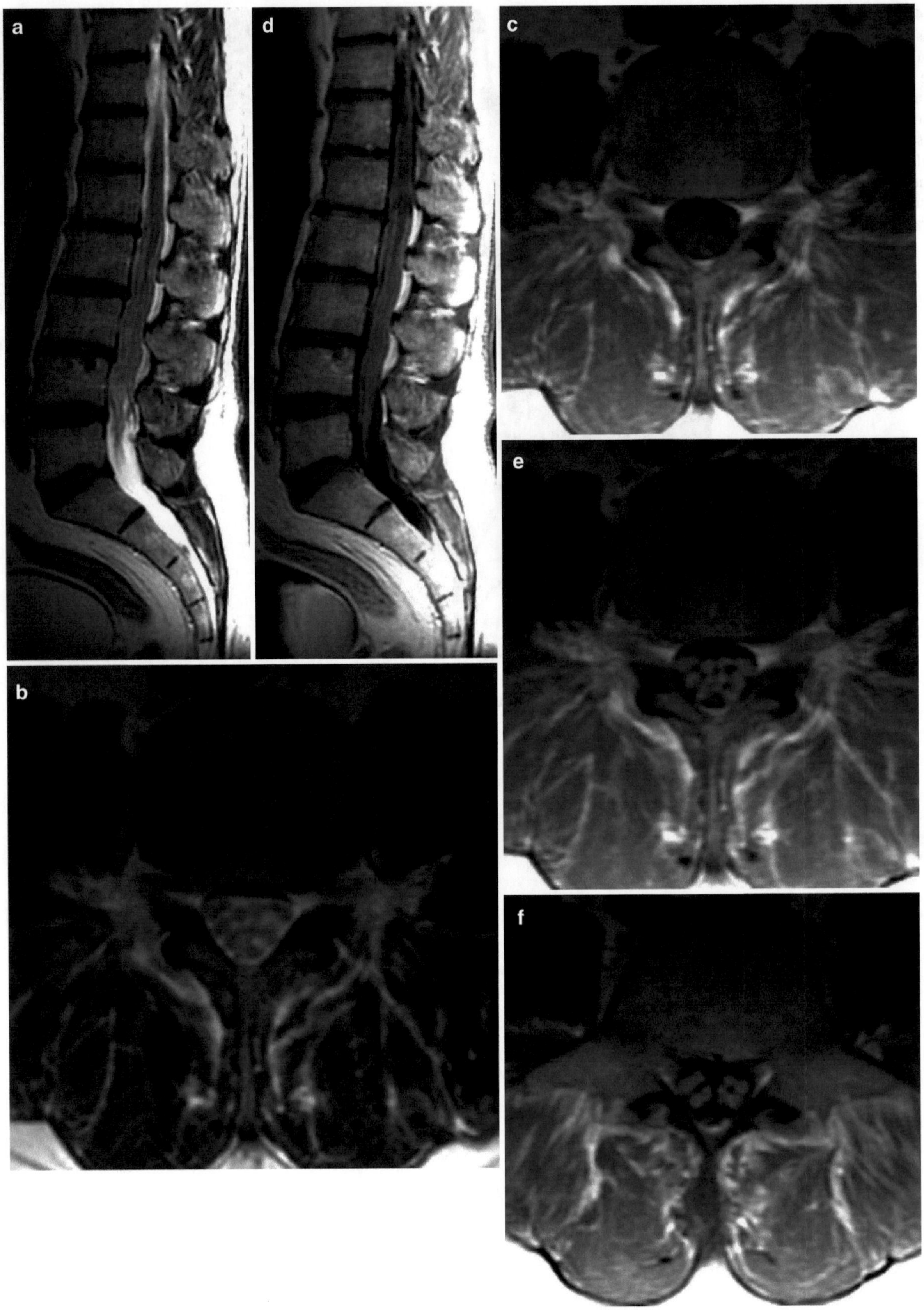

Fig. 4.34 Leptomeningeal metastases. Sagittal T2 (**a**), axial T2 (**b**), and axial T1 (**c**) weighted MR images demonstrate marked nodular thickening of the cauda equina nerve roots, which appear T1 isointense and mildly T2 hyperintense. Sagittal (**d**) and axial contrast T1 (**e** and **f**) weighted MR images demonstrate homogeneous enhancement of the nerve roots consistent with leptomeningeal spread of disease in this patient with Mantle cell lymphoma

Intramedullary Neoplasms

Ependymoma

Ependymomas are benign, intramedullary neoplasms accounting for 50–60 % of adult spinal cord tumors, typically presenting within the cervical cord, followed by the thoracic cord and conus medullaris [25]. These lesions are most common in young adulthood with a slight male predilection and a mean age at presentation of approximately 39 years [25]. They are classified into five histologic subtypes: cellular, papillary, epithelial, tanycytic, and myxopapillary. The myxopapillary subtype almost exclusively arises from the filum terminale, sometimes involving the conus medullaris [32]. As their name implies, ependymomas arise from ependymal cells within the central canal of the spinal cord leading to fusiform spinal cord expansion, sometimes associated with spinal canal widening and posterior vertebral body erosion and scalloping. They are central in location with characteristic, benign, noninfiltrating, well-circumscribed margins and a propensity to hemorrhage [32]. They are often associated with nontumoral or tumoral cystic changes. Tumoral cystic changes occur due to degeneration, necrosis, and liquefaction within the neoplasm and typically demonstrate peripheral contrast enhancement [32]. Nontumoral cystic changes typically occur rostral or caudal to the tumor and do not enhance peripherally. Tumoral cysts need to be surgically excised, as they may be lined with abnormal glial cells, whereas nontumoral cysts do not require surgical excision and may simply be aspirated and drained [32].

On MRI, ependymomas are most commonly T1 iso to hypointense relative to the spinal cord and T2 hyperintense with or without marginal T2 hypointensity related to hemosiderin deposition in the setting of repetitive hemorrhage. Following contrast administration, enhancement is typically homogeneous, although sometimes heterogeneous or rim enhancement may occur.

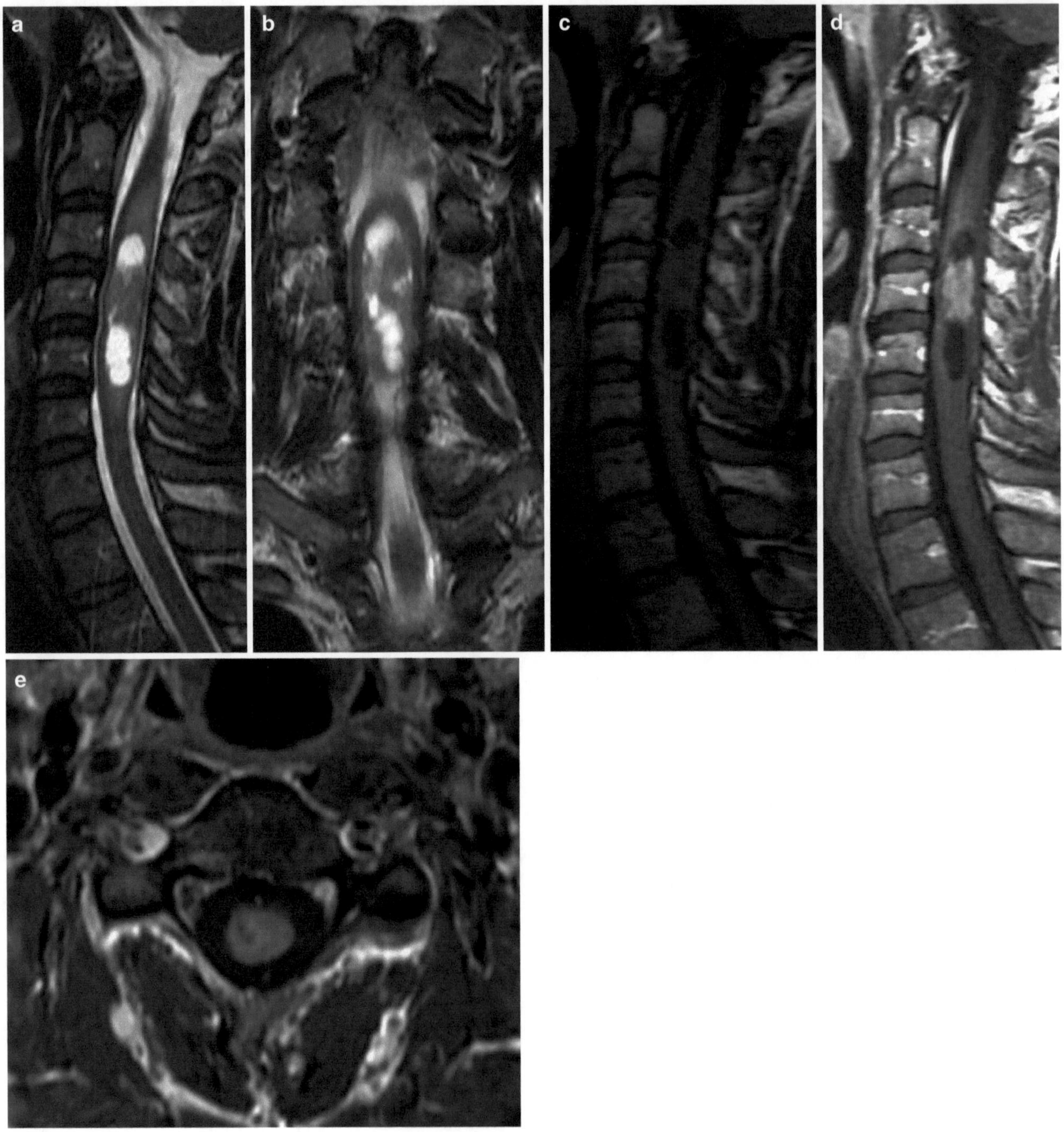

Fig. 4.35 Ependymoma. Sagittal and coronal T2 (**a** and **b**) and sagittal T1 (**c**) weighted MR images demonstrate a complex intramedullary lesion with an ovoid, solid, T1 isointense, T2 hyperintense component, as well as associated well-circumscribed, nontumoral versus tumoral cystic changes. The lesion causes symmetric cord expansion effacing the subarachnoid space and is associated with surrounding T2 hyperintense cord edema. Sagittal (**d**) and axial (**e**) contrast T1-weighted images demonstrate focal, well-circumscribed, homogeneous enhancement within the noncystic component of the lesion

Myxopapillary Ependymoma

Myxopapillary ependymomas are a histologic subtype accounting for 27–30 % of all ependymomas, typically presenting during the fourth decade of life with a mean age of 35 [32]. They are categorized as WHO grade 1 neoplasms without risk of malignant degeneration. Originating from the ependymal glia of the filum terminale, they arise almost exclusively within this location, often associated with extension into the conus and cauda equina. Morphologically, they are well-circumscribed, soft, round- or ovoid-shaped, slow growing lesions. They are prone to repetitive hemorrhage and superficial siderosis, particularly at the tumor margins. Sometimes, they may be a cause of diffuse subarachnoid hemorrhage.

On MRI, they are usually isointense relative to the spinal cord on T1 and hyperintense on T2. Occasionally, they may demonstrate hyperintense signal on both T1- and T2-weighted MR sequences due to their tendency to hemorrhage or their unique propensity to accumulate intracellular and perivascular mucin [25, 32]. Following intravenous contrast administration, avid enhancement is virtually always present.

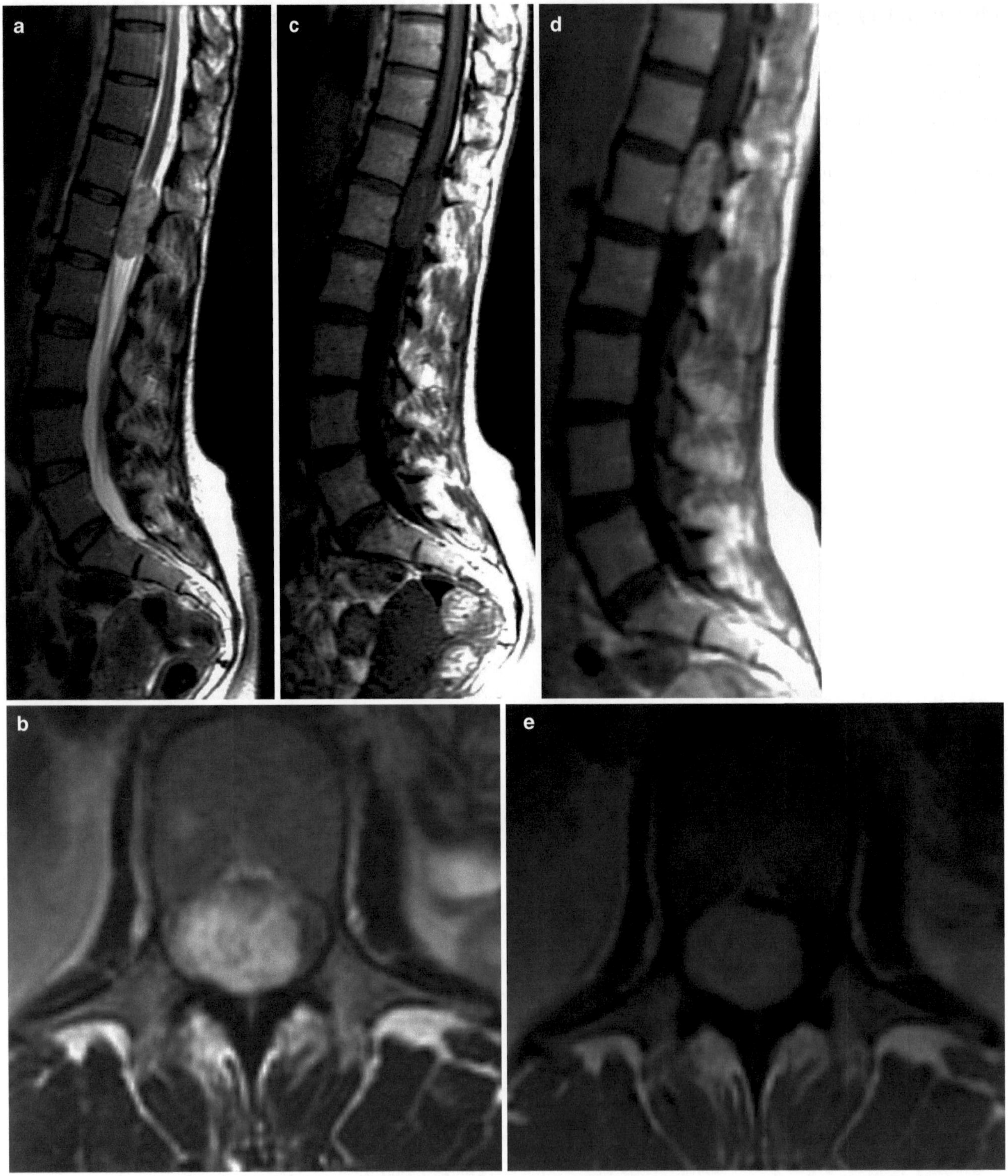

Fig. 4.36 Myxopapillary ependymoma of the conus medullaris. Sagittal T2 (**a**), axial T2 (**b**), and sagittal T1 (**c**) weighted MR images demonstrate a heterogeneous but predominantly T1 hypointense, T2 hyperintense ovoid lesion centered within the conus medullaris slightly expanding the spinal canal. Punctuate foci of intralesional pre-contrast T1 hyperintensity are noted with corresponding hypointense T2 signal suggesting hemorrhage. Following the administration of intravenous contrast, there is avid homogeneous enhancement (**d** and **e**)

Spinal Cord Astrocytoma

Spinal cord astrocytomas are primary malignant neoplasms of astrocytic glial cell origin considered the most common intramedullary tumors in the pediatric population and the second most common intramedullary tumors in adults after ependymoma [33]. The overall peak incidence of spinal cord astrocytomas is in the third and fourth decades of life. They are most commonly found within the cervical cord, followed closely by the thoracic cord and to a lesser extent the lumbar cord. Holocord involvement may also occur, most commonly in children. Isolated conus medullaris lesions occur in only 3 % of cases [25]. Filum terminale involvement is rare. The most common histologic subtypes are pilocytic astrocytoma (WHO grade I) and fibrillary astrocytoma (WHO grade II). Anaplastic astrocytoma (WHO grade III) is less common whereas glioblastoma (WHO grade IV) is rare, accounting for only 0.2–1.5 % of astrocytoma cases [33]. Astrocytomas typically span the length of less than four vertebral bodies and are eccentric in location, sometimes associated with caudal and rostral cysts. The pilocytic subtype tends to be well circumscribed, whereas higher grade II through IV astrocytomas tend to have poorly defined infiltrative margins. Unlike ependymomas, hemorrhage is very uncommon. Leptomeningeal dissemination may occur with higher-grade lesions but has also been reported with grade I astrocytomas.

On MRI, spinal astrocytomas are iso- to hypointense relative to the spinal cord on T1 and hyperintense on T2-weighted imaging. Contrast-enhanced imaging typically shows irregular patchy enhancement regardless of the histologic grade. Because of the infiltrative nature of the tumor and absence of a capsule, the margins are typically poorly defined.

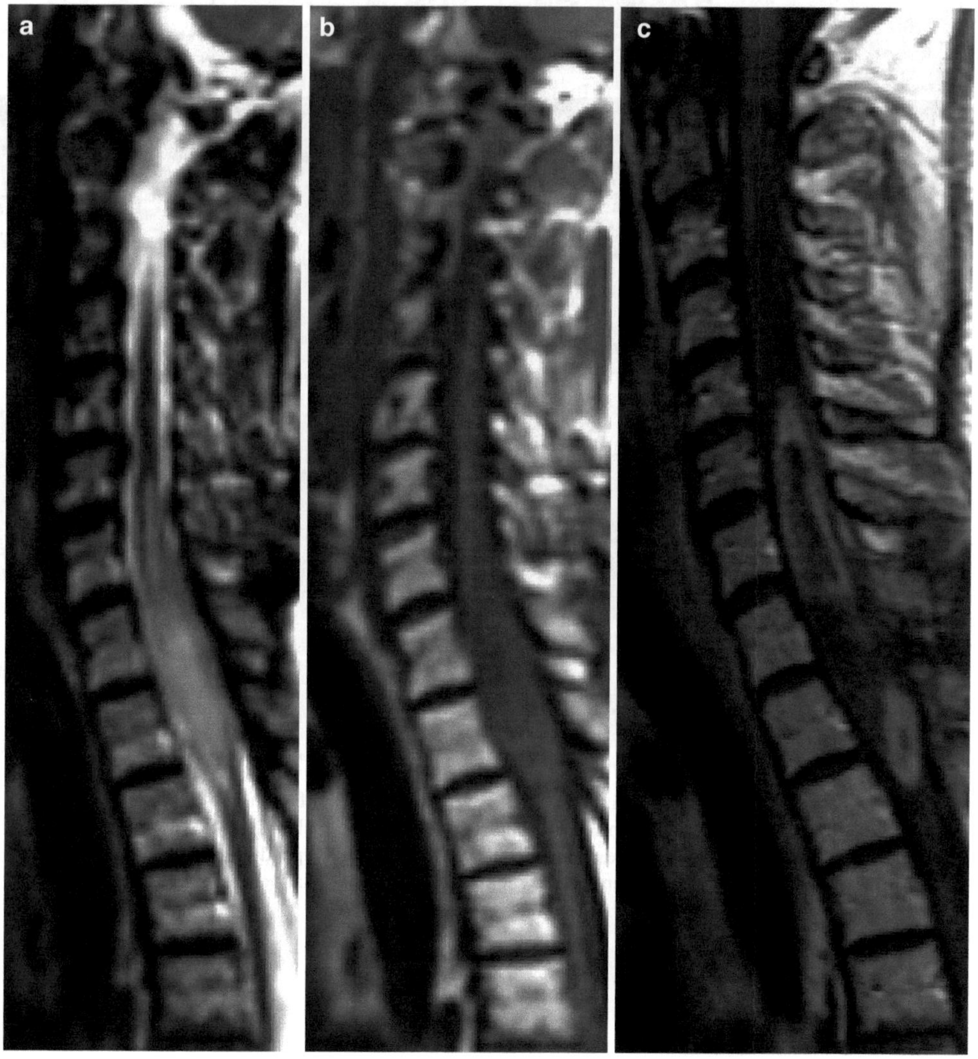

Fig. 4.37 Anaplastic astrocytoma following posterior decompression and surgical biopsy. Sagittal T2 (**a**) and sagittal T1 (**b**) weighted MR imaging depicts an infiltrative, T2 hyperintense, T1 hypointense mass expanding the cervical spinal cord spanning approximately four vertebral levels. The margins of the lesion are ill-defined and difficult to discern from the normal spinal cord making surgical resection difficult. This is in contrast to ependymomas, which tend to have circumscribed margins that help to delineate them from normal surrounding spinal cord parenchyma. Avid heterogeneous enhancement is evident following the administration of intravenous contrast (**c**)

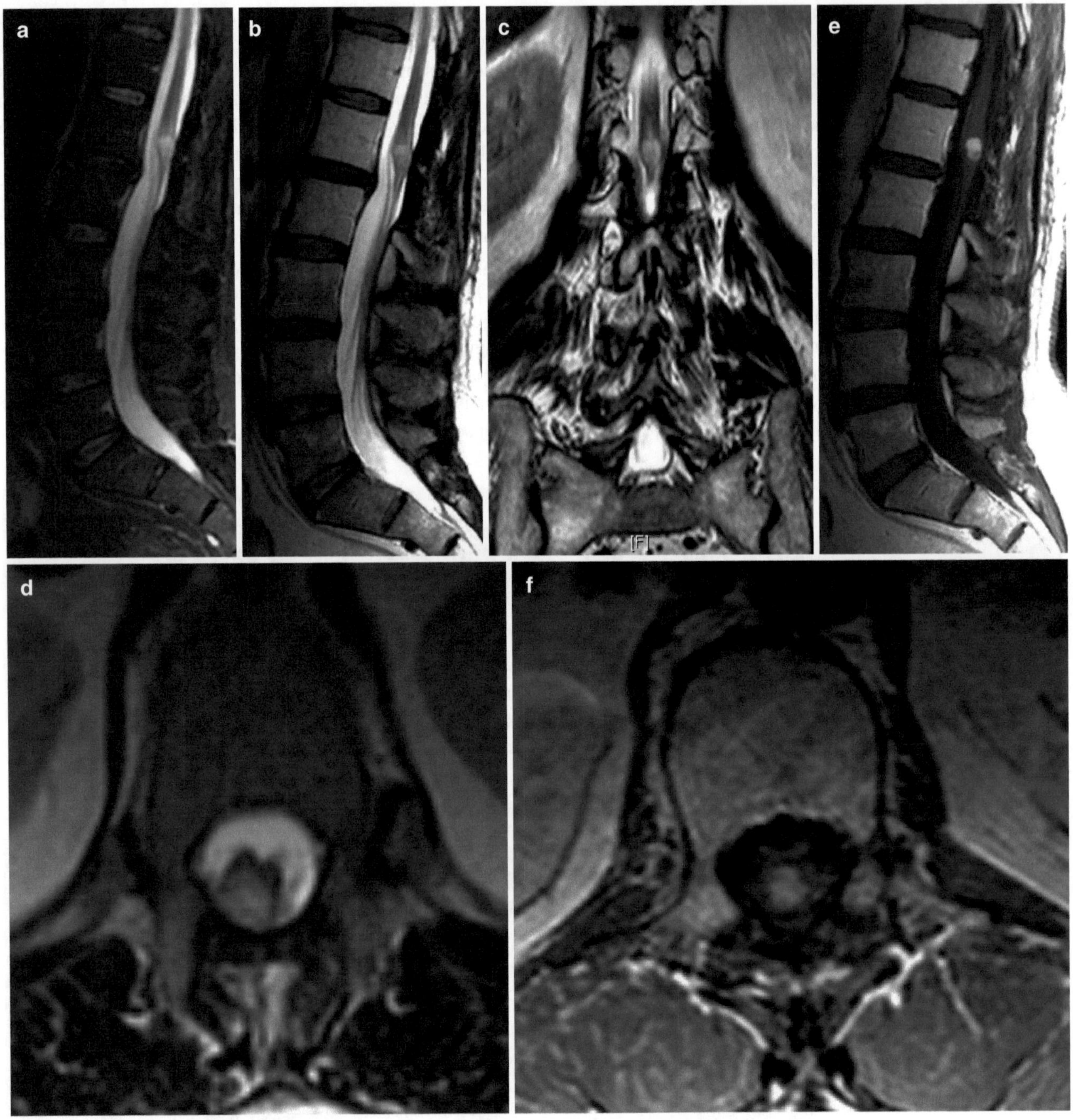

Fig. 4.38 Anaplastic astrocytoma. Sagittal STIR (**a**) as well as sagittal (**b**), coronal (**c**), and axial (**d**) T2-weighted MRI depicts a nodular T2 hyperintense expansile lesion within the conus medullaris. The lesion demonstrates homogeneous enhancement on the sagittal (**e**) and axial (**f**) contrast T1-weighted images. The location of the tumor is more characteristic of ependymoma; however, its homogeneity makes ependymoma less likely. Pathology was consistent with anaplastic astrocytoma WHO grade III

Pilocytic Astrocytoma

Spinal pilocytic astrocytoma is a histologic subtype of astrocytoma accounting for 21 % of intramedullary glial tumors characteristically affecting children and young adults [34]. They are among the most common intramedullary spinal cord tumors in the pediatric population and their incidence decreases with age with only a few cases described after the fourth decade of life [35]. Unlike astrocytomas of the brain, spinal cord pilocytic astrocytomas are usually low, WHO grade 1 lesions. They tend to occur eccentrically within the thoracic cord, followed by the cervical and lumbar spinal cord. Sometimes, they may be central in location or rarely present as holocord involvement. Unusually, multicentric medullary involvement may occur, typically in patients with neurofibromatosis type 1 or less commonly neurofibromatosis type 2. They tend to displace rather than infiltrate the cord and usually contain nonneoplastic intratumoral or rostral and caudal cysts [35]. Unlike ependymomas, hemorrhage is an uncommon feature. CSF dissemination may be present but is rare [36]. Canal widening or vertebral body scalloping may occur due to the expansile space occupying nature of the tumor.

On MRI, pilocytic astrocytomas are iso- to hypointense on T1 and hyperintense on T2. They may demonstrate peripheral or central enhancement of faint to avid intensity. Sometimes, the lesions may not enhance at all. Associated intratumoral and polar cysts may vary in signal intensity and may not always be of the same signal as CSF due to the presence of septa and cellular debris. Larger tumors will often be associated with syringomyelia at the tumor ends progressing in length over time. Hemorrhage may occur spontaneously and is best appreciated on T2 or gradient echo imaging depending on the age of hemorrhage and hemoglobin degradation products.

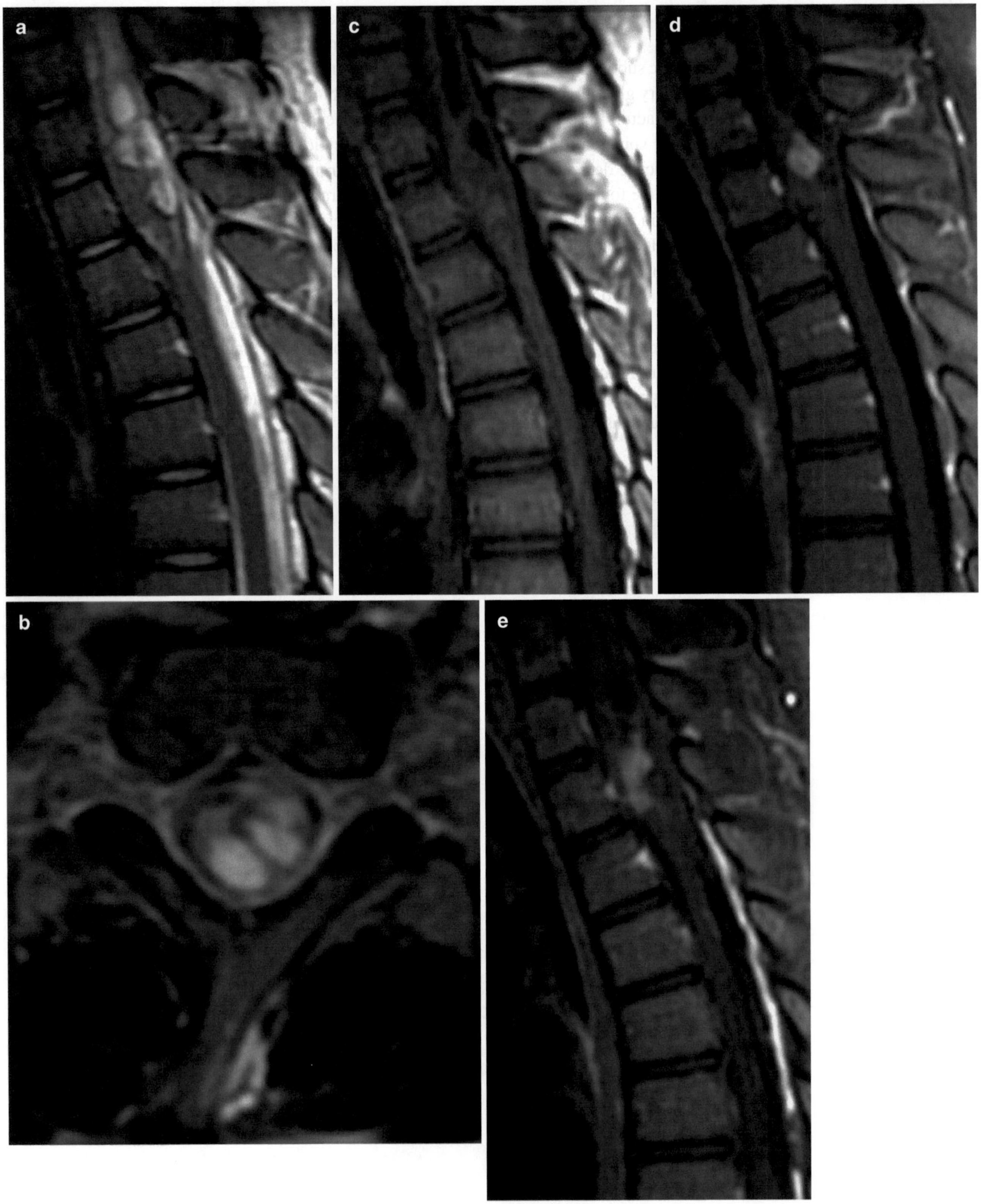

Fig. 4.39 Pilocytic astrocytoma. Sagittal and axial T2 (**a** and **b**), as well as sagittal T1 (**c**) weighted MRI sequences demonstrate an expansile, intramedullary lesion with solid and cystic components. Sagittal and axial contrast T1-weighted sequences (**d–f**) demonstrate the solid enhancing eccentric portion of the lesion with rostral and central non-enhancing T1 hypointense cysts

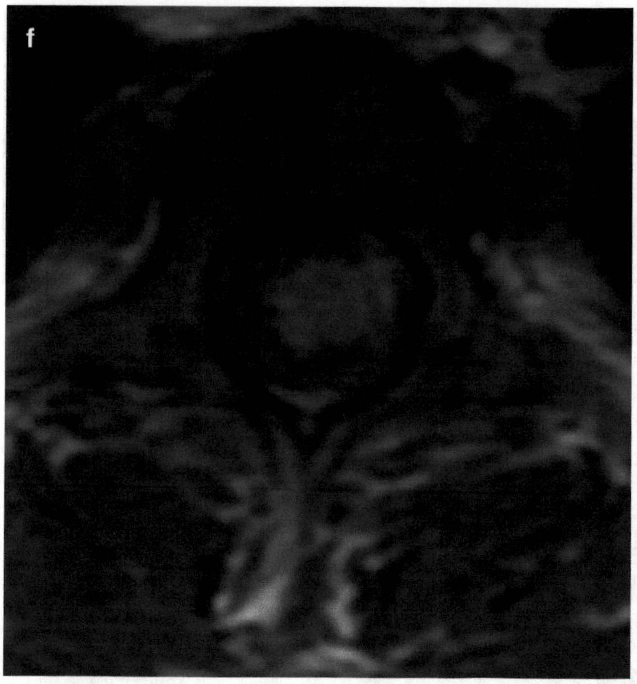

Fig. 4.39 (continued)

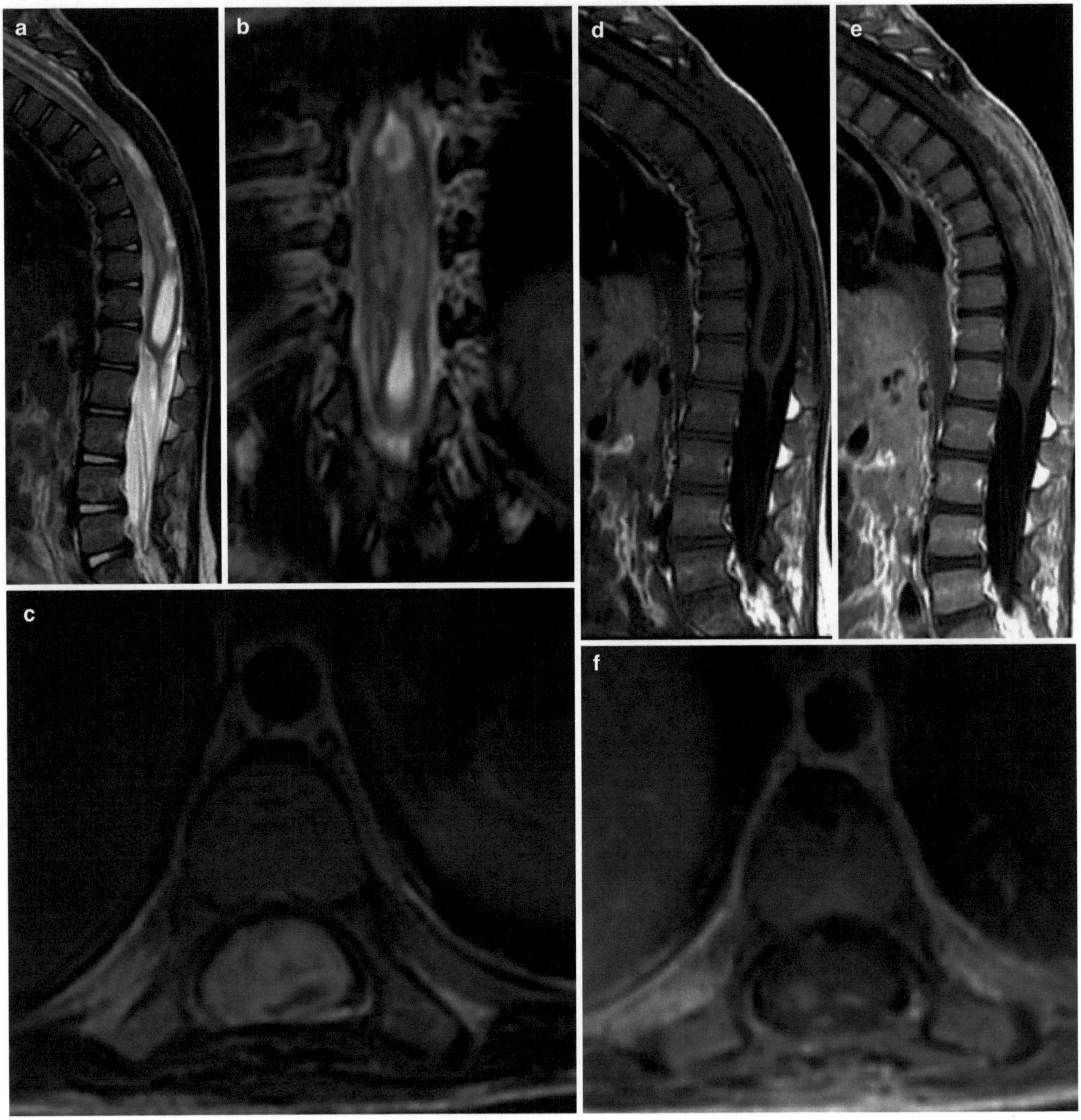

Fig. 4.40 Pilocytic astrocytoma. Sagittal (**a**), coronal (**b**), and axial (**c**) T2 as well as sagittal T1 (**d**) weighted MR images demonstrate expansion of the lower thoracic spinal cord by a heterogeneous, T2 hyperintense, T1 isointense mass widening the spinal canal. Sagittal (**e**) and axial (**f**) contrast T1-weighted images further delineate the margins of the heterogeneously enhancing solid portion of the tumor. There is associated expansion of the central canal following CSF signal intensity on all pulse sequences without associated enhancement consistent with a syrinx

Hemangioblastoma

Hemangioblastomas are rare, benign WHO grade 1 lesions representing 1.6–6.4 % of spinal tumors [37]. They occur sporadically or are associated with von Hippel-Lindau disease (VHLD) in approximately one third to one half of cases [25]. In sporadic cases, the lesions are usually solitary, whereas in VHLD they are often multiple. The number of cases associated with VHLD may be underestimated as the lesions tend to be smaller and often asymptomatic. Hemangioblastomas are most commonly intramedullary (60 %) but may also be extramedullary intradural (21 %), combined intra and extramedullary (11 %), or even extradural (8 %) [37]. They have a predilection for the thoracic spinal cord (51 %), followed by the cervical spinal cord (38 %) [37]. Less commonly, they may arise from the filum terminale, intradural nerve roots, extradural nerve roots or even exist independently.

On MRI, hemangioblastomas are typically T1 isointense and T2 hyperintense to the spinal cord with associated contrast enhancement representing dense vascular tumor parenchyma consisting of thin-walled, closely packed blood vessels within a background of large stromal cells. They are usually intramedullary subpial in location within the superficial dorsal spinal cord associated with a large syrinx. Intratumoral or peritumoral T2 vascular flow voids related to enlarged feeding arteries and or draining veins is a characteristic finding usually of larger tumors measuring 2.5 cm or greater. Flow voids are typically absent in smaller lesions measuring 1.5 cm or less [37]. Peritumoral cysts may be an associated finding, particularly with intramedullary lesions. These cysts may be of varying signal intensity depending on the relative amount of protein content. Cysts containing higher protein content will be of higher signal intensity than CSF on T1-weighted images and may be indistinguishable from the tumor nidus. Peritumoral edema is another common finding associated with intramedullary lesions, often out of proportion to the size of the tumor nidus, thereby mimicking metastatic disease.

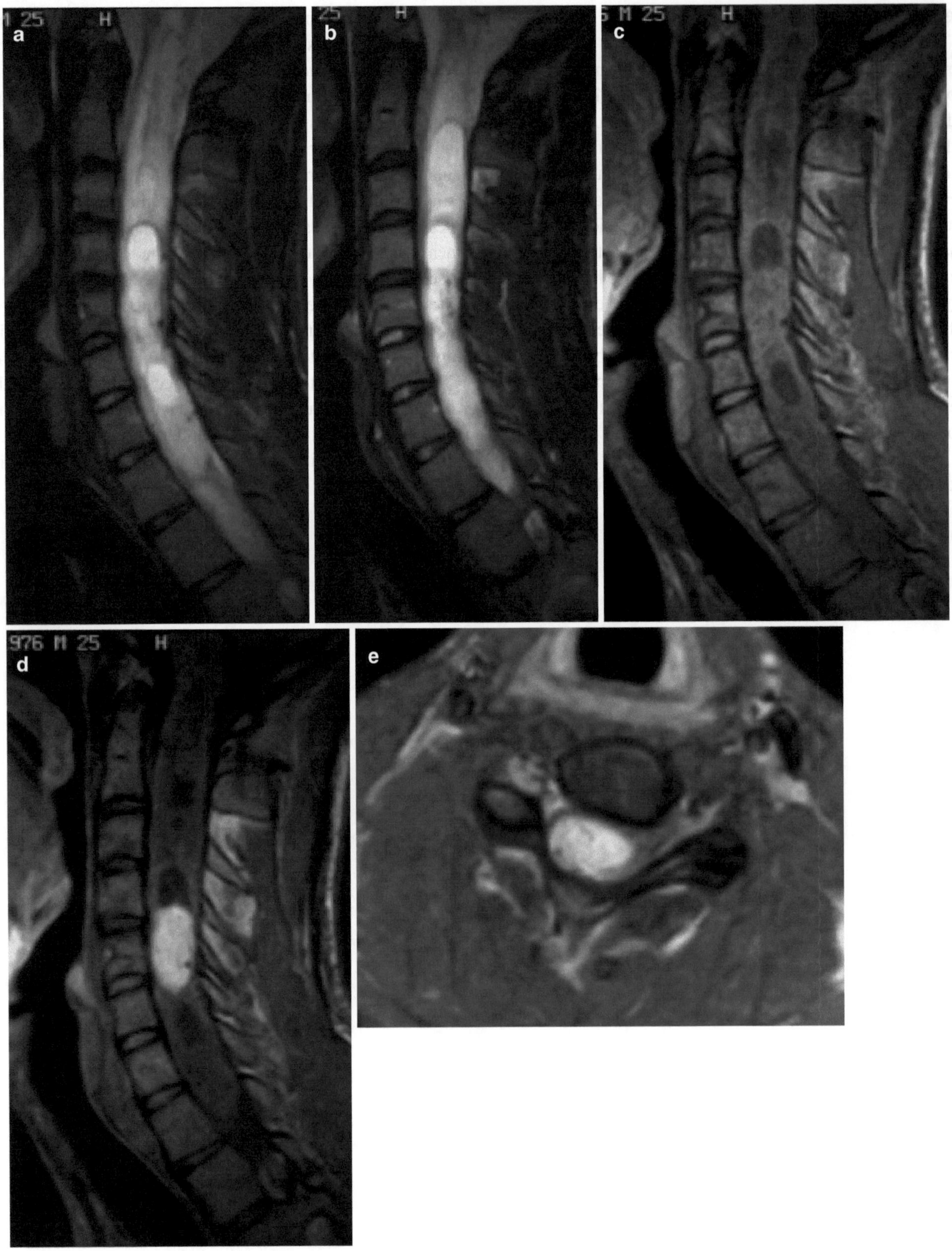

Fig. 4.41 Hemangioblastoma. Sagittal T2 (**a** and **b**), sagittal T1 (**c**), and sagittal and axial contrast T1-weighted (**d** and **e**) MR images demonstrate a T1 isointense, T2 hyperintense, homogeneously enhancing intramedullary tumor with associated T2 flow voids, as well as multiple nonenhancing peritumoral cysts of varying T1 signal intensity

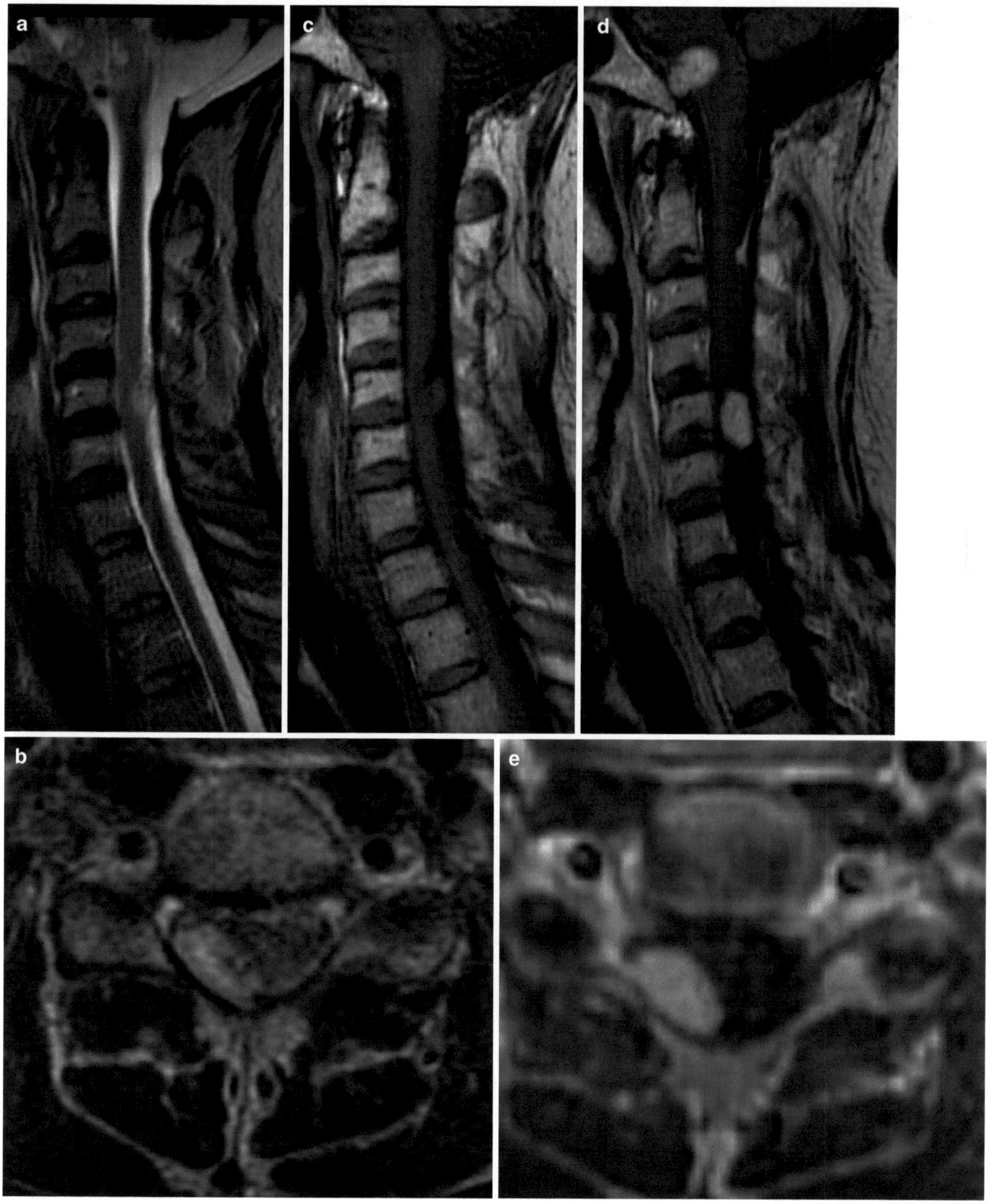

Fig. 4.42 Multiple hemangioblastomas in the setting of VHLD. Sagittal T2 (**a**), axial T2 (**b**), and sagittal T1 (**c**) weighted MR images demonstrate two well-circumscribed T2 hyperintense, T1 hypointense masses located within the ventral pons and superficial right dorsolateral portion of the cervical spinal cord at the C5 level. Several T2 hypointense flow voids are noted in association with these lesions. Sagittal (**d**) and axial (**e**) contrast T1-weighted images reveal avid homogeneous enhancement of the lesions as well as an additional smaller enhancing lesion located within the dorsal spinal cord at the C2/C3 level, inconspicuous on the nonenhanced images. The constellation of findings is characteristic of multiple hemangioblastomas in this patient with known history of VHLD

Intramedullary Lymphoma

Intramedullary spinal cord lymphoma may be primary or may be associated with systemic lymphoma or other CNS sites of involvement sequentially or concurrently [38]. Primary intramedullary spinal cord lymphoma is a rare entity accounting for only 3.3 % of primary CNS lymphoma [33]. Only a few cases are reported in the literature, with the cervical spinal cord being the most common site of disease, followed by the thoracic and lumbar spine. Intramedullary lymphoma is usually under diagnosed as it may mimic more common entities such as transverse myelitis, demyelinating disorders, or other primary neoplasms such as astrocytoma.

On MRI, CNS lymphoma of the spinal cord is strikingly T2 hyperintense, in contrast to primary CNS lymphoma of the brain, which is usually T2 iso- to hypointense [33]. On T1-weighted imaging, intramedullary lymphoma is typically isointense to the spinal cord and demonstrates homogenous or patchy contrast enhancement that in some cases may be multifocal [39].

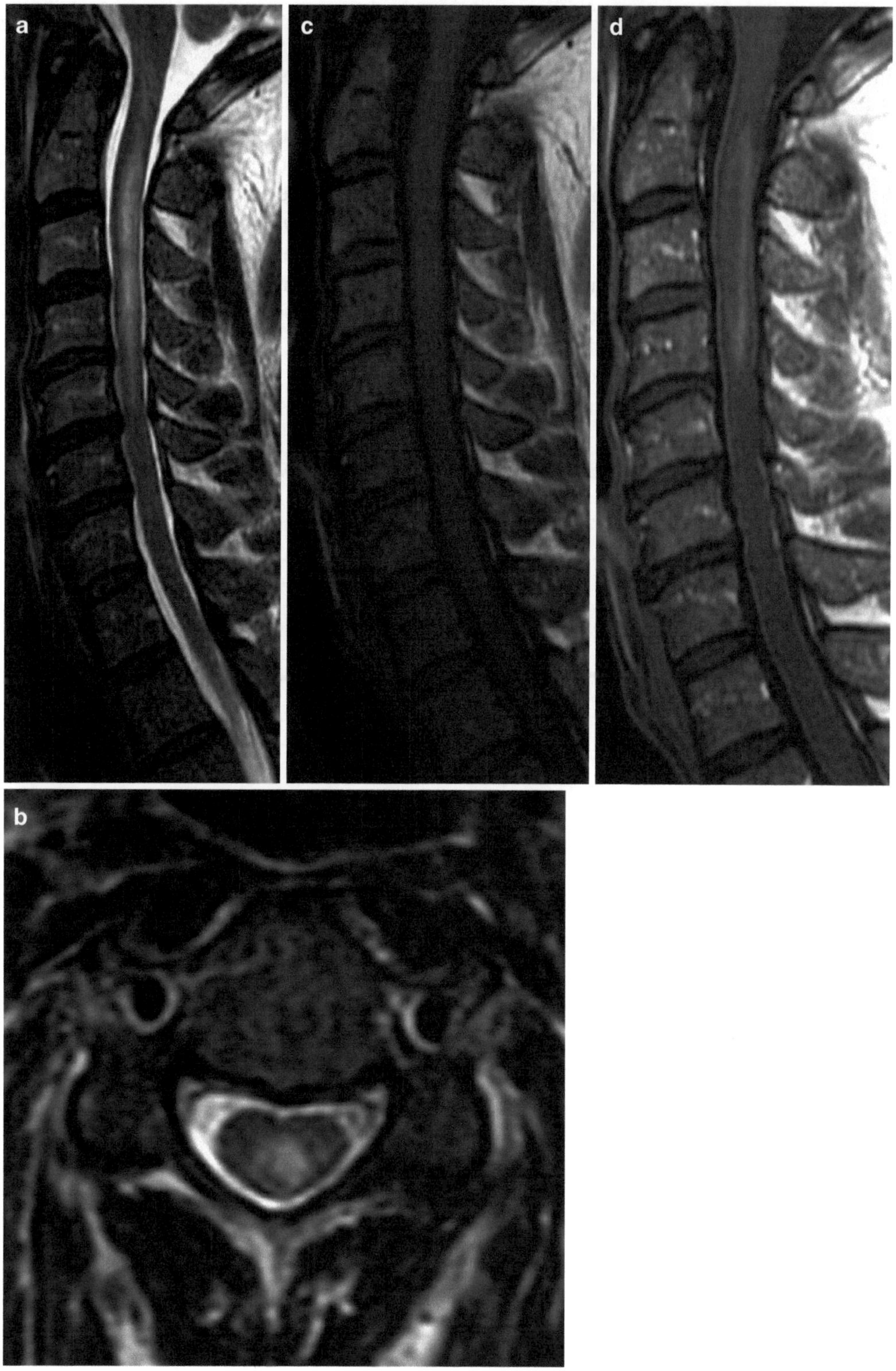

Fig. 4.43 Intramedullary spinal cord lymphoma. Sagittal (**a**) and axial (**b**) T2-weighted MR images demonstrate a central, intramedullary, T2 hyperintense, slightly expansile lesion spanning the C2–C5 vertebral levels. On the nonenhanced sagittal T1 (**c**) weighted sequence, the lesion is isointense to the rest of the spinal cord and inconspicuous. Following contrast administration, it demonstrates heterogeneous enhancement along its entirety (**d**)

Intramedullary Spinal Cord Metastasis

Intramedullary spinal cord metastases are rare, affecting 0.1–0.4 % of all cancer patients and comprising 1–3 % of all intramedullary spinal cord neoplasms [40]. They are often a result of hematogenous spread or direct invasion by disease tracking along the nerve roots or leptomeninges [41]. Lung carcinoma accounts for the most documented lesions, accounting for nearly 50 % of intramedullary metastases. The rest are accounted for by breast carcinoma, melanoma, lymphoma, colon, and renal cell carcinoma [42]. The thoracic spinal cord is the most commonly affected site, followed by the cervical and lumbar spinal cord [8].

MRI is essential for detection of intramedullary metastases, which typically manifest as homogeneously enhancing lesions with a disproportionate amount of surrounding edema. Peripheral ring enhancement may also occur often due to central tumor necrosis [41]. On T1-weighted MRI sequences, the metastatic deposits are usually isointense to the spinal cord whereas the surrounding edema is typically hypointense. On T2-weighted sequences, the deposits may be iso- to hyperintense with extensive surrounding hyperintense intramedullary edema that may span several levels, sometimes mimicking syringohydromyelia.

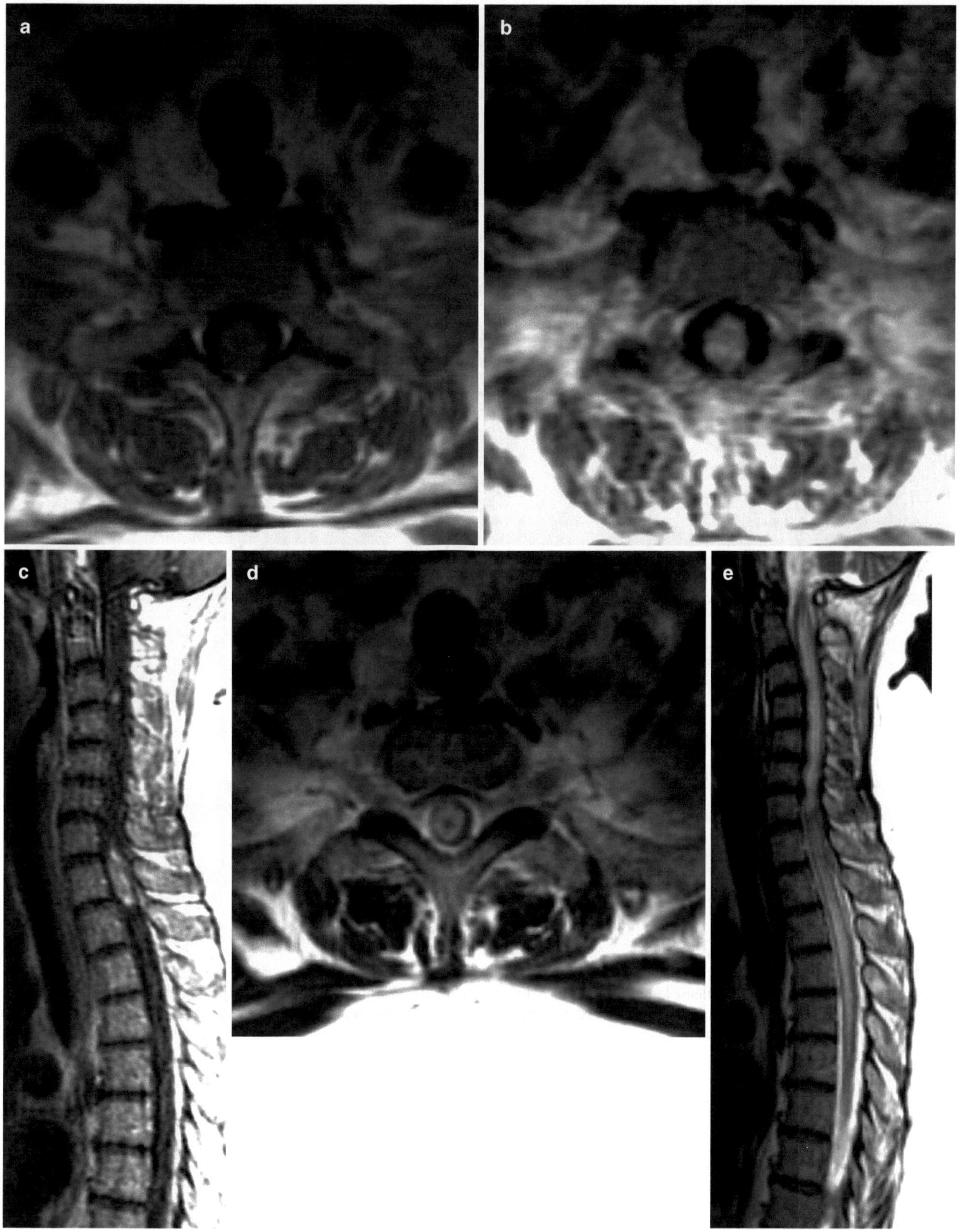

Fig. 4.44 Intramedullary metastases. Nonenhanced axial T1 (**a**) as well as axial (**b**) and sagittal (**c**) contrast T1-weighted images demonstrate two homogeneously enhancing intramedullary lesions centered at the C3 and T1 levels. The smaller enhancing nodular lesion at the C3 level corresponds to the T2 isointense nodule noted on the axial T2-weighted image (**d**). Sagittal T2-weighted imaging (**e**) demonstrates the degree of disproportionate surrounding T2 hyperintense intramedullary edema resulting in spinal cord expansion. The patient was known to have breast carcinoma

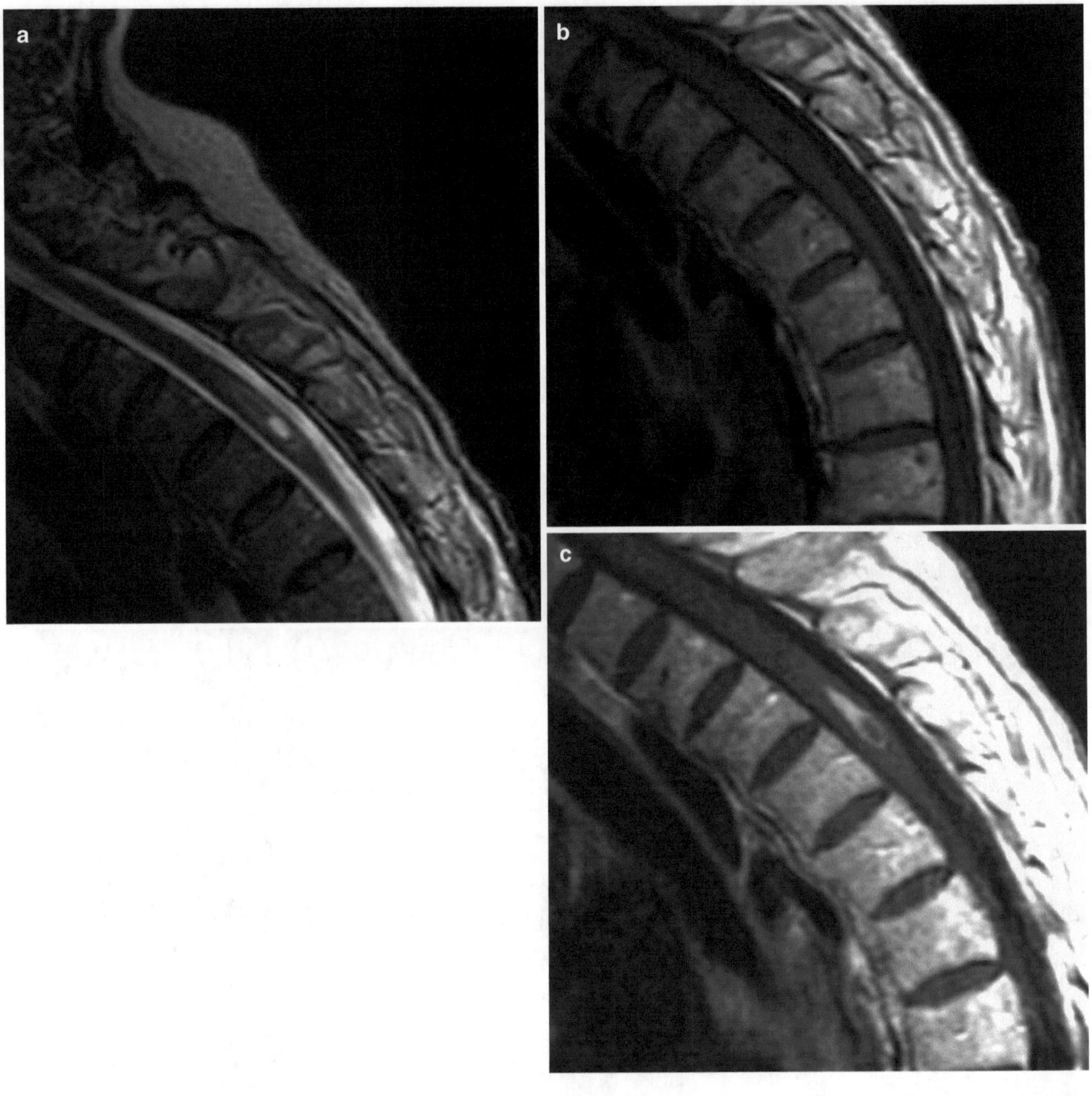

Fig. 4.45 Intramedullary metastasis. Sagittal T2 (**a**) weighted MRI demonstrates an ovoid-shaped T2 isointense lesion with an area of hyperintense central necrosis and surrounding intramedullary edema affecting the mid thoracic spinal cord. On the nonenhanced sagittal T1 sequence (**b**), the lesion is inconspicuous with the exception of the T1 hypointense centrally necrotic component. Sagittal contrast T1 (**c**) imaging demonstrates homogenous enhancement of the nonnecrotic portion of the lesion. The patient was known to have non–small cell lung carcinoma

Radiation-Induced Complications

Radiation-Induced Myositis

Striated muscle myositis is a rare complication occurring within the radiation field. It is thought to be the result of damage to small arteries, arterioles, and capillaries with ensuing ischemia and inflammation resulting from vascular injury [43]. In severe cases, muscle fibrosis may occur as a reactive repair mechanism leading to alteration in muscle parenchyma, architectural distortion, and chronic pain [43]. Acute changes on MRI are characterized by hyperintense T2 signal due to edema and inflammation within the treatment fields. Chronic changes typically include muscle fibrosis and atrophy.

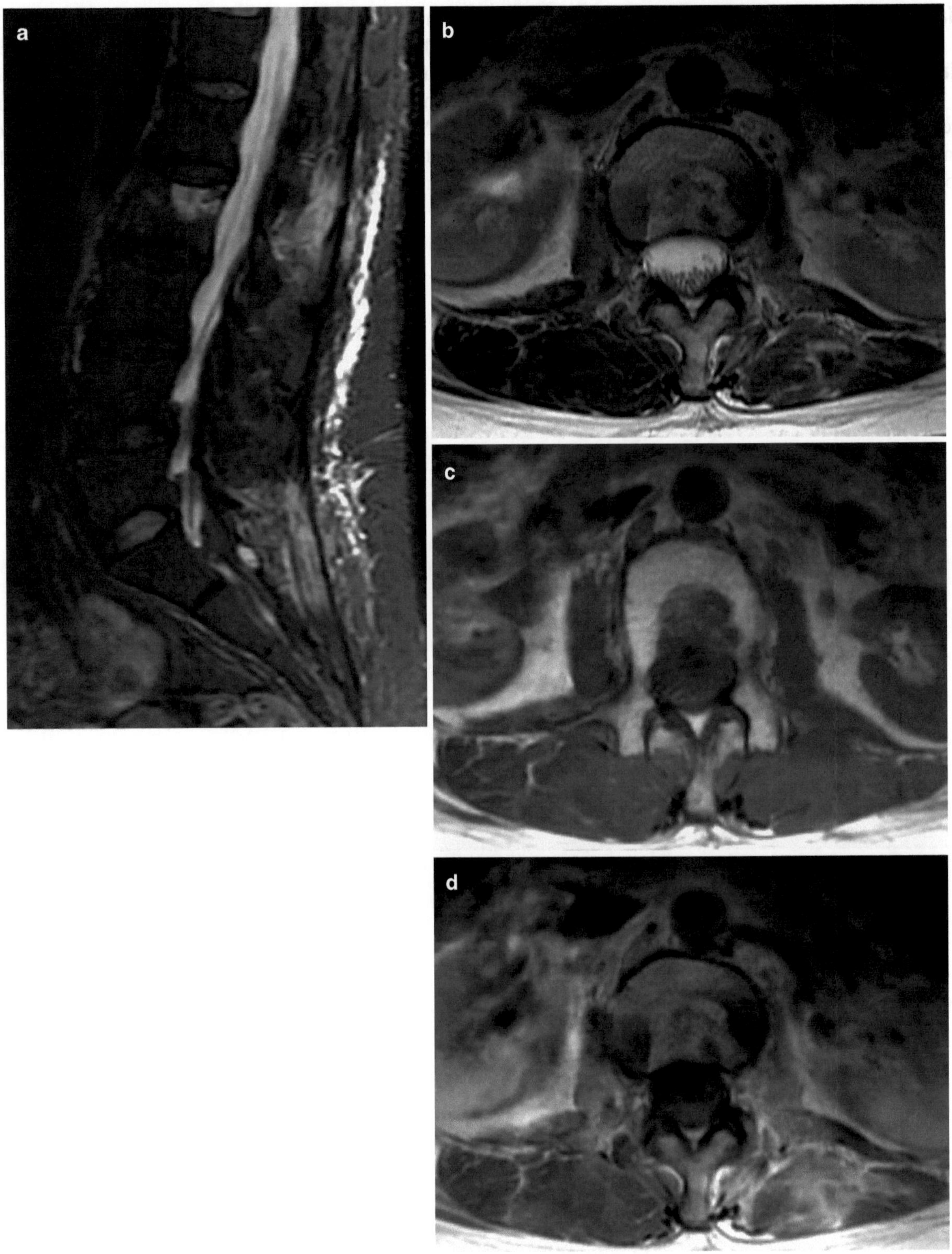

Fig. 4.46 Radiation-induced myositis. Sagittal STIR (**a**) and axial T2 (**b**) weighted MR images demonstrate patchy hyperintense signal within the dorsal and lateral paravertebral musculature. There is infiltration of the fascial planes and loss of the intervening T1 hyperintense intermuscular fat (**c**). Heterogeneous patchy enhancement of the musculature (**d**) is noted following contrast administration. A T2 hyperintense, T1 hypointense, enhancing, lytic metastasis is also noted involving the L2 vertebral body in this patient with known lung carcinoma

Sacral Insufficiency Fracture

The earliest radiation-induced changes seen on MRI are fatty replacement of normal marrow, occurring as early as 2 weeks following treatment and manifesting as markedly hyperintense T1/T2 marrow signal [44]. Secondary complications such as insufficiency fractures due to normal stress on abnormal bone may be seen as a later complication, particularly within the sacrum [45].

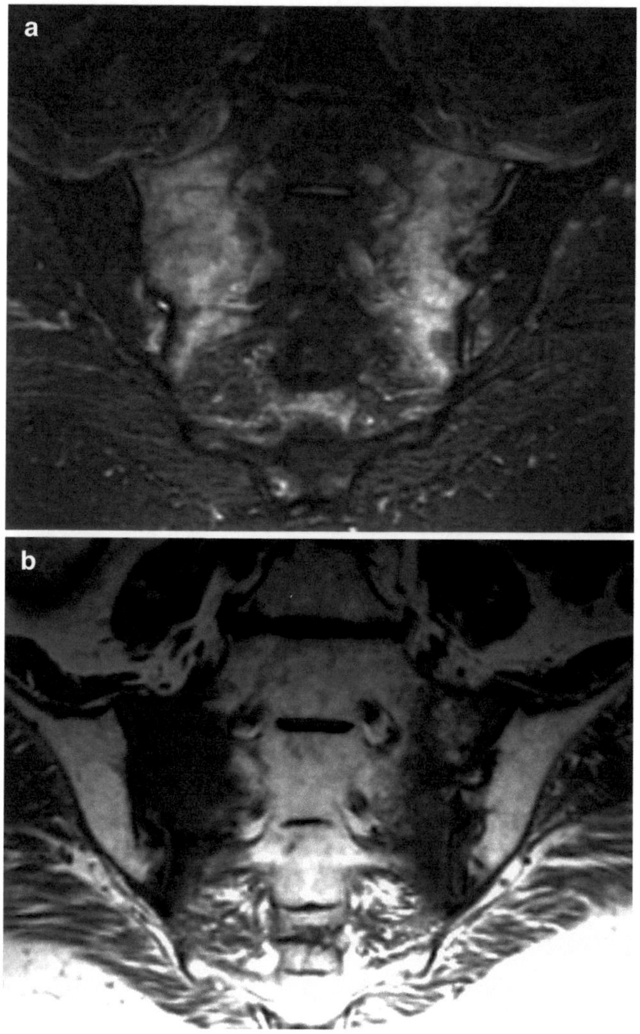

Fig. 4.47 Sacral insufficiency fractures. Coronal STIR (**a**) and coronal T1 (**b**) MR images of the sacrum demonstrate markedly STIR hypointense, T1 hyperintense fatty marrow replacement changes throughout the sacrum and iliac bones. Superimposed symmetric, vertically oriented, patchy, STIR hyperintense, T1 hypointense edema is noted along the sacral ala bilaterally in the setting of acute sacral insufficiency fractures

Radiation-Induced Lumbosacral Radiculopathy

Radiation-induced polyradiculopathy is a rare complication of radiotherapy that may mimic leptomeningeal carcinomatosis. Helpful distinguishing features are a stable MRI appearance over time with imaging findings restricted to the radiation field, coupled with a slowly progressive clinical course and repeatedly negative cerebrospinal fluid cytology analyses [46].

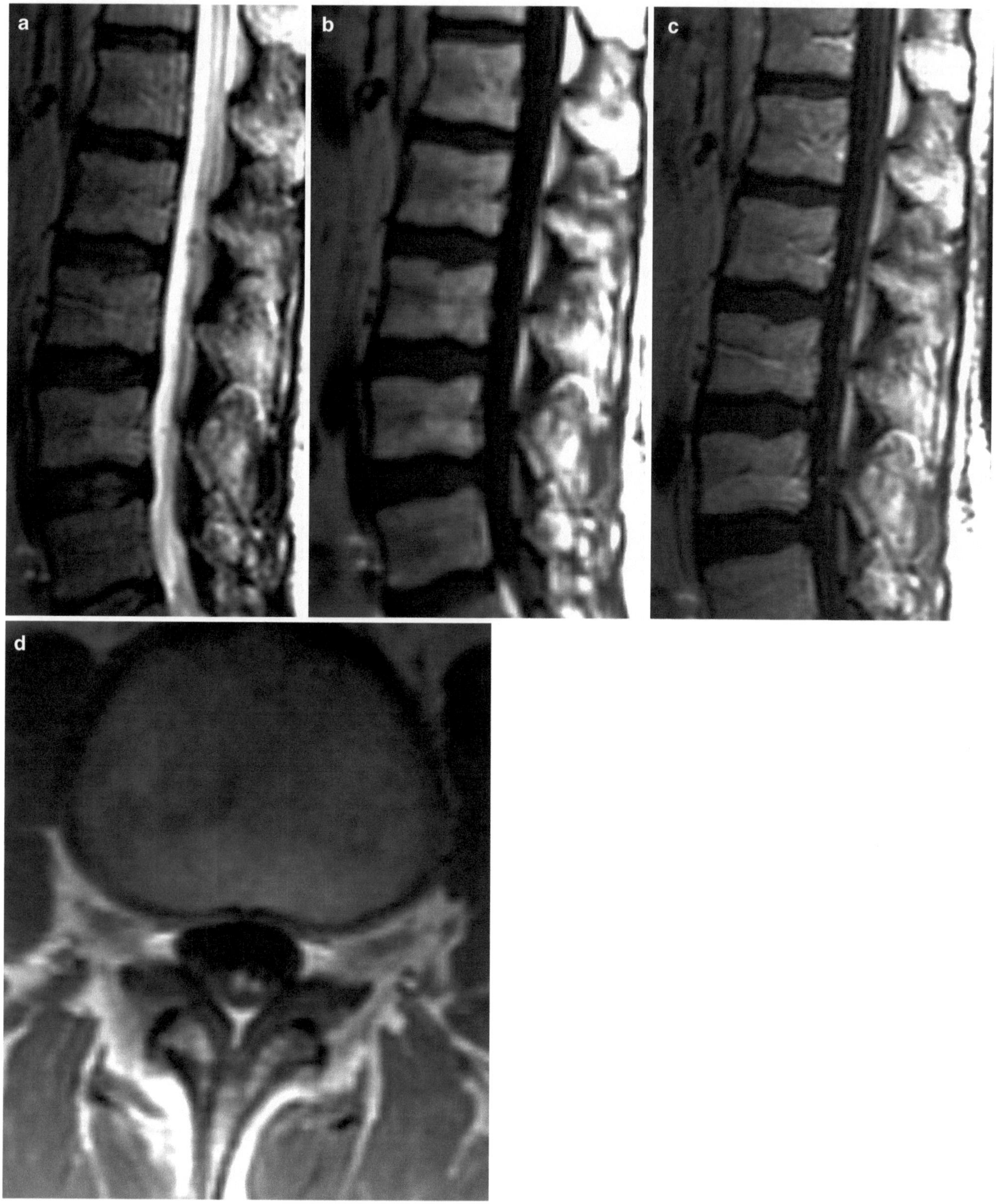

Fig. 4.48 Radiation-induced lumbosacral radiculopathy. Sagittal T2 (**a**), sagittal T1 (**b**), as well as sagittal and axial contrast T1 (**c** and **d**) weighted images demonstrate nodular, T1/T2 isointense, plaque-like lesions along the surface of the cauda equina, with associated avid enhancement following contrast administration. An appropriate clinical history led to the diagnosis of radiation-induced polyradiculopathy; however, the radiographic findings are indistinguishable from leptomeningeal carcinomatosis

Radiation Myelopathy

Radiation myelopathy is an irreversible process, usually occurring after high-dose radiation therapy with total doses at or just below 50 Gy or fraction doses above 2 Gy, typically following 6 months to 2 years after completion of therapy [47, 48]. It is estimated that doses of 45 Gy in 22–25 fractions yields an incidence of myelopathy of less than 0.2 %, whereas doses of 57–61 Gy yields a 5 % incidence [49]. Symptoms are usually paresthesias that may progress to total paralysis occurring in the setting of extensive demyelination and coagulation necrosis [47].

MRI findings depend on the timing of imaging. Imaging within 6 months following symptoms is characterized by fusiform expansion of the spinal cord with patchy or ring-like areas of intramedullary enhancement and surrounding T2 hyperintense, T1 hypointense intramedullary edema. Imaging performed approximately 3 years after the onset of symptoms is characterized by spinal cord atrophy, often at sites of previous enhancement and continued intramedullary T2 hyperintensity [47].

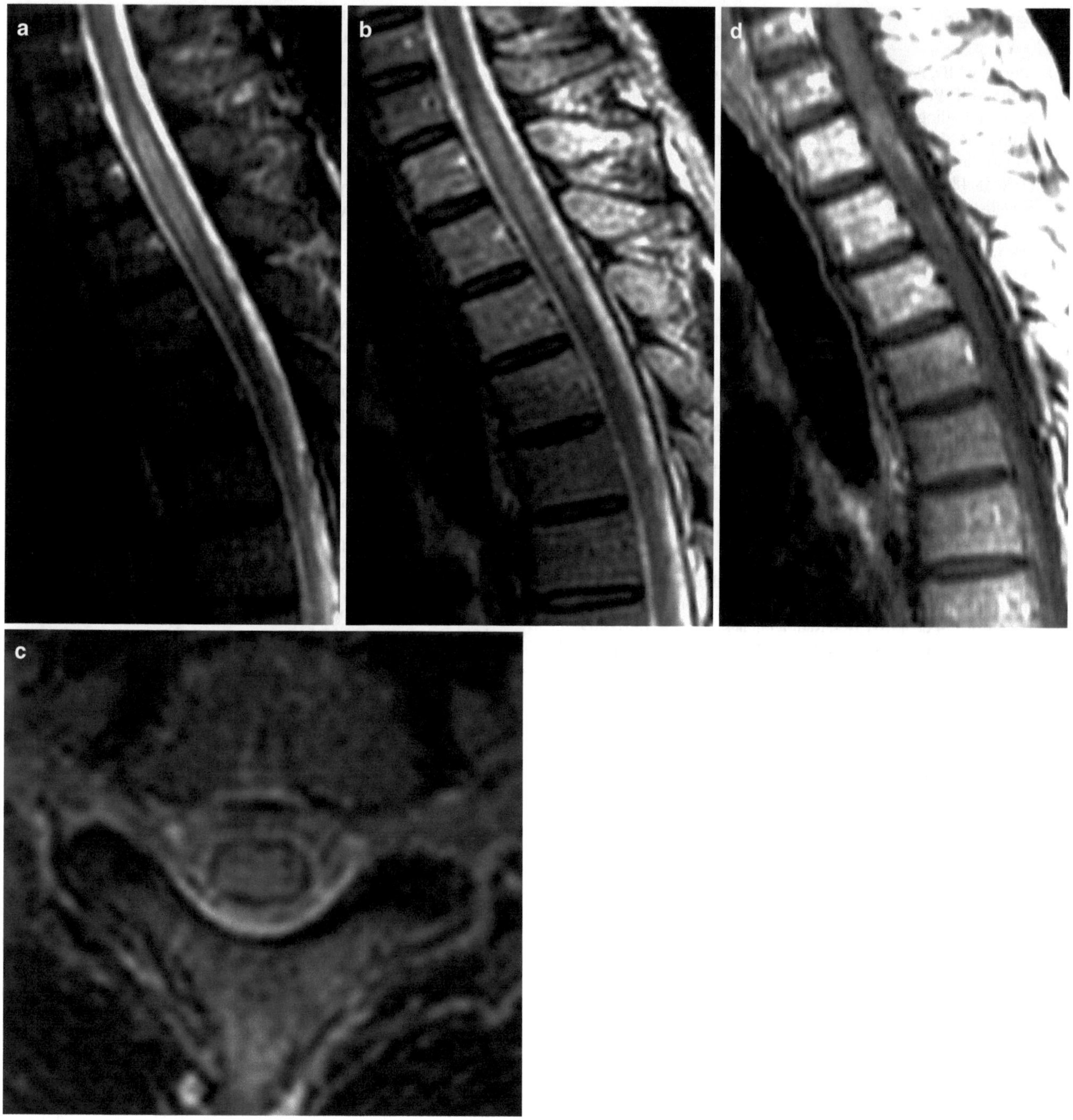

Fig. 4.49 Radiation myelopathy. Sagittal STIR (**a**), sagittal T2 (**b**), axial T2 (**c**), and sagittal contrast T1 (**d**) weighted MR images, demonstrate T2 hyperintensity within the central portion of the cervical cord, which appears slightly expanded. Patchy heterogeneous enhancement is present following contrast administration (**d**). Subtle T1/T2 hyperintense radiation-induced fatty marrow replacement is seen within the upper cervical vertebrae. The findings are relatively nonspecific and knowledge of a history of prior irradiation is essential to the diagnosis of radiation injury

References

1. Murphey MD, Andrews CL, Flemming DJ, et al. From the archives of the AFIP. Primary tumors of the spine: radiologic pathologic correlation. Radiographics. 1996;16:1131–58.
2. Erlman R. Imaging and differential diagnosis of primary bone tumors and tumor-like lesions of the spine. Eur J Radiol. 2006;58:48–67.
3. Rodallec M, Feydey A, Larousserie F, et al. Diagnostic imaging of solitary tumors of the spine: what to do and say. Radiographics. 2008;28:1019–41.
4. Boriani S, De Lure F, Campanacci L, et al. Aneurysmal bone cyst of the mobile spine. Spine. 2001;26:27–35.
5. Pennekamp W, Peters S, Schinkel C, et al. Aneurysmal bone cyst of the cervical spine. Eur Radiol. 2008;18:2356–60.
6. Rodriguez DP, Poussaint TY. Imaging of back pain in children. AJNR Am J Neuroradiol. 2010;31:787–802.
7. Harrop JS, Schmidt MH, Boriani S, Shaffrey C. Aggressive benign: primary spine neoplasms: osteoblastoma, aneurysmal bone cyst and giant cell tumor. Spine. 2009;34:539–47.
8. Atlas SW. Magnetic resonance imaging of the brain and spine, vol. 2. 4th ed. Philadelphia: Lippincott Williams and Wilkins; 2009. p. 1521–3.
9. Kwon JW, Chung HW, Cho EY, et al. MRI findings of giant cell tumors. AJR Am J Roentgenol. 2007;189:246–50.
10. Littrell LA, Wenger DE, Wold LE, et al. Radiographic, CT, and MR imaging features of dedifferentiated chondrosarcomas: a retrospective review of 174 de novo cases. Radiographics. 2004;24:1397–409.
11. Smolders D, Wang X, Drevelengas A, et al. Value of MRI in the diagnosis of non-clival, non-sacral chordoma. Skeletal Radiol. 2003;32:343–50.
12. Wippold FK, Koeller KK, Smirniotopoulos JG. Clinical and imaging features of cervical chordoma. AJR Am J Roentgenol. 1999;172:1423–6.
13. Sung MS, Lee GY, Kang HS, et al. Sacrococcygeal chordoma: MR imaging in 30 patients. Skeletal Radiol. 2005;34:87–94.
14. Nishiguchi T, Mochizuki K, Ohsawa M, et al. Differentiating benign notochordal cell tumors from chordomas: radiographic features on MRI, CT, and tomography. AJR Am J Roentgenol. 2011;196:644–50.
15. Yamaguchi T, Iwata J, Sugihara S, et al. Distinguishing benign notochordal cell tumors from vertebral chordoma. Skeletal Radiol. 2008;37:291–9.
16. Duffy S, Jhaveri M, Scudierre J, et al. MR Imaging of a posterior mediastinal ganglioneuroma: fat as a useful diagnostic sign. AJNR Am J Neuroradiol. 2005;26:2658–62.
17. Shah LM, Salzman KL. Imaging of spinal metastatic disease. Int J Surg Oncol. 2011;2011:769753.
18. Hanrahan CJ, Shah LM. MRI of spinal bone marrow: part 2, T1 weighted imaging-based differential diagnosis. AJR Am J Roentgenol. 2011;197:1309–21.
19. Cole JS, Patchell RA. Metastatic epidural spinal cord compression. Lancet Neurol. 2008;7:459–66.
20. Abdul-Kasim K, Thurnher M, McKeever P, Sundgren P. Intradural spinal tumors: current classification and MRI features. Neuroradiology. 2007;50:301–14.
21. Wippold II FJ, Lubner M, Perrin RJ, et al. Neuropathology for the neuroradiologist: antoni A and antoni B tissue patterns. AJNR Am J Neuroradiol. 2007;28:1633–8.
22. Ferner RE, Gutmann DH. International consensus statement on malignant peripheral nerve sheath tumors in neurofibromatosis 1. Cancer Res. 2002;62:1573–7.
23. Sandalcioglu IE, Hunold A, Müller O, et al. Spinal meningiomas: critical review of 131 surgically treated patients. Eur Spine J. 2008;17:1035–41.
24. Faro S, Turtz A, Koenigsberg R, et al. Paraganglioma of the cauda equine with associated intramedullary cyst: MR findings. AJNR Am J Neuroradiol. 1997;18:1588–90.
25. Koeller K, Rosenblum R, Morrison A. Neoplasms of the spinal cord and filum terminale: radiologic-pathologic correlation. Radiographics. 2000;20:1721–49.
26. Olsen WL, Dillon WP, Kelly WM, et al. MR imaging of paragangliomas. AJNR Am J Neuroradiol. 1986;7:1039–42.
27. Wang MY, Levi AD, Green BA. Intradural spinal arachnoid cysts in adults. Surg Neurol. 2003;60:49–55.
28. Kikuchi K, Miki H, Nakagawa A. The utility of diffusion weighted imaging with navigator-echo technique for the diagnosis of spinal epidermoid cysts. AJNR Am J Neuroradiol. 2000;21:1164–6.
29. Thurnher M. Diffusion-weighted MR imaging (DWI) in two intradural spinal epidermoid cysts. Neuroradiology. 2012:1–2. http://dx.doi.org/10.1007/s00234-012-1032-x.
30. Kukreja K, Manzano G, Ragheb J, Santiago M. Differentiation between pediatric spinal arachnoid-dermoid cysts: is diffusion-weighted MRI useful? Pediatr Radiol. 2007;37:556–60.
31. Shin M, Lee J, Cho WH, et al. Intradural epidermoid cyst at conus medullaris and cauda equina of the spine: a case report. J Korean Soc Radiol. 2012;66:113–6.
32. Kahan H, Sklar E, Post JD, Bruce JH. MR characteristics of histopathologic subtypes of spinal ependymoma. AJNR Am J Neuroradiol. 1996;17:143–50.
33. Smith AB, Soderlund KA, Rushing EJ, Smirniotopoulos JG. Radiologic-pathologic correlation of pediatric and adolescent spinal neoplasms: part I intramedullary spinal neoplasms. AJR Am J Roentgenol. 2012;198:34–43.
34. Horger M, Ritz R, Beschorner R, et al. Spinal pilocytic astrocytoma: MR imaging findings at first presentation and following surgery. Eur J Radiol. 2011;79:389–99.
35. Saad A, Tuli S, Ali E, et al. Pilocytic astrocytoma of the spinal cord in an adult. J Neurooncol. 2008;88:189–91.
36. Abel TJ, Chowdhary A, Thapa M, et al. Spinal cord pilocytic astrocytoma with leptomeningeal dissemination to the brain: a case report and review of the literature. J Neurosurg. 2006;105:508–14.
37. Chu BC, Terae S, Hida K, et al. MR findings in spinal hemangioblastoma: correlation with symptoms and with angiographic and surgical findings. AJNR Am J Neuroradiol. 2001;22:206–17.
38. Flanagan EP, O'Neill BP, Porter AB. Primary intramedullary spinal cord lymphoma. Neurology. 2011;77:784–91.
39. Caruso PA, Patel MR, Joseph J, Rachlin J. Primary intramedullary lymphoma of the spinal cord mimicking cervical spondylotic myelopathy. AJR Am J Roentgenol. 1998;171:526–7.
40. Lee SS, Kim MK, Sym SJ. Intramedullary spinal cord metastases: a single-institution experience. J Neurooncol. 2007;84:85–9.
41. Watanabe M, Nomura T, Toh E, et al. Intramedullary spinal cord metastasis: a clinical and imaging study of seven patients. J Spinal Disord Tech. 2006;19:43–7.
42. Schiff D, O'Neill BP. Intramedullary spinal cord metastases: clinical features and treatment outcome. Neurology. 1996;47:906–12.
43. Otake S, Mayr NA, Ueda T, et al. Radiation-induced changes in MR signal intensity and contrast enhancement of lumbosacral vertebrae: do changes occur only inside the radiation therapy field? Radiology. 2002;222:179–83.

44. Addley HC, Vargas HA, Moyle PL, et al. Pelvic imaging following chemotherapy and radiation therapy for gynecologic malignancies. Radiographics. 2010;30:1843–56.
45. Ducray F, Guillevin R, Psimaras D, et al. Postradiation lumbosacral radiculopathy with spinal root cavernomas mimicking carcinomatous meningitis. Neuro Oncol. 2008;10:1035–9.
46. Welsh JS, Torre TG, DeWeese TL, O'Reilly S. Radiation myositis. Ann Oncol. 1999;10:1105–8.
47. Becker M, Schroth G, Zbären P, et al. Long-term changes induced by high-dose irradiation of the head and neck region: imaging findings. Radiographics. 1997;17:5–26.
48. Koehler PJ, Verbiest H, Jager J, Vecht CJ. Delayed-radiation myelopathy: serial MR-imaging and pathology. Clin Neurol Neurosurg. 1996;98:197–201.
49. Gibbs IC, Patil C, Gerszten PC, et al. Delayed radiation-induced myelopathy after spinal radiosurgery. Neurosurgery. 2009;64:A67–72.

Index

A
Adult brain tumor
  extra-axial
    hemangiopericytoma, 59–61
    meningioma (*see* Meningiomas)
    schwannoma (*see* Schwannoma)
  infratentorial, hemangioblastoma, 41–43
  intra-axial
    GBM (*see* Glioblastoma multiforme (GBM))
    low-grade astrocytoma (*see* Low-grade astrocytoma)
    metastases (*see* Metastases)
  intraventricular
    central neurocytoma, 44–45
    subependymoma, 46–48
  supratentorial
    adult ependymoma (*see* Adult ependymoma)
    anaplastic astrocytoma (*see* Anaplastic astrocytoma)
    anaplastic oligodendroglioma (*see* Anaplastic oligodendroglioma)
    gliomatosis cerebri (*see* Gliomatosis cerebri)
    oligodendroglioma (*see* Oligodendroglioma)
    primary CNS lymphoma (*see* Primary central nervous system lymphoma)
Adult ependymoma
  characteristics, 38
  expansile right thalamic tumor, 39
  fourth ventricular outlet foramina, 40
  posterior fossa ependymoma, 38
  posterior third ventricle, 40
  supratentorial ependymoma, 39
Anaplastic astrocytoma, 209–210
  bifrontal-transcallosal infiltrating tumor, 22
  characteristics, 21
  left frontal lobe, 22
  left hemispheric, minimally enhancing, expansile tumor, 23
  left insular and peri-insular infiltrating tumor, 21
  multivoxel spectroscopy, 23
Anaplastic oligodendroglioma
  axil relative cerebral blood volume map, 27
  characteristics, 24
  expansile left insular and basal ganglia minimally enhancing tumor, 24
  large left frontal, 25
  large, right frontal, predominantly nonenhancing tumor, 24
  left paramedian nonenhancing tumor, 26
  SWAN, 27
Aneurysmal bone cysts (ABC), 147
Arachnoid cysts
  axial T2, 197–198
  characteristics, 194
  sagittal STIR, 195–196
  signal intensity, 194
ATRT. *See* Atypical teratoid rhabdoid tumor (ATRT)
Atypical teratoid rhabdoid tumor (ATRT)
  characteristics, 68
  expansile tumor, 68–69
  heterogeneously enhancing tumor, 70, 71

B
Benign notochordal cell tumors (BNCT), 168–170
Bone island, 142–144
Bone metastases
  breast, 176
  melanoma, 177
  osseous spine, 174
  prostate, 175
Brainstem glioma
  characteristics, 72
  heterogeneously enhancing tumor, 75, 77, 82
  multiloculated expansile tumor, 74
  nonenhancing tumor, 75
  reduced N-acetylaspartate, 76
  T2 hyperintense tumor, 73, 76

C
Central neurocytoma
  hydrocephalus, 44, 45
  lobulated nonenhancing tumor, 44
  solid tumor, 45
Cerebrospinal fluid (CSF), 141
Chondrosarcomas, 161–163
Chordomas
  amorphous calcification, 164
  cervical, 167
  prevalent, 164
  sacral, 165–166
Choroid plexus
  carcinoma
    characteristics, 104
    heterogeneously enhancing tumor, 104–105
  papilloma
    characteristics, 101
    enhancing tumor, 101
    lobulated tumor, 102
    posterior fossa tumor, 102
    T1-weighted, small, 103
Craniopharyngioma, 120–124

S. Karimi (ed.), *Atlas of Brain and Spine Oncology Imaging*, Atlas of Oncology Imaging,
DOI 10.1007/978-1-4614-5653-7, © Springer Science+Business Media New York 2013

D
Dysembryonic neuroepithelial tumor (DNET)
  anterior left frontal lobe, 64
  characteristics, 63
  corpus callosum, 65
  focal nodular enhancement, 66
  posterior enhancing nodule, 64

E
Ependymomas, 205–206. *See also* Subependymoma
  characteristics, 38
  expansile right thalamic tumor, 39
  fourth ventricular outlet foramina, 40
  posterior fossa ependymoma, 38
  posterior third ventricle, 40
  supratentorial ependymoma, 39
Epidermoid cysts, 199–201

G
Ganglioglioma
  characteristics, 63
  FLAIR hyperintense tumor, 67
  heterogeneous, partially calcified tumor, 66
  left mesial temporal lobe, 67
Ganglioneuroblastoma, 171
Ganglioneuroma, 171, 173
GBM. *See* Glioblastoma multiforme (GBM)
Germinoma
  characteristics, 86
  expansile tumor, 87
Giant cell tumors (GCTs)
  axial CT, 157–158
  osteolytic masses, 156
  sagittal and axial T2-weighted, 159
  T4 vertebra, 160
Glioblastoma multiforme (GBM)
  axial FLAIR, 9
  characteristics, 6
  cystic and necrotic components, 7
  left parietal lobe rim-enhancing, 6
  medial left temporal lobe, 7
  parenchymal and perivascular tumor, 8
  perivascular and leptomeningeal space, 7
  T1 hyperintense subacute blood, 8
Gliomatosis cerebri
  characteristics, 28
  hemispheric infiltrative nonenhancing tumor, left, 29
  insular and peri-insular hyperintensity, left, 30
  right parietal lobe infiltrative hyperintense tumor, 30
  subtle multifocal left frontal tumor, 30

H
Hemangioblastoma, 215–217
  characteristics, 41
  cystic tumors, 43
  left brachium pontis, 42
Hemangiomas, 145–146
Hemangiopericytoma
  characteristics, 59
  left frontal region, 60
  right occipital region, 59
  right posterior fossa, 61

I
Intramedullary metastases, 221–222
Invasive pituitary adenoma, 116–117
Ipilimumab hypophysitis, 132

J
Juvenile pilocytic astrocytoma (JPA)
  characteristics, 78
  cystic tumor, 80
  optic-hypothalamic tumor, 81
  single voxel spectroscopy, 78–79
  vermis, 78

L
Langerhans cell histiocytosis (LCH)
  characteristics, 134
  contrast coronal, 135
  infundibulum lymphoma, 136–137
Leptomeningeal metastasis, 202–204
Low-grade astrocytoma
  anterior paramedian frontal lobe nonenhancing tumor, left, 11
  characteristics, 10
  frontal lobe hypointense nonenhancing tumor, right, 14
  frontal lobe nonenhancing expansile tumor, left posterior, 12
  paramedian frontal lobe nonenhancing tumor, left posterior, 13
  paramedian frontal lobe tumor, left posterior, 15
Lymphocytic hypophysitis, 131

M
Medulloblastoma
  characteristics, 93
  heterogeneously enhancing midline tumor, 96
  multiple T2 hyperintense tumor, 97
  small midline enhancing tumor, 95
  T2 hyperintense heterogeneously enhancing tumor, 94
Meningiomas, 189–191
  burnt out tumor, 50
  characteristics, 49
  frontal convexity and mild hyperostosis, 53
  homogeneously enhancing tumor, 51
  right cerebellopontine angle cistern, 53
  subependymoma, 52
Metastases
  choroid plexus, 5
  craniotomy and postoperative changes, 3
  cystic, 5
  gray-white junction, 2
  non-small-cell lung carcinoma, 4
  parenchymal, 1
  radiation necrosis, 3
  temporo-occipital junction, 1
  vasogenic edema, 4
Metastatic epidural disease
  breast carcinoma metastase, 179, 181
  clincial complication, 178
  diagnostics, 178

neuroblastoma, 180
treatment, 178
Multiple hemangioblastomas, 217
Myxopapillary ependymomas, 207–208

N
Neoplastic disease
CSF, 141
extradural
ABC, 147–148
aggressive osteoblastoma, 153–154
BNCT, 168–170
bone island, 142–144
bone metastases (*see* Bone metastases)
chondrosarcomas, 161–163
chordomas, 164–167 (*see* chordomas)
enostoses, 142
epidural metastases (*see* Metastatic epidural disease)
ganglioneuroblastoma, 171
ganglioneuroma, 171, 173
GCTs (*see* Giant cell tumors (GCTs))
neuroblastomas, 142, 171
osteoblastomas, 152, 155
osteoid osteomas, 149–151
vertebral hemangiomas, 145–146
intradural extramedullary
arachnoid cysts (*See* Arachnoid cysts)
leptomeningeal metastasis, 202–204
meningiomas, 189–191
neurofibroma, 186–188
paragangliomas, 192–193
schwannoma (*see* Schwannoma)
spinal epidermoid cysts, 199–201
intramedullary
ependymomas, 205–206
hemangioblastoma, 215–217
myxopapillary ependymomas, 207–208
pilocytic astrocytoma, 211–214
spinal cord astrocytomas, 209–210
spinal cord lymphoma, 218–219
spinal cord metastasis, 220–222
radiation-induced complications
radiation-induced polyradiculopathy, 226–227
radiation myelopathy, 228–229
sacral insufficiency fracture, 225
striated muscle myositis, 223–224
spinal axis, 141
Neuroblastomas, 142, 171
Neurofibroma, 186–188

O
Oligodendroglioma
anterior corpus callosum, 18
axial non-contrast computed tomography, 20
characteristics, 16
cystic with tumor, 17
left posterior frontal nonenhancing, 19
peripheral tumour, 18
Optic pathway glioma
axial contrast T1-weighted image, 130
axial noncontrast CT, 129
axial T2-weighted, 126–127
coronal fat-saturated T2-weighted, 128
pediatric population, 125
Osteoblastomas, 152, 155
Osteoid osteomas, 149–151

P
Paracavernous sinus meningioma, 139
Paragangliomas, 192–193
PCNSL. *See* Primary central nervous system lymphoma (PCNSL)
Pediatric brain tumor
intra-axial
DNET (*see* Dysembryonic neuroepithelial tumor (DNET))
ganglioglioma, 63, 66–67
intratentorial
ATRT (*see* Atypical teratoid rhabdoid tumor (ATRT))
brainstem glioma (*see* Brainstem glioma)
JPA (*see* Juvenile pilocytic astrocytoma (JPA))
intraventricular
choroid plexus carcinoma, 104–105
choroid plexus papilloma, 101–103
medulloblastoma (*see* Medulloblastoma)
pediatric ependymoma, 90–92
pleomorphic xanthoastrocytoma, 106
subependymal giant cell tumor, 98–100
pineal
germinoma, 86–87
pineoblastoma, 83–85
pineocytoma, 88–89
Pediatric ependymoma
anterior lateral extension, 92
characteristics, 90
heterogeneously enhancing tumor, 91–92
Pilocytic astrocytoma, 211–214
Pineoblastoma
characteristics, 83
heterogeneous pineal gland tumor, 85
pineal region, 84
sagittal, 84
Pineocytoma, 88–89
Pituitary adenoma, 109
Pituitary cyst, 111
Pituitary hypophysitis, 131–132
Pituitary macroadenoma
coronal T2-weighted, 113–114
medical management, 112
sagittal preoperative, 115
Pituitary microadenoma, 109–110
Planum sphenoidale and tuberculum sella meningioma, 138
Pleomorphic xanthoastrocytoma, 106
Primary central nervous system lymphoma (PCNSL)
butterfly lymphoma, 32
characteristics, 31
cloud-like tumor, 35
coronal, 37
diffusion-weighted, 33–34
fat suppression, 37
left periatrial homogeneous-enhancing nodule, 36
periventricular white matter T2 hyperintensity, 36
subtle nonenhancing abnormal signal, 33

R

Rathke's cleft cyst (RCC), 118–119
Relative cerebral blood volume map (rCBV), 27

S

Schwannoma
  axial and coronal T2, 183–184
  brachium pontis, 56
  characteristics, 54
  enhancing intracanalicular tumor, 55
  expansile tumor, 58
  lesions, 182
  sagittal and axial T2, 185
  vestibular, 57
Sellar and parasellar masses
  anatomic location, 109
  craniopharyngioma, 120–124
  invasive pituitary adenoma, 116–117
  LCH (*see* Langerhans cell histiocytosis (LCH))
  meningioma, 138–139
  optic pathway glioma (*see* optic pathway glioma)
  pituitary adenoma, 109
  pituitary cyst, 111
  pituitary hypophysitis, 131–132
  pituitary macroadenoma (*see* pituitary macroadenoma)
  pituitary microadenoma, 109–110
  premenopausal women, 109
  RCC, 118–119
  tuber cinereum hamartoma, 133
Spinal axis, 141
Spinal epidermoid cysts, 199–201
Striated muscle myositis, 223–224
Subependymal giant cell tumor
  characteristics, 98
  heterogeneously enhancing tumor, 99
  nodular enhancing tumor, 98
  T2 hyperintense enhancing tumor, 99
  T2 hypointense calcification, 100
Subependymoma
  ependymoma, 47
  expansile hyperintense tumor, 48
  solid and cystic nonenhancing tumor, 46, 47
Susceptibility-weighted angiography (SWAN), 27

T

Tuber cinereum hamartoma, 133

W

World Health Organization (WHO), 182

MIX
Papier aus verantwortungsvollen Quellen
Paper from responsible sources
FSC® C105338

If you have any concerns about our products,
you can contact us on
ProductSafety@springernature.com

In case Publisher is established outside the EU,
the EU authorized representative is:
Springer Nature Customer Service Center GmbH
Europaplatz 3, 69115 Heidelberg, Germany

Printed by Libri Plureos GmbH
in Hamburg, Germany